**UCLA Symposia on Molecular and Cellular Biology
New Series**

Series Editor
C. Fred Fox

UCLA Symposia Published Previously

(Numbers refer to the publishers listed below.)

1972
Membrane Research (2)

1973
Membranes (1)
Virus Research (2)

1974
Molecular Mechanisms for the Repair
 of DNA (4)
Membrane (1)
Assembly Mechanisms (1)
The Immune System: Genes,
 Receptors, Signals (2)
Mechanisms of Virus Disease (3)

1975
Energy Transducing Mechanisms (1)
Cell Surface Receptors (1)
Developmental Biology (3)
DNA Synthesis and its Regulation (3)

1976
Cellular Neurobiology (l)
Cell Shape and Surface Architecture (1)
Animal Virology (2)
Molecular Mechanisms in the Control
 of Gene Expression (2)

1977
Cell Surface Carbohydrates and
 Biological Recognition (1)
Molecular Approaches to Eucaryotic
 Genetic Systems (2)
Molecular Human Cytogenetics (2)
Molecular Aspects of Membrane
 Transport (1)
Immune System: Genetics and
 Regulation (2)

1978
DNA Repair Mechanism (2)
Transmembrane Signaling (1)

Hematopoietic Cell Differentiation (2)
Normal and Abnormal Red Cell
 Membranes (1)
Persistent Viruses (2)
Cell Reproduction: Daniel Mazia
 Dedicatory Volume (2)

1979
Covalent and Non-Covalent Modulation
 of Protein Function (2)
Eucaryotic Gene Regulation (2)
Biological Recognition and Assembly
 (1)
Extrachromosomal DNA (2)
Tumor Cell Surfaces and Malignancy
 (1)
T and B Lymphocytes: Recognition and
 Function (2)

1980
Biology of Bone Marrow
 Transplantation (2)
Membrane Transport and
 Neuroreceptors (1)
Control of Cellular Division and
 Development (1)
Animal Virus Genetics (2)
Mechanistic Studies of DNA
 Replication and Genetic
 Recombination (2)

1981
Immunoglobulin Idiotypes and Their
 Expression (2)
Structure and DNA-Protein Interactions
 of Replication Origins (2)
Genetic Variation Among Influenza
 Viruses (2)
Developmental Biology Using Purified
 Genes (2)

Publishers

(1) Alan R. Liss, Inc.
    150 Fifth Avenue
    New York, NY 10011

(2) Academic Press, Inc.
    111 Fifth Avenue
    New York, NY 10003

(3) W.A. Benjamin, Inc.
    2725 Sand Hill Road
    Menlo Park, CA 94025

(4) Plenum Publishing Corp.
    227 W. 17th Street
    New York, NY 10011

Symposia Board

C. Fred Fox, Director
Molecular Biology Institute
UCLA

Members

Ronald Cape, Ph.D., MBA
Chairman
Cetus Corporation

Pedro Cuatrecasas, M.D.
Vice President for Research
Burroughs Wellcome Company

Luis Glaser, Ph.D.
Professor and Chairman
of Biochemistry
Washington University School
of Medicine

Donald Steiner, M.D.
Professor of Biochemistry
University of Chicago

Ernest Jaworski, Ph.D.
Director of Molecular Biology
Monsanto

Paul Marks, M.D.
President
Sloan-Kettering Institute

William Rutter, Ph.D.
Professor and Chairman
of Biochemistry
University of California Medical
Center

Sidney Udenfriend, Ph.D.
Director
Roche Institute

The members of the board advise the director in identification of topics for future symposia.

RATIONAL BASIS FOR CHEMOTHERAPY

RATIONAL BASIS FOR CHEMOTHERAPY

Proceedings of the UCLA Symposium
held at Keystone, Colorado
April 18–23, 1982

Editor

BRUCE A. CHABNER
National Institutes of Health
Bethesda, Maryland

Alan R. Liss, Inc. • New York

Address all Inquiries to the Publisher
Alan R. Liss, Inc., 150 Fifth Avenue, New York, NY 10011

Copyright © 1983 Alan R. Liss, Inc.

Printed in the United States of America.

Library of Congress Cataloging in Publication Data
Main entry under title:

Rational basis for chemotherapy.

(UCLA symposia on molecular and cellular biology; new ser., v. 4)
Includes bibliographical references and index.
1. Cancer--Chemotherapy--Congresses. 2. Antineo-plastic agents--Congresses. I. Chabner, Bruce.
II. UCLA Symposium on the Rational Basis for Chemotherapy (1982: Keystone, Colo.) III. University of California, Los Angeles. IV. Series.
RC271.C5R37 1983   616.99'4061   82-24921
ISBN 0-8451-2603-2

Contents

Contributors

Edward M. Acton [119]
SRI International, Menlo Park, CA 94025

G.E. Adams [389]
Radiobiology Unit, Institute of Cancer Research, Sutton, Surrey, England

Kenneth C. Anderson [211]
Division of Tumor Immunology, Sidney Farber Cancer Institute, Boston MA 02115

Christopher C. Badger [295]
Pediatric Oncology, Fred Hutchinson Cancer Research Center, Seattle, WA 98104

Michael P. Bates [211]
Division of Tumor Immunology, Sidney Farber Cancer Institute, Boston, MA 02115

Irwin D. Bernstein [295]
Pediatric Oncology, Fred Hutchinson Cancer Research Center, Seattle, WA 98104

June L. Biedler [71]
Cellular and Biochemical Genetics, Sloan-Kettering Institute for Cancer Research, Rye, NY 10580

Suzanne Bourgeois [153]
The Salk Institute, Regulatory Biology Laboratory, San Diego, CA 92138

N. Bruchovsky [23]
Division of Cancer Endocrinology, Cancer Control Agency of B.C., Vancouver, B.C., Canada V5Z 3J3

Ed Cadman [93]
Departments of Medicine and Pharmacology, Yale School of Medicine, New Haven, CT 06510

Desmond N. Carney [1]
NCI-Navy Medical Oncology Branch, Division of Cancer Treatment, National Cancer Institute and National Naval Medical Center, Bethesda, MD 20814

The boldface number in brackets following each contributor's name indicates the opening page of that author's paper.

Tien-ding Chang [71]
Cellular and Biochemical Genetics, Sloan-Kettering Institute for Cancer Research, Rye, NY 10580

D. Colcher [315]
National Cancer Institute, National Institutes of Health, Bethesda, MD 20205

A.J. Coldman [23]
Division of Epidemiology and Biometrics, Cancer Control Agency of B.C., Vancouver, B.C., Canada V5Z 3J3

Franklin Cuttitta [1]
NCI-Navy Medical Oncology Branch, Division of Cancer Treatment, National Cancer Institute and National Naval Medical Center, Bethesda, MD 20814

G.L. DeNardo [379]
UCD Medical Center, Division of Nuclear Medicine, Sacramento, CA 95817

S.J. DeNardo [379]
UCD Medical Center, Division of Nuclear Medicine, Sacramento, CA 95817

Juliana Denekamp [407]
Gray Laboratory, Mount Vernon Hospital, Northwood, Middlesex, HA6 2RN, England

Nancy Dillon [475]
Laboratory of Medicinal Chemistry and Biology, National Cancer Institute, Bethesda, MD 20205

K.L. Erickson [379]
Department of Anatomy, School of Medicine, Davis, CA 95616

John F. Fowler [407]
Gray Laboratory, Mount Vernon Hospital, Northwood, Middlesex, HA6 2RN, England

Richard M. Fox [239, 291]
Ludwig Institute for Cancer Research (Sydney Branch), University of Sydney, N.S.W. 2006, Australia

Arnold Fridland [261]
Division of Biochemical and Clinical Pharmacology, St. Jude Children's Research Hospital, Memphis, TN 38101

Richard Fuller [475]
Laboratory of Medicinal Chemistry and Biology, National Cancer Institute, Bethesda, Md 20205

Judith C. Gasson [153]
Regulatory Biology Laboratory, The Salk Institute, San Diego, CA 92138

Adi F. Gazdar [1]
NCI-Navy Medical Oncology Branch, Division of Cancer Treatment, National Cancer Institute and National Naval Medical Center, Bethesda, MD 20814

J.H. Goldie [23]
Division of Advanced Therapeutics, Cancer Control Agency of B.C., Vancouver, B.C., Canada V5Z 3J3

James E. Griffin [137]
Department of Internal Medicine, The University of Texas Health Science Center, Dallas, TX 75235

Adeline J. Hackett [119]
Peralta Cancer Research Institute, Oakland, CA 94609

George M. Hahn [427]
Department of Radiology, Stanford University, Stanford, CA 94305

Rosemary E. Hall [177]
Ludwig Institute for Cancer Research (Sydney Branch), University of Sydney, Sydney, N.S.W. 2006, Australia

P. Horan Hand [315]
National Cancer Institute, National Institutes of Health, Bethesda, MD 20205

Timothy D. Heath [437]
Cancer Research Institute, University of California Medical Center, San Francisco, CA 94143

Robert Heimer [93]
Departments of Medicine and Pharmacology, Yale School of Medicine, New Haven, CT 06510

Fred J. Hendler [309]
Division of Hematology/Oncology, Department of Internal Medicine, University of Texas Health Science Center, Dallas, TX 75235

G.H. Heppner [41, 107]
Department of Immunology, Michigan Cancer Foundation, Detroit, MI 48201

Michael S. Hershfield [249, 275]
Department of Medicine, Duke University Medical Center, Durham, NC 27710

Margaret Hinchliffe [407]
Gray Laboratory, Mount Vernon Hospital, Northwood, Middlesex, HA6 2RN, England

H.H. Hines [379]
Division of Nuclear Medicine, UCD Medical Center, Sacramento, CA 95817

Pamela J. Hodson [177]
Ludwig Institute for Cancer Research (Sydney Branch), Sydney, N.S.W. 2006, Australia

Janet A. Houghton [61]
Department of Biochemical and Clinical Pharmacology, St. Jude Children's Research Hospital, Memphis, TN 38101

Peter J. Houghton [61]
Department of Pharmacology, St. Jude Children's Research Hospital, Memphis, TN 38101

Richard F. Kefford [239]
Ludwig Institute for Cancer Research (Sydney Branch), University of Sydney, N.S.W. 2006, Australia

D. Kufe [315]
National Cancer Institute, National Institutes of Health, Bethesda, MD 20205

Joanne Kurtzberg [249]
Department of Medicine, Duke University Medical Center, Durham, NC 27710

Robert C.F. Leonard [211]
Division of Tumor Immunology, Sidney Farber Cancer Institute, Boston, MA 02115

Amitabha Mazumder [359]
Surgery Branch, National Cancer Institute, Bethesda, MD 20205

Nicholas J. McNally [407]
Gray Laboratory, Mount Vernon Hospital, Northwood, Middlesex HA6 2RN, England

Peter W. Melera [71]
RNA Synthesis and Regulation, Sloan-Kettering Institute for Cancer Research, Rye, NY 10580

Marian B. Meyers [71]
Cellular and Biochemical Genetics, Sloan-Kettering Institute for Cancer Research, Rye, NY 10580

B.E. Miller [107]
Department of Immunology, Michigan Cancer Foundation, Detroit, MI 48201

F.R. Miller [107]
Department of Immunology, Michigan Cancer Foundation, Detroit, MI 48201

John D. Minna [1]
NCI-Navy Medical Oncology Branch, Division of Cancer Treatment, National Cancer Institute and National Naval Medical Center, Bethesda, MD 20814

Leigh C. Murphy [195]
Ludwig Institute for Cancer Research (Sydney Branch), University of Sydney, Sydney, N.S.W. 2006, Australia

Charles E. Myers [423]
Clinical Pharmacology Branch, COP, DCT, National Cancer Institute, Bethesda, MD 20205

Lee M. Nadler [211]
Division of Tumor Immunology, Sidney Farber Cancer Institute, Boston, MA 02115

M. Nuti [315]
National Cancer Institute, National Institutes of Health, Bethesda, MD 20205

Demetrios Papahadjopoulos [437]
Cancer Research Institute, University of California Medical Center, San Francisco, CA 94143

Edward K. Park [211]
Division of Tumor Immunology, Sidney Farber Cancer Institute, Boston, MA 02115

Robert H.F. Peterson [71]
Cellular and Biochemical Genetics, Sloan-Kettering Institute for Cancer Research, Rye, NY 10580

Barbara J. Petro [475]
Laboratory of Medicinal Chemistry and Biology, National Cancer Institute, Bethesda, MD 20205

Varinder S. Randhawa [407]
Gray Laboratory, Mount Vernon Hospital, Northwood, Middlesex, HA6 2RN, England

Roger R. Reddel [177]
Ludwig Institute for Cancer Research (Sydney Branch), University of Sydney, Sydney, N S W 2006, Australia

Steven A. Rosenberg [359]
National Cancer Institute, Bethesda, MD 20205

J. Schlom [315]
National Cancer Institute, National Institutes of Health, Bethesda, MD 20205

Stuart F. Schlossman [211]
Division of Tumor Immunology, Sidney Farber Cancer Institute, Boston, MA 02115

Joan R. Shapiro [41,45]
Department of Neurology, Memorial Sloan-Kettering Cancer Center, New York, NY 10021

William R. Shapiro [45]
Department of Neurology, Memorial Sloan-Kettering Cancer Center, New York, NY 10021

Helene S. Smith [119]
Peralta Cancer Research Institute, Oakland, CA 94609

Barbara A. Spengler [71]
Cellular and Biochemical Genetics, Sloan-Kettering Institute for Cancer Research, Rye, NY 10580

Fiona A. Stewart [407]
Gray Laboratory, Mount Vernon Hospital, Northwood, Middlesex, HA6 2RN, England

I.J. Stratford [389]
Radiobiology Unit, Institute of Cancer Research, Sutton, Surrey, England

Robert L. Sutherland [177, 195]
Ludwig Institute for Cancer Research (Sydney Branch), University of Sydney, Sydney, N.S.W. 2006, Australia

Ian W. Taylor [177]
Ludwig Institute for Cancer Research (Sydney Branch), University of Sydney, Sydney, N.S.W. 2006, Australia

Y.A. Teramoto [315]
National Cancer Institute, National Institutes of Health, Bethesda, MD 20205

Vernon L. Verhoef [261]
Division of Biochemical and Clinical Pharmacology, St. Jude Children's Research Hospital, Memphis TN 38101

David T. Vistica [475, 487]
Laboratory of Medicinal Chemistry and Biology, National Cancer Institute, Bethesda, MD 20205

Colin K.W. Watts [195]
Ludwig Institute for Cancer Research (Sydney Branch), University of Sydney, Sydney, N.S.W. 2006, Australia

John N. Weinstein [441]
National Institutes of Health, Bethesda, MD 20205

D. Wunderlich [315]
National Cancer Institute, National Institutes of Health, Bethesda, MD 20205

Dorothy Yuan [309]
Department of Microbiology, University of Texas Health Science Center, Dallas, TX 75235

Preface

The UCLA Symposium on the Rational Basis for Chemotherapy was itself an experiment. Cancer chemotherapy has for many years been the province of the biochemist and the specialist in chemical synthesis; the traditional objectives for drug design have been enzyme inhibition or the synthesis of analogs of active antibiotics or plant derivatives. In the past few years, the rapid development of our understanding of basic processes related to cancer biology has opened potential new avenues for cancer treatment. This conference addressed the question of whether the time is ripe for utilizing our growing knowledge of such topics as: mechanisms of drug transport and resistance, the biochemical basis of hormone action, drug interactions, and the potential of monoclonal antibodies as therapeutic tools. A further concern was whether a meaningful dialogue could be established between the basic scientists and the clinicians, and among basic workers in such widely divergent fields.

The conference proved to be a most stimulating event. To a person we left with a sense of exhilaration, realizing the vast possibilities and opportunities we faced. A true synthesis of disciplines occurred. Ling's membrane glycoprotein P-170 (a likely factor in antibiotic resistance) became the target of Schlom's monoclonal antibody linked to Youle's ricin. Was P-170 another example of gene amplification as described by Schimke? Was it amplified in Minna's drug-resistant cell lines derived from human cases of small cell carcinoma? Could drug resistance be detected in human tumor material by transfection of DNA into recipient cell lines, as proposed by Chabner? All these questions seemed answerable, and, of course, highly relevant to the goal of establishing a rational basis for chemotherapy. As the conference progressed, recurrent themes surfaced. We realized more fully that the task of placing chemotherapy on a rational basis depends on identifying mechanisms of drug action in model systems and determining mechanisms of drug resistance in human material. Finally, it was reaffirmed that having human tumor cell lines is an indispensable part of the problem for all types of new cancer therapeutics.

Thus, Minna's opening plenary talk on the biology of human lung carcinoma was a fitting introduction to the best-studied example of a human malignancy cultured and studied *in vitro*. Succeeding sessions considered the genetic, biochemical, and cytokinetic basis of drug resistance, a topic which was introduced by Goldie and colleagues. Their theories regarding the spontaneous mutation to drug-resistant status melded admirably with the studies of gene amplification in response to methotrexate as discussed by Schimke and Biedler, and the P-170 mediated resistance as described by Ling. We learned that tumor heterogeneity, as identified by Heppner and Shapiro, tends to confirm the spontaneous genetic "drift" of tumor cell populations as predicted by Goldie. Griffin, Bourgeois, and Lippman discussed the multiple biochemical steps in the action of androgens, glucocorticoids, and estrogens, and identified the missing steps in steroid resistance syndromes and steroid-resistant tumor cells. The interaction of hormone-receptor complex with DNA was highlighted as an important area for future work.

Nadler described the complex maturation cycle of the T and B lymphocytes, as dissected by monoclonal antibodies, while Fox, Hirschfield, Fridland, and colleagues examined the unique sensitivity of T-lymphocyte malignancies to inhibitors of adenosine deaminase and other purine/pyrimidine antimetabolites, possibly related to the cell's deficiency in nucleotide-degrading enzymes.

Immunologic targeting of therapy through the use of monoclonal antibodies was described in experimental systems by Bernstein, and the specificity and cytotoxicity of antibodies to human breast cancer cell lines was examined by Hendler and Schlom. Others described the coating of lysosomes with antibodies in an effort to improve the selectivity of drug distribution. DeNardo examined the radio-isotopic characteristics of various alpha emitters.

Adams and Fowler reviewed the principle considerations behind the development of hypoxic cell sensitizers and their poorly understood, paradoxical enhancement of response to certain alkylating agents such as cis-platinum. The importance of glutathione depletion in determining sensitivity to alkylating agents, and free-radical-producing agents such as adriamycin, was a recurrent theme of these talks and the discussion by Myers. The final sessions concerned the importance of pharmacokinetic parameters (distribution, transmembrane transport) and the influence of liposomal encapsulation on these factors.

We all look forward to a renewal of this meeting a few years hence to determine whether the experiment will bear fruit. I have every confidence that it will, and that cancer therapeutics in the present decade will undergo significant changes as these new ideas become realities. The conference was generously supported by a grant from the National Cancer Institute (USPHS CA 31746-01) and by support from Smith Klein and French Laboratories.

Bruce A. Chabner

Rational Basis for Chemotherapy, pages 1–22
© 1983 Alan R. Liss, Inc., 150 Fifth Avenue, New York, NY 10011

THE BIOLOGY OF LUNG CANCER

John D. Minna, Desmond N. Carney,
Franklin Cuttitta and Adi F. Gazdar
NCI-Navy Medical Oncology Branch
Division of Cancer Treatment
National Cancer Institute and
National Naval Medical Center
Bethesda, Maryland   20814

In discussing the biology of lung cancer, it is useful to review the results of countless treatment trials of lung cancer in patients (1). First, local therapy such as surgery or radiotherapy fails to cure patients in the great majority of cases. This is because microscopic metastatic disease is usually present at the earliest time the primary lung cancer is discovered. Next, small cell lung cancer is usually quite sensitive to chemotherapy and radiotherapy while the non-small cell varieties of adenocarcinoma, squamous and large cell carcinomas are usually relatively resistant to chemo-therapy and radiotherapy. The chemoradio-sensitivity of small cell lung cancer is such that approximately 10% of patients may actually be cured by appropriate combinations of these two modalities. However, exactly which patients will be cured and how best to do this is not clear. Finally, paraneoplastic syndromes suggesting the production of hor-mones by tumor cells are quite frequent in lung cancer (2).

The origin of the malignant cells for the different histologic types of lung cancer remains unclear. One plan for the differentiation of bronchial epithelial cells is a unitarian hypothesis. Under this hypothesis all epithelial cells are thought to arise from a common precursor stem cell rather than from bronchial epithelial stem cells of different embryonic lineage (3,4,5,6). The stem cell then undergoes several divisions yielding various sublines committed to different biochemical and morphologic pathways of differen-tiation.

One pathway would give rise to a ciliated cell, another
to a mucous secreting cell, a third to keratinizing squamous
cells, and a fourth to cells with endocrine properties
potentially of multiple types. It should be stressed, however, that a unitarian hypothesis is controversial. Some
workers would feel that the pulmonary endocrine cells in
particular would arise from stem cells of distinct embryologic lineage. (See References 3 and 4 for review).
To understand human lung cancer, one of our major goals has
been to isolate in clonal form, tumors as well as normal
cells in various stages of differentiation along these putative pathways. This will allow the study of the biology of
bronchial epithelial cells of both the normal as well as the
neoplastic cell.
    This work represents a collaborative effort within
our own group formally the NCI-VA and now the NCI-Navy
Medical Oncology Branch and in addition with a series of
investigators at other institutions.

In Vitro Culture And Biology Of Human Lung Cancer

    Methods to culture lung cancer cells have been previous-
ly described (7). In brief, primary and metastatic lung
carcinomas are obtained from patients and introduced either
directly into tissue culture or into athymic nude mice as
heterotransplants. The tissue culture lines are then serially propagated and can be injected into nude mice to test
for tumorogenicity and maintainence of histology. Likewise
the nude mouse heterotransplants can be introduced into
tissue culture for study at various time intervals. This
dual system is very useful for maintaining cell lines and
provides a means for a constant check on tumorigenecity and
histology. However, while lung cancer grows well in patients it is quite difficult to grow in tissue culture
direct from the patient unless specific conditions are
used. However, once we have a nude mouse heterotransplant
it is always possible to establish a tissue culture cell
line (7). Using this approach our group has been able to
establish a large number of human lung cancer cell lines
and heterotransplants (7). In addition to liquid culture of
fresh clinical specimens, it is also possible to prepare a
tumor sample from a patient and then to directly clone the
tumor cells in soft agarose (8,9). Because of the striking
clinical differences between small cell and non-small cell
lung cancer (1), cell lines of these tumors have provided

useful tools for comparing and contrasting the biologic properties of each type.

The typical culture of small cell lung cancer grows in suspension cultures as aggregates of cells forming organoid bodies. This aggregates will reform immediately after dis-aggregation and the cells grow best in this form suggesting cross feeding of the tumor cells. When the aggregates become very large they usually undergo central necrosis. In contrast a typical culture of non-small cell carcinoma grows attached to the culture surface and often can be seen to be producing mucin or attempting gland formation. Thus, it is possible to distinguish the two major classes of lung cancer by appearance in tissue culture. When the cell lines are injected into nude mice tumors form and these tumors maintain the histologic appearance of the original tumor (3,7) even after several years of heterotransplanta-tion. While lung cancers metastasize widely in humans, in nude mice all human tumors including lung cancers grow as locally expansive masses and rarely metastasize. The exact reasons for this are not yet known.

We have conducted a series of studies of both the cell lines and the primary lung cancer colonies. In beginning these studies we have of course been aided by all the prior work done on normal and fetal bronchial epithelium as well as lung cancer. A major guiding factor has been the informa-tion gained from studies of pulmonary endocrine cells of the amine precursor uptake and decarboxylation (or APUD) system of Pearse (3,5,6,10). From a variety of histologic studies, small cell lung cancers were thought to arise from these pulmonary endocrine or Kulchitzky cells. In addition, since some of the lung tumors may be racapitulating steps in fetal development, we have looked in tumors for markers thought to be expressed in fetal as well as adult pulmonary endocrine cells. Studies by Dr. John Guccion of the Washington VA Medical Center have demonstrated neurosecretory granules in all of our typical small cell lung cancer cell lines but not in the non-small cell lung cancer varieties (7).

Another key APUD marker is the enzyme L-dopa decarboxyl-ase (11). Small cell lung cancer cell lines all express high levels of this enzyme while non-small cell lung cancer lines express very low or no detectable levels (7). Dr. Stephen Baylin of Johns Hopkins our collaborator in these studies has pointed out that the occasional occurrence of a non-small cell lung cancer tumor expressing even low levels of

L-dopa decarboxylase is one piece of evidence in support of the unitarian origin of lung neoplasms (5). This expression indicates that cells committed to one pathway of differentiation, for example adenocarcinoma gland formation may in part retrace their steps and begin expressing markers of the small cell endocrine pathway.

Biochemical markers we have compared in our small cell versus non-small cell lung cancer lines are shown in Table 1. These are all markers which are expressed in high amounts in small cell lung cancer and at much lower or undetectable levels in non-small cell lung cancer.

TABLE 1

BIOCHEMICAL MARKERS DISTINGUISHING
SMALL CELL LUNG CANCER FROM
NON-SMALL CELL LUNG CANCER

Marker	SCLC/Non-SCLC (Fold Difference)*
L-DOPA Decarboxylase	2,800
Creatine Kinase BB	75
Neuron Specific Enolase	20
Bombesin	140

* Fold difference of mean levels

Data from References: 7,11,12,13,14

These observations have potential clinical application. If a lung cancer sample is tested for these panel of biochemical markers, and they are all elevated, the diagnosis of small cell lung cancer is assured.

With a series of collaborators we have tested for many peptide hormones reported to be made by human lung cancers. (Table 2)

TABLE 2

EXPRESSION OF APUD SYSTEM PEPTIDE
HORMONES BY LUNG CANCER CELL LINES

Hormone	Fraction Lines Positive	
	Small Cell	Non-Small Cell
Bombesin	15/15	0/10
Calcitonin	12/15	6/8
ACTH	6/15	1/8
AVP	2/15	0/8
Somatostatin	(+)	?
Neurophysin	(+)	?

Absent or seldom present: met enkephalin,
CCK/Gastrin, LHRH, insulin, glucagon, VIP.

(+) = found to be positive by other investigators,
not yet confirmed by us.

We stress that we have found bombesin in all the small
cell lung cancer cell lines we have tested while we have not
detected it in any of the non-small cell lung cancers tested
so far (14). In contrast, calcitonin was frequently found in
both small cell and non-small cell lung cancer. ACTH was less
frequently expressed in both, and arginine vasopressin, while
probably specific for small cell lung cancer was infrequently
expressed. Other groups notably Dartmouth Medical Center and
several groups in Japan have reported on the expression of
somatostatin and neurophysin by small cell lung cancer as well.
Again the expression of calcitonin and ACTH by non-small cell
lung cancers provides evidence for a unitarian stem cell of
origin.
     Hormone receptors represent other potential markers dis-
tinguishing small cell from non-small cell lung cancer and
also provide a clue to new methods to regulate lung cancers
growth in vitro and in patients. Table 3 summarizes our data
as to expression of hormone receptors in lung cancer types
based on binding of radiolabeled hormones to lung cancer cell
lines, the use of specific antibodies against hormone receptors,
and the growth factor requirements of the lung cancer cells
(vide infra).

TABLE 3

HORMONE RECEPTORS DISTINGUISHING
SMALL CELL LUNG CANCER FROM
NON-SMALL CELL LUNG CANCER

Receptor	SCLC	Non-SCLC
Bombesin	+	-
AVP	+	-
NGF	LOW +	-
EGF	-	+
Insulin	+	+
Transferrin	+	+

EGF and NGF data from References 15,16;
Rest is unpublished.

Small cell lung cancer is characterized by the expression of receptors for bombesin, arginine vasopressin, low levels of receptors for nerve growth factor (NGF), and receptors for insulin and transferrin but not for epidermal growth factor (EGF). In contrast non-small cell lung cancer expresses EGF, insulin and transferrin receptors but not the other receptors found on small cell lung cancer. With further development of reagents, particularly specific anti-receptor antibodies, histologic typing of lung tumors should be possible.

Another approach is to identify all the proteins, for example of the cell membrane by two dimensional gel electrophoresis (17). In studies performed in collaboration with Dr. Baylin and Joel Shaper of Johns Hopkins using iodinated cell membranes followed by iso-electric focusing in the horizontal axis, and then molecular weight size fractionation by SDS gel electrophoresis in the vertical axis, small cell lung cancers have a typical phenotype with 12 protein spots distinguishing small cell from non-small cell lung cancers.

The non-small cell lung cancers have a very similar protein spot compared to one another and this is very distinct from the small cell cancer phenotype. There are a series of 16 high molecular weight proteins expressed in non-small cell lung cancer membranes not found in small cell lung cancer.

TABLE 4

^{125}I LABELED MEMBRANE PROTEIN PHENOTYPES
OF LUNG CANCER CELLS DETERMINED BY
2-DIMENSIONAL GEL ELECTROPHORESIS PATTERNS

Number of Protein Spots	SCLC	NSCLC	Lymph.	Fib.	Neurobl.
Small Cell Lung Cancer Associated					
5	+	-	-	-	-
3	+	-	-	-	+
4	+	-	+	-	+
Non Small Cell Lung Cancer Associated					
5	-	+	-	-	-
11	-	+	-	?/low	-
Present on many cell types or lymphocyte selective					
10	+	+	+	+	+
5	-	-	+	-	-

* SCLC = small cell lung cancer; NSCLC = non-small cell
lung cancer; Lymph = lymphoblastoid cell lines;
Fib. = fibroblast cell lines; Neurobl. = neuroblastoma cell lines.
Data from reference 17, Baylin et al.

Table 4 summarizes the number of different membrane protein spots which distinguish small cell lung cancer from non-small cell lung cancer as well as from other cell types. Five proteins were unique to small cell lung cancer. Three were expressed on small cell lung cancer and human neuroblastomas but not on other cell types. Four proteins were expressed on small cell lung cancer, neuroblastomas, and on human lymphoblastoid cells but not on other cell types. In contrast, five proteins were expressed on non-small cell lung cancers but not on other cell types, and 11 other proteins that were not expressed on small cell lung cancers, neuroblastomas or lymphoid cells, but may be expressed at low levels on fibroblasts. In addition, there were 10 proteins expressed on all cell types, and other proteins found on lymphoid cells but not on the lung cancers. Thus, there are 12 proteins which are present on small cell but not on non-small cell membranes, and 16 proteins expressed on non-small cell but not on small cell lung cancer membranes. In addition, small cell cancers share most of their distinguishing proteins with human neuroblastomas. Cells of ectodermal origin express many neuroendocrine features in common with small cell lung cancer. Thus, the two dimensional gel electrophoresis system provides a new way of biochemically typing human lung cancers and also indicates that while the system is complex there are only relatively few membrane proteins to be identified and characterized.

The DNA content of human lung cancers determined by cell sorter analysis has demonstrated that approximately 60-70% of all human lung cancers have aneuploid DNA contents. However, there is no significance difference between small cell and nonsmall cell lung cancer. These DNA content analysis provide a stable signature of the tumor cell lines for periods of over two years.

However, there are genetic differences which distinguish lung cancer types. In collaboration with Dr. Jacqualine Whang-Peng of the Medicine Branch of the NCI we have studied banded karyotypes of our lung cancer cell lines. A specific chromosomal defect has been found in small cell lung cancer, a deletion of the short arm of human chromosome 3 (18). This deletion has been found in all metaphases of all small cell lung cancer lines, short term cultures, or direct tumor preparations we have studied. While the deletion can be small or large, shortest region of overlap analysis shows the minimal deletion so far detected to be deletion of the 3p interband (14-23). While there is one deleted chromosome in every tumor cell metaphase there are also at least one and often multiple copies of a normal appearing chromosome 3 (18). The deletion is not found in lymphoblastoid or normal cells taken from these patients. Thus, the defect is an acquired somatic deletion. Similar defects have not been consistently found in non-small cell lung cancers. Thus, the defect appears specific for small cell lung cancer. This defect has been found it in tumors from Japan as well as from other institutions in the United States. The central question is whether the deletion allows the expression of a mutant, probably recessive, gene on the normal appearing chromosome 3 as is the case in the Wilm's tumor aniridia syndrome. Alternatively the fragment of 3 could have been translocated to another chromosome and thus act aberrantly as is possible for translocations seen in Burkett's lymphoma. While it is possible the 3p deletion is only associated and not in some way causal of the malignant state the constancy of the appearance of the deletion in tumor cells speaks against this.

One of the major problems of applying the findings of human tumor cell biology to clinical situations is determining the degree of heterogeneity of tumor markers from cell to cell within individual patient's tumors. To study this question we have cloned small cell lung cancer and studied the clones for expression of the APUD markers.

TABLE 5

CLONAL EXPRESSION OF APUD MARKERS IN
SMALL CELL LUNG CANCER LINE NCI-H128

Marker	Phenotype Parent Line	Clone 1	2	3	4
L-DDC, NSE, CK-BB	+	+	+	+	+
Bombesin	+	+	+	+	+
ACTH	+	+	+	+	-
AVP	+	+	+	-	-
Calcitonin	+	+	-	-	-

* L-DDC = L- dopa decarboxylase; NSE = neuron specific enolase; CK-BB = BB isozyme of creatine kinase (not a true APUD selective marker but distinguishes small cell from non-small cell lung cancer); ACTH = adrenocorticotrophic hormone; AVP = arginine vasopressin. APUD = amine precursor uptake and decarboxylation system.

In Table 5 the expression of several of markers in the parental cell line and four clones is shown. The parent and all the clones expressed high levels of L-dopa decarboxylase, neuron specific enolase, bombesin, and the BB isozyme of creatine kinase. In contrast the peptide hormones ACTH, AVP, and calcitonin were only expressed in some of the clones. Thus,

clonal heterogeneity with respect to peptide hormone production occurs. Obviously, if one was following the production of the peptide hormone as a tumor marker erronous conclusions could be drawn dependent on which clone was predominant in the patient's tumor at any one time. While all
of the clones expressed bombesin, if one of the small cell
lung cancer cell lines or tumors is stained with an anti-
bombesin antiserum using immune peroxidase technology variations in the amount of immune reactive bombesin were seen
from one cell to the next. Thus, even within a tumor where
all of the clones express bombesin there is variation in the
level of bombesin expressed from one cell to the next.

We have also tested clonal derivatives for their tumorigenicity in nude mice. The parent line had a latency period
of 4-5 weeks after 5×10^6 cells were injected. Several of
the clones had a similar latency period, two clones had a
longer latency period of 10 weeks and three clones failed to
form tumors. While there could be multiple reasons for
this difference in tumoigenicity it is intriguing to know
that clonable cells within a tumor differ greatly in their
ability to grow in vivo.

Primary Cloning Of Lung Cancer

In our laboratory much effort has been devoted to
the drug sensitivity testing of human lung cancer specimens
using an agarose clonogenic assay to measure the surviving
fraction of clonable tumor cells after exposure to various
drugs (8,9). Tumor cells taken directly from patients were
exposed to 1, 10, or 100% of the peak achievable human plasma
concentration for one hour and then cloned in soft agarose.
In addition to these fresh specimens, established lung cancer
cell lines were tested and results of in vitro sensitivity
or resistance with the clinical status of the patient at the
time the biopsy for starting the cell line was obtained.
As shown in Table 6 cell line NCI-H187 obtained from an untreated patient was sensitive to all the drugs tested, all
of which have known clinical activity against small cell lung
cancer. In addition, some of the drugs gave over three logs
of cell kill.

In contrast, cell line NCI-H146 obtained from a patient
at the time of clinical relapse was relatively resistant to
all the drugs with the exception of VP-16 a drug which the
patient had not yet been treated with. Thus, the small cell
lung cancer cell lines also maintained the drug sensitivity

and resistance phenotypes of the tumors expressed in the
patients.

In contrast to cell lines of small cell lung cancer,
cell lines of non-small cell lung cancer were relatively or
absolutely resistant to all of the drugs tested in vitro as
single agents. Thus, previously untreated non-small cell
lung cancer is resistant to chemotherapy in vitro compared
to small cell lung cancer and this mirrors the situation seen
in patients.

TABLE 6

COLONY FORMATION OF SMALL CELL
LUNG CANCER LINES AFTER DRUG
THERAPY IN VITRO*

DRUG TESTED	UNTREATED NCI-H187	RELAPSED NCI-H146
	(% OF CONTROL)	
Melphelan	1	100
Methotrexate	1	100
BCNU	1	70
Vincristine	2	70
Adriamycin	0.1	50
VP-16	0.1	10
Vindesine	2	70

* 1 hour exposure to 10% of
  peak obtainable plasma level.

Overall, in vitro chemosensitivity studies on direct
tumor biopsy specimens and tumor cell lines of small cell
lung cancer showed that for both clinical specimens and cell
lines the in vitro results showing chemosensitivity were correlated with the clinical results 72 and 90% of the time respectively. Likewise, in all cases where the tumor cells
were resistant to the chemotherapy in vitro they were also
resistant in the patient. All of these tumors were obtained
from patients treated by us so we could directly correlate,
albeit in a retrospective fashion the response of the tumor
in vitro in the agarose cloning assay with that seen in vivo
in the patient. It should be stressed that while the in vitro
testing was done with single agent chemotherapy, that in the

patients was done usually with combination chemotherapy as is standard practice. Nevertheless, it is data like this that strongly suggests to us that the in vitro clonogenic assays for drug sensitivity and resistance may eventually be used for selecting therapy for individual patients. What is needed in this regard are prospective randomized trials. In the case of small cell lung cancer because the tumor cells from untreated patients are sensitive to all drugs the randomization would be between a standard combination chemotherapy versus combinations of drugs showing the most sensitivity in the assay. Our prediction is that the 10% of patients that currently are cured, by chance receive drugs to which their tumor is very sensitive. In the case of non-small cell lung cancer the randomization could be between no chemotherapy but necessary radiotherapy and surgery and the same treatments with combination chemotherapy selected by the assay. In addition, the lung cancer cell lines can be used to screen for new drugs which subsequently could be tested in patients, as models to study the biochemical pharmacology of drug resistance, and as sources of DNA to isolate genes coding for drug resistance.

While drug and radiation resistance has usually been thought of in terms of biochemical changes independent of differentiation we would like you to consider another mechanism of developing resistance. A pattern of small cell plus large cell elements is found in approximately 6% of diagnostic biopsies (13). However, we and others have found similar mixtures of small cells and large cells or small cells and other histologic types like squamous carcinoma in over 30% of cases at necropsy. In addition, we have found that these patients have a lower complete response rate to combination chemotherapy and shorter survival compared to patients with pure small cell lung cancer (13). Thus, clinically we can detect histologically an interconversion of small cell and large cell lung cancer and find that this is associated with resistance to cytotoxic therapy.

We and others have seen this interconversion in nude mouse heterotransplants and in tissue culture. In addition, to the histologic changes, biochemical changes such as loss of L-dopa decarboxylase, neurosecretory granules and peptide hormone production were also seen. These histologic interconversions we feel are additional evidence in favor of a unitary origin of lung cancer.

In collaboration with Dr. Mitchell and Dr. Kinsella of the NCI Radiation Oncology Branch we have studied the radiobiology of small cell carcinoma and the large cell con-

vertors. The small cell carcinoma lines shown have a D_0's
of 51-140 and an extrapolation or "hit" number of ranging
from 1 - 3. In contrast the large cell converters have a
similar D_0's of 80-91 but extrapolation numbers of from 5
- 11. Thus, they appear to have developed radioresistance
via a repair process.

Associated with this large cell conversion Dr. Whang-
Peng has found the development of a homogeneously staining
chromosome region or HSR. In other situations where such
chromosomal regions are found they are associated with gene
amplification. Thus, our prediction is that the large cell
convertors will have an associated gene amplification. It
is natural to also consider that the gene(s) amplified will
be related to some process like improved growth or radiation
repair.

If we want to use the tumor agarose colony forming cells
for drug and radiation sensitivity testing we must be able
to reproducibly clone the tumor cells. Using standard culture conditions get colony formation in agarose in 15 observed in 86% of small cell carcincinomas and 64% of non-
small cell lung cancers (8). However, one needs at least
30 colonies per plate to test even one drug. With standard
growth conditions, only 22% of small cell cancers, and 18%
of non-small cell cancers gave enough colonies for testing
even a few drugs.

The reason for this is found in the low cloning
efficiencies of the primary lung cancers. In the case of
aneuploid tumors one can use the DNA content to accurately
estimate the number of tumor cells in the sample used for
cloning. The colony forming efficiency per plated tumor cell
ranged from 0.2 to 1.5% for all types of lung cancer. Thus,
only 1% or less of the tumor cells in clinical specimen actually form colonies. Whether this represents the true phenotype of tumor cells without self renewal capability or some
defect in the culture system remains to be determined. Nevertheless we set out to develop new ways to culture human lung
cancer. We have done this primarily by developing serum free,
hormone and growth factor supplemented media for the culture
of human lung cancer. The strategy we have used is to develop
such formulae for our lung cancer cell lines and then to apply
these media to fresh clinical tumor samples (16,20).

TABLE 7

SERUM FREE MEDIA FOR THE GROWTH
OF LUNG CANCER CELL LINES AND
FRESH CLINICAL TUMOR SPECIMENS OF
LUNG SMALL CELL AND ADENOCARCINOMA

Growth Factor	SCLC	ACL
Insulin	+	+
Transferrin	+	+
Selenium	+	+
Hydrocortisone	+	+
17 Beta Estradiol	+	-
T3	-	+
EGF	-	+
BSA	(+)	+
Ethanolamine, Phospho Ethanolamine	(+)	+

(+) = stimulatory but not essential.
Reference 20,21.

Shown in Table 7 are the two media for small cell carcinoma and adenocarcinoma. While many of the factors for the
growth of small cell lung cancer are found in the adenocarcinoma formula, adenocarcinoma cells also require T3 and
epidermal growth factor as well as attachment factors such as
fibronectin or collagen. While BSA and ethanolminephospho-
ethanolamine are not required for the continued growth of small
cell lung cancer they stimulate it. While neither of these
formulas may yet be optimal they are both better than serum
containing medium for the growth of fresh lung cancer specimens.
In serum supplemented medium we see growth in 20-40% of cases
while in the serum free growth factor supplemented medium this
is increased to 66-75%.
        In searching for ways to improve the serum free formula
Dr. Carney has turned to cloning in serum free medium. In
the original serum free growth factor supplemented formula
very poor or no colony formation is seen.
        When the peptide hormones bombesin and arginine vasopres-
sin are added colony formation occurs. Both of these hormones
are produced by small cell lung cancer and both when added to
the basal serum free formula will stimulate growth. Following

this approach Dr. Herbert Oie in our laboratory has developed a new formula which improved the liquid culture of cell lines of small cell lung cancer. This medium, containing the prior growth factors and is supplemented with bombesin, arginine vasopressin, bovine serum albumin, and ethanolamine-phosphoethanolamine, (SCLC-2 medium) also support the in vitro agarose cloning of these cells.

If the small cell lung cancers produce their own growth factors why can't they clone in the original serum free medium? Recall there is clonal heterogeneity for the production of the peptide hormones arginine vasopressin and bombesin both of which are growth factors for small cell lung cancer. Imagine two tumor cells [A and B] occuring within the same patient. Both have receptors for AVP and bombesin and require these hormones for their clonal growth. Cell of clone A makes AVP while that of clone B makes bombesin. The hormones thus cross feed the cells and the tumor cell clones live in symbiosis within the patient. In the serum free tumor cell culture cloning situation the tumor cells are situated far apart in the agarose and cannot cross feed one another and thus require exogenously added hormones. While this is currently only a hypothesis the data is mounting in its favor and it is subject to further direct tests.

Monoclonal Antibodies and Lung Cancer

Another new approach to studying lung cancer is the preparation of monoclonal antibodies with specificity for lung cancer cells. We have screened many thousands of antibody producing clones for antibodies that would react with lung cancer cells but not with B lymphoblastoid cell lines often from the same patient (22,23). At present we have 81 candidate antibodies representing about 0.5% of all the hybrids screened. In radioimmunoassays and immunohistochemical reactions these antibodies react with tumor taken from the patient but not a variety of normal adult tissues. However, some of the tumor nodules seen on the H and E stained sections do not react with the antibody indicating heterogeneity of antigen expression within an individual patient's tumor (23).

In preparing monoclonal antibodies against small cell and non-small cell lung cancer we have found at least 6 major classes of antigenic determinants as shown in Table 8.

TABLE 8

MAJOR GROUPS OF MONOCLONAL ANTIBODIES AGAINST HUMAN LUNG CANCER

Type	Prototype Monoclonal Antibody	Originator
SCLC-1	534F8 (LNFP III)*	Cuttitta
SCLC-2	604A9 (Glycolipid)	Rosen
SCLC-3	2HH7 (p120)	Fargion
AC-1	503D8 (p86,p130)	Abrams
AC-2	505C12(?)	Abrams
LC-1	311 (?)	Mulshine

*LNFP III = lacto N fucopentaose III

Small cell lung cancer antigen -1 discovered by Dr. Frank Cuttitta is a glycolipid and recent work by Dr. Laura Huang and Victor Ginsberg of NIH shows that the glycolipid is lacto N fucopentose III. This same glycolipid is found on colon and breast cancer cells and early mouse embryo cells. Small cell antigen -2 discovered by Dr. Stephen Rosen now at Northwestern University is against another as yet uncharacterized glycolipid. Small cell antigen -3 was prepared by Dr. Sylvia Fargion against a large cell variant of the small cell tumors and she has shown that it is a protein of 120,000 molecular weight. Adenocarcinoma antigen -1 was found by Dr. Paul Abrams now of the Biologic Response Modifiers Program of the NCI and is a protein of 86,000 molecular weight in the cell and when secreted 130,000 molecular weight. Adenocarcinoma antigen -2 is uncharacterized, as is large cell antigen -1 produced by Dr. James Mulshine.

Because we wanted to have a panel of monoclonal antibodies that would react with all of our small cell lung cancer lines we have first focused on generating a large number of antibodies against different determinants of this cell type. In addition to the three small cell antigens shown we have other monoclonal antibodies which detect 15 different specificities on the surface of small cell lung cancer. We know that at least 12 of these are not found in normal lung or liver. While we would like to have monoclonal antibodies that only react with small cell and not non-small cell lung cancer none of our antibodies yet meet that criteria. All react with at least some non-small cell lung cancers. Of great interest we have found that most of our monoclonal antibodies against small cell lung cancer also react with human neuroblastoma and breast cancer but are only rarely found on melanoma, glioblastoma, or fibroblasts. These results are similar to those found by Dr. Baylin in the 2 dimensional gel electrophoresis analysis of membrane proteins.

Because one wants to be able to detect all lung cancers of a given histologic type we have been interested in whether any specific lung cancer line will react with at least one of the antibodies. Because the antigenic determinants are common to many of the small cell lung and cancers, for this histologic type at least it appears we have at least one antibody that will detect it. However, within individual tumors tests with any one antibody show tumor cell heterogeneity for the antigen expression. Thus, it will probably be necessary to use "cocktails" of antibodies. Finally, we have noted with Dr. Ginsburg group that within our group of monoclonal antibodies selected against small cell lung cancer that glycolipid determinants were commonly detected. In particular the glycolipid lacto N fucopentaose III was immunodominant and we selected several antibodies which turn out to react with this determinant.

Another approach is to take an already identified marker and prepare monoclonal antibodies to gain even better reagents for immunologic detection. Dr. Frank Cuttitta using a monoclonal antibody he has prepared in collaboration with Dr. Terry Moody against the peptide hormone bombesin has developed a radioimmunoassay that can detect as little as 1 fmol of added bombesin. Thus, the monoclonal antibody should be useful for typing tumors in radio-immune and immune histochemical assays for bombesin as well as provided a means for searching for bombesin in patients' plasma.

While there are many potential uses for monoclonal antibodies for specificity for human lung cancer I would like to interject a note of caution in using them therapeutically. Using immune histochemical stains, we have found some of the antibodies react with normal human kidney. While this cross reaction may pose no problem for the antibody's use in immune histochemical stains or nuclear medicine scanning, obviously if one wished to target with the antibody drugs, toxins or radiotherapy to the tumor, the reaction with the kidney tubules would be of major concern. Thus, our group is first trying to conduct detailed immune histochemical staining studies before administration of the antibodies to patients.

Mechanisms of Malignancy in Lung Cancer

I return now to the uniterian schema of bronchial epithelial differentiation. We have presented data of interconversions of small cell cancer to other cell types, and uncommon
but interesting occurences of the expression of certain APUD
markers by non-small cell carcinomas which suggest that the
uniterian scheme may actually be true. However, the fundamental problem remains of why the cells differentiating along
any of the pathways becomes malignant. Let me suggest three
possible mechanisms all of which may play a role. First, a
tumor cell may produce a hormone or hormones which after secretion from the tumor cell bind to receptors on the tumor
cell's own surface and act to stimulate the growth of the
tumor cell in a so-called "autocrine" fashion. I have already given you two examples of this in the peptide hormones
bombesin and arginine vasopressin for small cell lung cancer.
In addition, in studies done in collaboration with Dr.
Stephen Sherwin and George Todaro of the NCI we have found
that all of the lung cancer cell lines tested make factors
which will cause normal rat kidney cells to form tumor like
colonies in agarose (15). If one plates 1,000 normal rat
kidney cells in agarose without any added lung cancer factor
no colonies form. However, using feeder layers of epidermoid,
adenocarcinoma, large cell or small cell carcinoma up to 30%
of the normal cells will form colonies. Dr. Todaro calls such
factors transforming growth factors or "TGF's". Whether the
factors produced by lung cancer are similar or different from
other TGF's Dr. Todaro has discovered remains to be determined. However, recently Dr. Sherwin has reported on finding similar factors in the urine of lung cancer patients (24).
While we have also investigated whether the small cell
lung cancer made any thing in addition to AVP and bombesin
which would stimulate their clonal growth. Dr. Carney grew
one line NCI-N592 under serum free conditions and harvested
the medium. He previously had found that this line cloned
easily and grew without problems directly from the patient
and thus he suspected that it might be making a lot of putative growth factors. He then added this "conditioned" medium
to a series of basal media and cloned small cell lung cancer
cells. In all cases the addition of the 592 growth factor
stimulated the clonal growth of the lung cancer cells. This
was seen when it was added to serum containing medium, or
the various growth factor supplemented serum free media including our newest small cell lung cancer -2 medium which
contains bombesin and arginine vasopressin. Thus, this factor

or factors does not appear to be in these growth media. We have therefore concluded that small cell lung cancer makes a series of peptide hormones or growth factors which act to stimulate its own growth.

Recently the techniques of DNA transfection have been applied to the study of human lung cancer (25,26,27). In experiments conducted in the laboratory of Dr. Michael Wigler at Cold Spring Harbor by Dr. Manuel Perucho, DNA was taken from two cases of lung adenocarcinoma lines and transfected into non-malignant mouse NIH 3T3 cells. A few colonies arose that display malignant behavior. If the DNA is isolated from these colonies, cut with a restriction enzyme, electrophoresed and then probed for human repetitive DNA sequences the results showed incorporation of many bands of human DNA. If DNA is isolated from these primary transfectants, retransfected, and selection for malignant cells again made a series of secondary transfectants are obtained. They contain much less human DNA. This allows one to ask if there are any DNA bands in common between all of these secondary clones. The answer is yes and these common bands represent human DNA from adenocarcinoma of the lung which is capable of transferring the property of malignancy to a non-malignant cell and thus potentially represent the primary genetic defect in these tumor cells. The gene or genes appears to be large approximately 30-40 kilobases in length. While this was exciting, several other pieces of information have also recently come to light. First in similar experiments several labs have found that at least some colon cancers also have an identical gene (27). Second, the laboratories of Dr. Geoffory Cooper of Harvard, Robert Weinberg of MIT, and Dr. Michael Wiglar and Manuel Perucho of Cold Spring Harbor and the State University of New York have found that this gene is very closely related to the Kirsten sarcoma virus p21 gene first found in rats. Thus, it is possible that adenocarcinoma of the lung has as its primary genetic defect the activation of a sarcoma virus like gene. The proof that such a gene really causes lung cancer will be eagerly awaited and obviously would provide a major new clue into dealing with lung cancer.

Finally, because of this new interest in genetics and rodent genes it is relevant to ask if there are genetic studies of lung cancer in mice? One recently published study by Dr. Nomura of Japan is very interesting (28). Dr. Nomura treated mice with several carcinogens including x-rays, 4-nitroquinoline, and urethane, bred the mice and identified the progeny who developed lung tumors most of which were lung adenomas.

He then bred mice who had tumors with other littermate mice but who did not have tumors as well as interbreeding mice who had never had lung cancers. These F2 progeny were then examined for the development of lung tumors. He found that the tumor bearing mice had progeny with a greatly increased chance of developing lung tumors compared to the control animals. Thus, he identified a dominant, mendelian gene induced by the carcinogen treatment several generations before. As the accompanying editorial in Nature pointed out this has grave implications if cigarette smoking could also cause heritable genetic changes which coded for lung cancer.

REFERENCES

1. Minna JD, Higgins GA, Glatstein EJ (1981): Cancer of the Lung. In Principles and Practice of Oncology In DeVita, VT, Hellman S, Rosenberg SA (eds): "Principles and Practice of Oncology: Philadelphia: J. B. Lippincott, p 396.
2. Minna JD, Bunn PA, Jr. (1981): Paraneoplastic Syndromes. In Principles and Practice of Oncology. In DeVita VT, Hellman S, Rosenberg SA (eds): Philadelphia, J.B. Lippincott, p 1477.
3. Gazdar AF, Carney DN, Minna JD (1981): In vitro study of the biology of lung cancer. Yale J Biol and Med 54:187.
4. Gazdar AF, Carney DN, Minna JD (1982). The biology of non-small cell lung cancer. Seminars in Oncology (In press)
5. Baylin SB, Gazdar AF (1981): Endocrine biochemistry in the spectrum of human lung cancer: implications for the cellular origin of small cell carcinoma. In Greco A, Bunn PA, Oldham R (eds): "Small Cell Lung Cancer" New York: Grune and Stratton, p 123.
6. Gazdar AF, Carney DN, Guccion JG, Baylin SB (1981). Small cell carcinoma of the lung: cellular origin and relationship to other pulmonary tumors. In Greco A, Bunn PA, and Oldham R (eds): "Small Cell Lung Cancer." New York: Grune and Stratton, p 145.
7. Gazdar AF, Carney DN, Russell, EK, Sims HL, Baylin SB, Bunn PA, Guccion JG, Minna JD (1980). Establishment of continuous, clonable small cell carcinomas of the lung cultures having amine precursor uptake and decarboxylation properties. Cancer Res 40: 3502.
8. Carney DN, Gazdar AF, Minna JD (1980). Positive correlation between histologic tumor involvement and generation of tumor cell colonies in agarose in specimens taken directly from patients with small cell carcinoma of the lung. Cancer Res 40: 1820.

9. Carney DN, Gazdar AF, Bunn PA, Guccion JG (1981). Demonstration of the stem cell nature of clonogenic tumor cells from lung cancer patients. Stem Cell 1 (3):149.
10. Pearse AG (1969). The cytochemistry and ultrastructure of polypeptide hormone producing cells of the APUD series, and the embryologic, physiologic and pathologic implications of the concept. J Histochem Cytochem 17:303.
11. Baylin SB, Abeloff MD, Goodwin G, Carney DN, Gazdar AF (1980) Activities of L-dopa decarboxylase and diamine oxidase (histaminase) in human lung cancers and decarboxylase as a marker for small (oat) cell cancer in cell cultures. Cancer Res 40: 1990.
12. Gazdar AF, Zweig MH, Carney DN, Van Stierteghen AC, Baylin SB, Minna JD (1981). Levels of creatine kinase and its BB isozyme in lung cancer specimens and cultures. Cancer Research 41:2773.
13. Marangos PJ, Gazdar AF, Carney DN (1982). Neuron specific enolase in human small cell carcinoma cultures. Cancer Letters 15:67.
14. Moody TW, Pert CB, Gazdar AF, Carney DN, Minna JD (1981). High levels of intracellular bombesin characterize human small cell lung carcinoma. Science 214:1246.
15. Sherwin SA, Minna JD, Gazdar AF, Todaro GJ (1981). Expression of epidermal and nerve growth factor receptors and soft agar growth factor production by lung cancer cells. Cancer Res 41:3538.
16. Sims E, Gazdar AF, Abrams P, Minna JD (1980). Growth of human small cell (oat cell) carcinoma of the lung in serum-free growth factor supplemented medium. Cancer Research 40: 4356.
17. Baylin SB, Gazdar AF, Minna, JD, Shaper HH (1982). Cell surface protein phenotype of human lung cancer in culture. Identification of common and distinguishing cell surface proteins on the membranes of different human lung cancer cell types. Proc Natl Acad Sci. (In press)
18. Whang-Peng J, Kao-Shan CS, Lee EC, Bunn PA, Carney DN, Gazdar AF, Minna JD (1982). Specific Chromosome defect associated with human small cell lung cancer: Deletion 3p(14-23). Science 215:181.
19. Radice PA, Matthews MJ, Ihde DC, Gazdar AF, Carney DN, Bunn PA, Cohen MH, Fossieck BE, Makuch RW, Minna JD (1982). The clinical behavior of "mixed" small cell/large cell bronchogenic carcinoma compared to "pure" small cell subtypes. Cancer (in press)
20. Carney DN, Bunn PA, Gazdar AF, Pagan JF, Minna JD (1981).

Selective growth in serum-free hormone supplemented medium of tumor cells obtained by biopsy from patients with small cell carcinoma of the lung. Proc Natl Acad Sci USA 78:3185.
21. Brower M, Carney D, Oie H, Matthews M, Minna J (1982). Growth of human adenocarcinoma of the lung cell lines and clinical specimens in serum-free defined medium. Proc Amer Assoc Clin Oncol 1:140.
22. Cuttitta F, Rosen S, Gazdar AF, Minna JD (1981). Monoclonal antibodies which demonstrate specificity for several types of human lung cancer. Proc Natl Acad Sci USA 78:4591.
23. Minna JD, Cuttitta F, Rosen S, Bunn PA, Jr, Carney DN, Gazdar AF, Krasnow S (1982). Methods for production of monoclonal antibodies with specificity for human lung cancer cells. In Vitro 17:1058.
24. Sherwin S, Twardzik D, Bohn W, Cockley K, Todaro G (1982). Tumor associated transforming growth factor activity in the urine of patients with disseminated cancer. Proc Amer Assoc Cancer Res 23:41.
25. Perucho M, Goldfarb M, Shimizu K, Lama C, Fogh J, Wigler M (1981). Human-tumor-derived cell lines contain common and different transforming genes. Cell 27:467.
26. Krontiris TG, Cooper GM (1981). Transforming activity of human tumors DNAs. Proc Natl Acad Sci USA 78:1181.
27. Murray MJ, Shilo BZ, Shih C, Cowing D, Hsu HW, Weinberg RA (1981). Three different human tumor cell lines contain different oncogenes. Cell 25:355.
28. Nomura. Nature 296: 575, 1982.

Rational Basis for Chemotherapy, pages 23–39
© 1983 Alan R. Liss, Inc., 150 Fifth Avenue, New York, NY 10011

A QUANTITATIVE MODEL FOR DRUG RESISTANCE IN
CANCER CHEMOTHERAPY

J.H. Goldie,[1] A.J. Coldman,[2] N. Bruchovsky,[3]

Cancer Control Agency of British Columbia
2656 Heather Street, Vancouver, B.C., Canada V5Z 3J3

ABSTRACT   A quantitative model for the emergence of
drug resistant cells in tumors is described. It is assumed
that drug resistant phenotypes arise as a consequence of
random, spontaneous mutations in accordance with the basic
relationships first described by Luria and Delbruck. Such
a model allows one to simulate the behaviour of neoplasms
developing resistance to chemotherapy and to make inferences
in how treatment strategy can be more effectively implement-
ed.

INTRODUCTION

A fundamental problem in cancer chemotherapy, at both
the experimental and clinical level, is the extent to which
neoplastic cell populations can display resistance to the
whole range of chemotherapeutic drugs available. In a number of types of neoplasms significant progress has been
made over the last ten to fifteen years in achieving long
term remission or cure, but despite these impressive achieve-
ments the great majority of patients who receive cancer
chemotherapy can expect to receive only temporary remission
with treatment.
A number of explanations have been advanced to account

[1]Division of Advanced Therapeutics, Cancer Control
Agency of British Columbia
[2]Division of Epidemiology and Biometrics, C.C.A.B.C.
[3]Division of Cancer Endocrinology, C.C.A.B.C.

for the refractoriness to drug treatment of human neoplasms.
These include, variations in host immune responses against
the tumor, pharmacokinetic differences in individuals resulting in variable levels of effective drug concentration,
and the overall growth kinetic properties of the tumor cell
populations themselves.[1,2,3] The processes resulting in drug
treatment failure in cancer are undoubtedly multifactorial,
and we do not wish to suggest that the phenomena mentioned
above might not be expected to contribute to ultimate end
results in cancer treatment. However, it seems to us that
taken individually or together the kinetic and host defence
explanations by themselves are inadequate to account for
many of the observed phenomena that are seen in cancer
chemotherapy in both the experimental and clinical situations. As will be described in detail in this paper, we
believe that genetic variability resulting in a great range
of tumor cell heterogeneity with respect to drug sensitivity
and resistance constitutes an extremely important consideration
as to whether or not a tumor cell population can be erradi-
cated by drug treatment. A quantitative model based on
such assumptions provides a heuristically useful explanation
for many phenomena that would be otherwise extremely
difficult to understand. In addition, such an approach
provides possible directions which can be explored for
improving the effectiveness of current chemotherapeutic
programs.

The Spontaneous Origin of Drug Resistant Phenotypes

In 1943, Luria and Delbruck published their now famous
paper on the phenomenon of mutations to resistance in
bacterial populations[4]. This landmark work provided a
means of distinguishing between the two alternative explanations for the phenomenon of acquired resistance. If
such resistance   comes about as a consequence of the specific
acquisition of resistant phenotypy which is then transmitted
to the resistant cells' progeny, then one can consider such
a process to be essentially Lamarckian in nature. The
alternative view, ie. Darwinian, would be that any population
of cells, eukaryotic or prokaryotic, are continuously giving
rise spontaneously and randomly to a broad range of phenotypic variants. Physical and chemical processes operating
in the environment will act to select for those spontaneous
variants that by chance are better adapted to particular environmental circumstances. If the environmental selection
pressure is extreme, ie. high concentrations of a toxic

chemical, then the result will be rapid elimination of
sensitive phenotypes leaving behind only a small population
of genetically resistant variants, assuming they were
present at the time that the selection phenomenon occurred.

If subjected to experimental test, then these two
competing explanations will yield different results under
appropriate circumstances. Luria and Delbruck devised the
so-called fluctuation test to distinguish between these
different postulates. Essentially, what was found was that
when subclonal populations derived from an initially
homogeneous clonal population, are subjected to environmental
selection, then each of the subclones will display a
substantial variation in the number of phenotypic variants
present per clone. This variation or fluctuation is much
greater than what would be anticipated due to simple
technical mixing errors or what would be expected if the
selecting agent simply acted on the wild cell population
to specifically transfer inheritable phenotypic resistance.
Since the classical studies of Luria and Delbruck were reported, many investigators have repeated their basic experiment on a wide range of microbial and mammalian tumor cell
populations. The results of such tests are summarized in
two recent comprehensive reviews, and they are totally
consistent with the hypothesis that phenotypic variation
arises as a consequence of spontaneous random changes in the
target cell population.[5,6] Although a positive result in a
fluctuation test does not constitute proof of the genetic
origin of such variants, it is completely consistent with
the mutational origin of the phenotypes. More recent
studies, in which the genetic material or the gene products
of drug resistant phenotypes has been examined directly,
[7,8,9] confirms that drug resistant phenotypy, at least in
the vast majority of cases, can be confidently attributed to
spontaneous mutations.

Stochastic processes such as spontaneous mutations
lend themselves to modelling by the use of appropriate
probability theory. The mathematical relationships derived
therefrom can in turn lend themselves to computer simulation
techniques, which can examine the effect of a number of
simultaneously interacting variables.

THEORY

We have previously published a mathematical model of
the emergence of drug resistant phenotypes which allows one
to examine in detail the implications for cancer chemotherapy

that randomly arising mutations produce.[10] In this initial
basic model of tumor growth and cancer chemotherapeutic
effect a number of simplifying assumptions were made. It
was assumed in the first instance that at time zero (ie.
when the size of the tumor population N = 1) that the
number of resistant cells = 0. The situation where resistance
is manifested at time 0 will be dealt with in a later section
in this paper. It was further postulated that each of the
constituent cells within the tumor had stem cell function
(ie. the cloning efficiency was 100% or that cell loss as a
consequence of loss of stem cell function did not occur).
It was assumed in the initial minimal model that we had only
one form of chemotherapeutic treatment available to us and
that the emergence of a drug resistant phenotype to this
modality would constitute a condition of incurability.
Resistant cells are then assumed to arise spontaneously and
randomly from the sensitive population with a certain
frequency, α, which we will call the mutation rate. The
mutation rate is in effect a measure of the probability of
one of the sensitive phenotypes converting to a resistant
state at its next division. It is not synonymous with the
measured percentage or fraction of resistant cells in a
tumor population of a given size.

From these basic assumptions an expression can be
developed which defines the fraction F of resistant cells,
$F = (1-N^{-\alpha})$.[10]

From this relationship it is apparent that both the
proportion and absolute numbers of resistant cells will
increase with increasing size of the total tumor cell
population. This occurs because the expansion in size of
the resistant population occurs as a consequnce of two processes. As each new resistant cell is formed it will undergo its own clonal expansion. In addition to this there will
be a continuous addition of new resistant cells to the
resistant cell pool arising as a consequence of further
mutations in the sensitive cell population. If we assume
that the resistant cells are kinetically identical to
sensitive cells (that is they have the same doubling time)
and that the back mutation rate is no greater than the forward mutation rate, then there will be an inevitable increase
in proportion and   absolute number of resistant cells as
the tumor population expands.

The consequences of this increased rate in accumulation
of resistant cells with time becomes amplified if one
examines the consequences of subsequent mutations arising
in the initial resistant cell population to double levels of

resistance.[11] Double resistant mutants will occur at a frequency of one hundred to a thousand times greater than would be anticipated by the simple product of their individual mutation rates. Again this is because of the consequence of the fact that the growth of the single resistant compartments will be greater than that of the tumor cell population as a whole. It can be demonstrated that if one assumes the existence of n classes of resistant cells that there will be a progressive acceleration of this effect so that multiple levels of resistance can be expected to develop at a disproportionately higher frequency than would be anticipated from examination of individual mutation rates.

This disproportionate increase in resistance with expansion of tumor size would be in addition to the significant effects that might be attributed to classes of mutants (pleotropic) which are known to exhibit cross resistance to a broad range of different antineoplastic agents.[12,13]

From this relationship it is apparent that large tumor cell populations will be extremely difficult to erradicate by chemotherapeutic agents because of their substantial populations of singly and multiply level resistant mutants.

The probability distribution of resistant mutants within a family of tumor clones can be expected to be highly skewed with the mean value being substantially larger than the mode. Although the size of the resistant fraction in any individual tumor cell population will clearly have implications for the duration of treatment response in that individual case, a more important quantity to be estimated is a probability of there being zero resistant cells in a given tumor population.

If one assumes that the probability of a new mutation occurring during a total population increase of ΔN is distributed approximately as a poisson process then it is possible to calculate an expression for the probability of there being zero resistant cells present in a tumor of a given size.[10] The form of this expression is P (probability of zero resistant cells) = exp $(-\alpha \, (N-1))$.

In other words, the lower the mutation rate and the smaller the size of the tumor, the greater will the probability be on average of their being zero resistant cells in a given tumor colony.

If we assume that the absence of resistant cells constitutes the minimum conditions required for drug induced curability then this expression can be considered as a

relationship between tumor burden, mutation rate and
potential cure. It is obvious from this relationship that
the smaller the tumor population, on average, the greater
the likelihood of the induction of drug induced cure. Likewise, the lower the mutation rate to resistance for a particular drug (or drug combination) the greater the
probability of cure.

These basic mathematical relationships can be seen to
have three obvious implications with respect to both
experimental and clinical cancer chemotherapy. Firstly,
because of the probabilistic nature of the process whereby
drug resistant cells appear one would not expect to find
in a given series of otherwise identical tumors an indentical
proportion of drug resistant cells. This is, essentially,
the nature of the Luria Delbruck fluctuation phenomenon. In
clinical terms this would translate into a variable response
by apparently histologically identical tumors of equal
stage to identical chemotherapy. One might anticipate a
range of responses from little or transient effect to
sustained remission to under some circumstances complete
cure of the tumor. This prediction corresponds to what is
consistently observed in clinical and experimental systems
(14), and this phenomenon would be difficult to explain by
resorting to purely kinetic explanations for tumor response
and behavior.

The next inference that can be developed from the above
relationships has to do with the relationship between tumor
burden and curability. It is readily apparent, that on
average, small tumor populations will be disproportionately
more easily curable than will be large ones. This can be
more easily visualized if one plots the function $P = \exp -\alpha$
$(N-1)$ for a given value for alpha and with increasing size
of tumor. This is depicted in figure 1 where it is seen
that the probability of there being zero resistant clones
falls off very steeply with increasing size of tumor. The
likelihood of there being zero resistant cells present goes
from a state of near 100% to close to zero over an approximately two log increase in tumor size.

This relationship between tumor burden and curability
has long been recognized in experimental tumors, and might
be considered to be one of the reasons for enhanced effectiveness of adjuvant chemotherapy in the clinical situation.
What is not intuitively obvious is the steepness of which
the probability of cure falls off with tumor expansion.
This suggests that in the growth of any tumor there will be
a critical transition time during which its likelihood of

FIGURE 1.

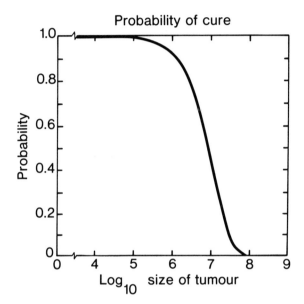

FIGURE 1.   Plot of the function $P = \exp(-\alpha(N-1))$
for increasing values of N and $\alpha = 10^{-7}$.

being cured by a given drug or drug combination will change
relatively rapidly. The broad inference of such a phenomenon
would be that the institution of adjuvant chemotherapy should
not be subject to undue delay. Indeed a strong case can be
made for the initiation of such treatment during the pre-
or perioperative period. The effectiveness of early adjuvant
chemotherapy can be readily demonstrated in experimental
systems, though hard evidence on what the critical delay
times would be in clinical situations is lacking at the
present time. It is self-evident, however, that adjuvant
chemotherapy cannot be postponed indefinitely and that there
would seem to be a strong case for critically examining the
effect of early chemotherapeutic intervention by the
appropriate clinical trials.

Just as there is a strong inverse relationship between
tumor burden and curability there will be a similar relationship between the net mutation rate to resistance for the
system for a tumor of a given size. That is, the lower the
mutation rate then the greater the likelihood of cure.
Although the mutation rate for a population of cells is
obviously related to some intrinsic property of these cells,
the measured value for this rate will be in a sense dictated
by the particular probe that the experimentalist uses. In
this sense, the outcome of the mutation rate measurement is
to a degree under the control of the experimentalist or the
therapist. To choose an extreme example we could say that
the mutation rate to resistance to boiling sulphuric acid
for nearly all cell populations is virtually zero. The mutation rate to resistance to, for example 10^{-20} molar
methotrexate would be virtually one. These are deliberate
extreme examples of course, but it is apparent that choice
of agents and dosage by the therapist will have a significant
impact on what the mutation rate to resistance for the
system will be. Thus a clear cut rationale for combination
chemotherapy emerges if one assumes that with the choice of
non-cross resistant agents that the mutation rate to resistance
to the combination will be lower than that of to the individual single agents. Combination chemotherapy would
then be considered to have a much greater potential for cure
than single agents, even given in maximum tolerated dosages.
For this effect to be achieved one must assume that the
individual agents on their own have significant effect and
at least to a degree are non-cross resistant.

There are other arguments that can be put forward for
the use of multiple agent therapy in tumors, including
pharmacokinetic differences between the various agents,

different effects on the cell cycle, biochemical synergism and, hopefully, in some circumstances increased collateral sensitivity between the agents. This latter effect would be equivalent to having a lower net mutation rate to the drug combination.

Combinations of Hormones and Cytotoxic Drugs

There are a number of classes of clinical tumors which are known to be sensitive to hormonal manipulations of various types. These are primarily the malignancies of the breast, endometrium and prostate which respond to estrogenic or androgenic steroids, and many types of tumors of the lymphoid system which are sensitive to glucocorticoids. If one makes the assumption that tumor cells may mutate to drug resistance without necessarily at the same time acquiring the properties of steroid hormone resistance then a case can be made for the simultaneous use of cytotoxic chemotherapy and the appropriate steroid hormone.(15) In those tumors where this option is available, such combinations are attractive because steroid hormones have generally little in the way of acute toxicity and this does not overlap with the side effects of most chemotherapeutic agents. Although there is not a large body of data from either the experimental or clinical level with respect to these treatment modalities, such information as available does tend to favor the conclusion that combinations of effective drugs and hormones when given concurrently may be more effective than the sequential application of such therapies.(16,17)

A possible therapeutic approach that has received attention in recent years, involves the deliberate use of stimulatory hormones to increase drug sensitivity by a) increasing the growth fraction of the tumor and b) shortening the mean generation time of component cells and c) possibly recruiting cells from a cell cycle inactive stage to a proliferative state where they become much more vulnerable to cytotoxic drug effect. While this approach has some theoretical attractions, we believe it should be explored with considerable caution. Firstly, there is the implicit assumption in such an approach that it is purely or at least primarily the cell kinetic state of the target tissue that is going to determine its drug sensitivity. If the target tumor cells were uniformly highly drug sensitive then it is possible that by increasing their growth rates their sensitivity to a number of chemotherapeutic agents could be enhanced. On the other hand, however, it could be argued

that if the cells are in fact uniformly sensitive then they
should be susceptible to progressive cytoreduction in any
event, although perhaps at a slower rate. Furthermore it
seems highly improbable to us, that in tumor cell populations
of any significant size that there would not be at least
some drug resistant phenotypes present. Certainly this
would appear to be the case for such tumors as breast and
prostate which do not appear to be curable in the advanced
stage with existing chemotherapeutic modalities. The
deliberate induction of enhanced growth potential of drug
resistant clones likely to be present in such tumor cell
populations, it seems to us, is clearly fraught with many
risks. It might seem to be a wise precaution to have
available considerably more in the way of experimental data
from appropriate animal model systems to determine the
relative effectiveness of hormone suppressive therapy versus
hormone stimulative therapy in combination with appropriate
chemotherapy. A tumor cell that is genetically drug
resistant is unlikely to be converted to a state of drug
sensitivity by the simple manoevre of increasing its growth
rate. In some patients, serious clinical consequences such
as increased rate of tumor growth and dissemination which
cannot be impeded by drug therapy might be the result.

Intrinsic drug resistance

     In the minimal model described above we have assumed
an initial condition of drug sensitivity, and that drug
resistance arises as the consequence of spontaneous mutations
occurring within a sensitive population. Therapy, by eliminating sensitive counterparts, will leave behind a totally
resistant tumor. This state of affairs clearly seems to
operate in many experimental and clinical tumors. However,
it is also apparent that individual tumors of different
histological type show a broad range of differences in
their basic sensitivity to the numbers of chemotherapeutic
drugs that we have available to us. In nearly all circumstances, it has required painstaking empirical clinical
testing to determine which drugs have useful effects against
which tumors. Thus, the agent 6-mercaptopurine appears to
have no useful clinical activity against a neoplasm such as
malignant melanoma. Furthermore the data that are becoming
available from the in vitro cloning assays of drug sensitivity
(18) show a great range in drug responsiveness to chemotherapeutic agents for virtually all neoplasms. Furthermore,
numerous examples can be found of tumor clones that appear

to be totally resistant to given chemotherapeutic agents,
even without prior treatment and selection.

That this phenomenon should occur, should not be totally
surprising, as the normal cell systems of the body do not
exhibit a uniform marked sensitivity to all chemotherapeutic
agents. The most broadly sensitive normal cells to
chemotherapeutic drugs in general appear to be those of the
hemopoietic and lymphoid systems. It may not be surprising
therefore that neoplasms derived from such tissues tend also
to display a broad range of sensitivity to many classes of
chemotherapeutic drugs. On the other hand, the rapidly
dividing cells of the oral and pharangeal mucosa appear to
be quite resistant to the effects of a variety of alkylating
agents such as cyclophosphomide and nitrogen mustard. This
is despite the essentially rapid growth kinetics that these
normal cell systems exhibit. Clearly the sensitivity of a
tumor population may in part be determined by the range of
sensitivity of the normal tissues from which it was
originally derived.

Compounding this problem, are recent observations
suggesting that the actual process of neoplastic transformation itself may be associated with genetic and chromosomal
changes (such as gene amplification) which increase the
probability of drug resistance being present.(19) Thus, some
cell populations may actually transform into a drug resistant
state at the same time as they acquire their properties of
neoplastic growth.

Thus the initial assumptions in the basic model that
one postulates the value of the resistance cells R = 0 at
the time when N = 1 cannot be expected to be true for every
class of tumor and every drug. However it does seem that
for most tumors and for many drugs the initial conditions
of R = 0 and N = 1 likely will be met. There does not appear
to be any apriori method of predicting which class of tumor
is going to be sensitive to which class of chemotherapeutic
agents, other than by direct measurement, either in vitro
or in vivo. The selection of specific drugs or drug
combinations for particular classes of tumors is an issue
that cannot be dealt with by the somatic mutation model of
drug resistance. For the time bieng, it appears that only
empirical testing can provide answers to these questions.

The Phenomenon of Repeated Remission Induction With the Same
Agents in the Same Tumor

A criticism of the somatic mutation model of resistance

that is frequently voiced is that it does not account for the occasionally observed clinical phenomenon of the ability to reinduce second (and sometimes many more) remissions in the same patient with the same drugs after initial relapse. This is a valid objection because, while such instances appear to be the exception rather than the rule for most tumors, they do occur under some circumstances, and any comprehensive theory of drug resistance must be able to account for this phenomenon in a reasonably satisfactory fashion.

We believe that there are basically two processes whereby the above observed phenomenon might come about. In the first set of circumstances, what is commonly observed is that it is possible to induce second remissions of shorter duration with the same drugs that produce the initial response. In a recent monograph Skipper(20) has addressed this question using the somatic mutation model and appropriate computer simulations. One of the inferences of the somatic mutation theory is that there will be a variable proportion of drug resistant cells to a given class of agents in individual patients. In some patients, this proportion may be very small though not zero. Following a fixed number of courses of therapy resulting in complete remission one would anticipate that substantial regression of tumor, but short of cure, would be achieved. If the surviving burden of tumor cells at the end of therapy still had a relatively high sensitive to resistant ratio, then on relapse such a tumor would again be expected to display drug responsiveness, at least to a limited extent. One would not expect however, such remissions to be of equivalent durability as the first group and it would not be expected that the neoplasm could be cured by courses of therapy that were ineffective in curing the tumor the first time. Generally speaking, this expectation conforms to what is commonly seen in the re-induction of second remissions. Thus, this type of phenomenon is still consistent with the basic minimal model of somatic mutations to resistance.

It must be conceded, however, that there are clinical instances known where it is possible to repetitively induce fairly durable complete remissions with essentially the same treatment on a number of occasions with the remissions lasting very close to the same period of time. Despite this however, it is not possible to cure these patients by intensification of the basic treatment regimen. Such phenomena are uncommon, and are primarily confined to certain tumors of the lyphoid system such as acute lymphoblastic

leukemia of children and nodular well differentiated
lymphocytic lymphoma. It is, moreover, far from being
universally observed in all instances of these tumors.

It must be conceded that there is no firm scientific
evidence that would at the present time provide a definitive
explanation for these types of phenomena. However, such
processes would not be inconsistent with the behavior of
certain classes of drug resistant cells that are known to
develop in experimental systems. Thus, a number of investigators have recently (21,22) demonstrated in in vitro
systems the occurrence of so-called unstable resistant
phenotypes that are characterized by extremely high
reversion rates to the wild sensitive state. Moreover, an
observed property of such unstably resistant phenotypes
which has been seen in a number of instances, is the fact
that they have significantly slower growth rates than that
of their wild sensitive counterparts. In the initial mutation
to resistance model we assumed that the kinetic properties
of the resistant and sensitive phenotypes were similar, if
not identical. If one postulates a situation whereby
unstably resistant phenotypes occur which have a kinetic
disadvantage compared to sensitive cells and which have a
high reversion rate (in the absence of selection) to a
sensitive state then this provides the basis for possible
explanation of the phenomenon of tumors repetitively
recurring after therapy in a predominantly drug sensitive
mode. One would predict (and this is observed in experimental systems) that eventually a stable drug resistant
phenotype would arise, abolishing the phenomenon of repeated
remission inducibility.
      At the present time we are not aware of any evidence
from clinical or in vivo systems that would allow one to
say with any confidence that such unstable resistant phenotypes do occur and are the basis for recurrent drug sensitive
tumors. However, their existence in in vitro systems appears
to be well established and such phenotypes appear to have
the properties that would go some distance towards explaining
this otherwise very baffling clinical phenomenon. It would
be of great interest in the future, to see whether direct
evidence can be obtained of the existence of such unstable
phenotypes in clinical neoplasms.

The Relationship Between Doubling Time and Curability

      Although there are many individual exceptions to the

observation that rapidly growing tumors are more drug
sensitive and curable than slow growing ones, it does appear
that as a general rule this relationship holds true.   It has
been primarily this observation that has tended to support
the belief that growth kinetics on their own played the
dominant role in determining drug curability. Without
minimizing the likely significant contribution of overall
kinetics to inherent sensitivity, it is useful to point out
that tumors that recur in the face of continuing drug
treatment generally have not altered their growth kinetics
to any significant degree.(23) This has also been observed
in in vitro cloning systems where the drug resistant phenotypes that develop appear if anything to have shortened
doubling times and increased growth fraction. Likewise,
those neoplasms that undergo a terminal accelerated phase
such as the blast cell crisis of chronic myelogenous
leukemia, tend to be much more refractory to drug treatment
than tumors that present initially with rapid growth kinetics.

This paradox may be resolved if one postulates some
real time dependent process which influences the probability
of drug resistant mutants arising. A slow growing neoplasm
that reaches clinical dimensions will be much older in a
biological sense than a rapidly growing tumor of the same
clinical stage. This enhanced elapsed time interval may in
itself increase the probability of unfavourable mutations
arising within the tumor cell population. For instance, one
putative cause of spontaneous mutations are the interactions
between living cells and background radiation and cosmic
rays. The dosages of these mutagens tends to be constant
with time and might therefore increase the likelihood of
mutagenic events in a tumor cell population that requires
a long elapsed time interval to reach the point where it
can be diagnosed and treatment started. Other time dependent
mutagenic processes may be operative as well, all tending
towards making the more slowly growing system more likely
to have undergone mutations and phenotypic diversity.

The above, however, can only be considered as speculative
and the problem as to why neoplasms with long doubling times
generally, as well as why certain broad classes of tumors
exhibit significant degrees of drug resistance without having
undergone prior drug treatment and selection is clearly of
the utmost importance and will need to be resolved if
significant improvements in the chemotherapy of many types
of malignancies are to be improved.

SUMMARY

We have described in this paper briefly, how the somatic mutation theory can be applied to account for a number of perplexing phenomena that are observed during the drug treatment of both experimental and clinical neoplasms. Such a theory makes a number of unambiguous predictions as to how chemotherapy might be more rationally and effectively utilized, but the predictions of the theory await verification by appropriate clinical experiments.

REFERENCES

1. Harris JE, Bogoi RC, Stewart THM (1973). Serial monitoring of immune reactivity in cancer patients receiving chemotherapy as a means of predicting anti-tumor response. In Daguillard S (ed): "Proc /th Leukocyte Culture Conf," New York: Academic Press.

2. Livingston RB, Sukes A, Thirwell MP, Murphy WK, Hart JS (1977). Cell kinetic parameters: Correlation with clinical response. In Derwinko B, Humphrey RM (eds): "Growth Kinetics and Biochemical Regulation of Normal and Malignant Cells," Baltimore: William and Wilkins, pp 767-85.

3. Simpson-Henen L (1977). Growth kinetics as a function of tumor size. In Derwinko B, Humphrey RM (eds): "Growth Kinetics and Biochemical Regulation of Normal and Malignant Cells," Baltimore: William and Wilkins, pp 547-59.

4. Luria SE, Delbruck M (1943). Mutations of bacteria from virus sensitivity to virus resistance. Genetics 28:491.

5. De Mars R (1974). Resistance of cultured human fibroblasts and other cells to purine analogues in relation to mutagenesis detection. Mutat Res 14:335.

6. Siminovitch L (1976). On the nature of hereditable variation in cultured somatic cells. Cell 7:1.

7. Beaudet AL, Rougin DJ, Caskey CT (1973). Mutations affecting the structure of hypoxanthine: Guanine phosphoribosyl transferase in cultured Chinese hamster cells. Proc Natl Acad Sci USA 70:320-24.

8. Cline MJ, Stang H, Mercola K, Morse L, Ruprecht R, Browne J, Salser W (1980). Gene transfer in intact animals. Nature (London) 284, 3:422-25.

9.   Chan VL, Whitmore GF, Siminovitch L (1972). Mammalian cells with altered forms of RNA polymerase II. Proc Natl Acad Sci USA 69:3119-23.

10. Goldie JH, Coldman AJ (1979). A mathematic model for relating the drug sensitivity of tumors to their spontaneous mutation rate. Cancer Treat Rep 63, 11-12:1727-33.

11. Goldie JH, Coldman AJ, Gudauskas GA (1982). A rationale for the use of alternating non-cross resistant chemotherapy. Cancer Treat Rep 66:439-49.

12. Brockman RW, Yung-Chi C, Schabel FM Jr, Montgomery JA (1980). Metabolism and chemotherapeutic activity of 9-B-D- Arabinofuranosyl-2-fluoroadenine against murine leukemia L1210 and evidence for its phosphosylation by deoxycytidine kinase. Cancer Res 40:3610.

13. Ling V (1978). Genetic aspects of drug resistance in somatic cells. In Schoenfeld H (ed): "Antibiotics and Chemotherapy," Basil, Switzerland: Karger, vol 23, pp 191.

14. Skipper HE (1980). Some thoughts regarding a recent publication by Goldie and Coldman entitled "A Mathematical Model for Relating the Drug Sensitivity of Tumors to Their Spontaneous Mutation Rate". Booklet 9, Southern Research Institute, Birmingham, Alabama.

15. Goldie JH, Bruchovsky N, Coldman AJ, Gudauskas GA (1981). Steroid receptors in adjuvant hormonal therapy for breast cancer. Can J Surg 24:3.

16. Drago JR, Goldman LB, Gershwin ME (1980). Chemotherapeutic and hormonal considerations of the NB rate prostatic adenocarcinoma model. In: "Models for Prostate Cancer" New York: Alan R. Liss, p 325.

17. Nischer B, Plotkin D, Bowman D, et all (1981). The benefits of 1-pam + 5-FU + tamoxifen adjuvant therapy in stage II breast cancer patients. Proc Amer Soc Clin Oncol 22:C-412.

18. Salmon SE, Alberts DS, Meyskens FL Jr, Durie BGM, Jones SE, Srehalen B, Young L, Chen HS, Moon TE (1980). Clinical correlations of in-vitro drug sensitivity. In Salmon SE (ed): "Cloning of Human Tumor Stem Cells," New York: Alan R. Liss, pp 223-46.

19. Varshavsky A (1981). Phorbol ester dramatically increases incidence of methotrexate-resistant mouse cells: Possible mechanisms and relevance to tumor promotion. Cell 25:561-72.

20. Skipper HE (1981). Computer simulations of chemotherapeutic end results IV. Some thoughts on second

remissions with the same drugs. Booklet 12, Southern
Research Institute, Birmingham, Alabama.

21. Kaufman RJ, Brown PC, Schimke RT (1979). Amplified
dihydrofolate reductase genes in unstably methotrexate-
resistant cells are associated with double minute
chromosomes. Proc Natl Acad Sci USA 76:5669-73.

22. Tischfield JA, Trill JJ, Lee YI, Coy K, Tylor MW
(1982). Genetic instability at the adenine
phosphoribosyltransferase locus in mouse L cells.
Molecular and Cellular Biology 2:250-57.

23. Durie BGM, Salmon SE (1980). Cell kinetic analysis of
human tumor stem cells. In Salmon SE (ed): "Cloning
of Human Tumor Stem Cells," New York: Alan R. Liss,
pp 153-163.

Rational Basis for Chemotherapy, pages 41–43
© 1983 Alan R. Liss, Inc., 150 Fifth Avenue, New York, NY 10011

WORKSHOP SUMMARY: TUMOR HETEROGENEITY

G.H. Heppner and J.R. Shapiro

Department of Immunology
Michigan Cancer Foundation
110 East Warren Avenue
Detroit, Michigan 48201

Department of Neurology
Memorial Sloan-Kettering Cancer Center
1275 York Avenue
New York, New York 10021

G. Heppner opened the workshop by discussing various
kinds of tumor heterogeneity. The most overwhelming type
is that seen between different patients with the same
disease. For example, human breast cancer is notoriously
variable among different patients. A second type of
heterogeneity derives from consideration of tumor "geogra-
phy"; vasculature, supporting tissue, and cellular infil-
trates are not evenly distributed within a tumor. Furthermore, tumor cells are not synchronous populations, and,
consequently, are heterogeneous for cell-cycle dependent
phenomena. Recent attention has been focussed on yet
another type of heterogeneity, that which is due to the
existence of clonal subpopulations within individual
cancers. Such tumor subpopulations have been shown to
differ in many characteristics, including sensitivity to
chemotherapeutic agents. There is evidence that these subpopulations are distributed "zonally" within a tumor, a
point which can contribute to sampling error. There is
also evidence that certain subpopulations are relatively
unstable and give rise to new variants at varying frequencies. Variation in metastatic phenotype seems particularly
common. Thus, intra-tumor heterogeneity is a dynamic phenomenon, with a more-or-less continual evolution of new
variant subpopulations. Tumor heterogeneity is dynamic in
another sense also: although individual subpopulations

may differ in many characteristics, they can also interact with each other to influence growth, metastasis, and sensitivity to drugs. Examples of different interactions were described. Some depend on host, some on tumor factors; some require tumor cell contact and some act systemically. Thus, tumors are ecosystems in which the individual subpopulations contribute to the over-all behavior but do not define it completely.

B. Miller described progress in the development of a new in vitro assay for drug sensitivity which attempts to accomodate the heterogeneous nature of neoplasms and the ability of individual subpopulations to alter each other's drug response. Since, in this view, all tumor cells within a cancer may influence therapeutic response, the new assay is not a clonogenic one but, instead, aims to be as non-selective as possible. The assay is being developed for breast cancer and involves growth within a collagen gel matrix. Individual pieces of tumor are embedded in the matrix. The pieces grow out in a variety of morphologically distinguishable, three-dimensional patterns which reflect, at least to some extent, the heterogeneity of the starting tumor. Growth is quantitated by planimetry using images of the pieces projected by a camera lucida attached to an inverted microscope. Subpopulations of a single mouse mammary tumor are differentially sensitive to methotrexate in this assay, but the degree of sensitivity is up to two orders of magnitude less than that shown by the same populations grown as monolayers.

P. Houghton described how some cells within childhood rhabdomyosarcomas grown as xenografts in immune-deprived mice demonstrate differential sensitivities to classes of agents with different mechanisms of cytotoxicity. The patterns of cross-resistance of such instrinsically resistant cells differ from those seen among cells selected by previous exposure to drugs. Thus, the mechanisms of intrinsic resistance may differ from those described for "acquired" resistance. Since some cells are already intrinsically resistant to a given drug, Dr. Houghton was able to readily select a stable vincristine-resistant line, which carried an altered karyotype, from one rhabdomyosarcoma which was apparently heterogeneous for drug sensitivity prior to any chemotherapy.

H. Smith described a clonogenic assay which has been developed for human breast tissues. Dose-response curves for adriamycin are biphasic, indicating a differential sensitivity of some populations within the breast tissues. Interestingly, such heterogeneity was seen both with malignant and normal samples, suggesting that tumor heterogeneity is a reflection of normal tissue heterogeneity, and can arise through the same processes of development and differentiation.

J. Shapiro demonstrated that the near-diploid subpopulations within human gliomas often become more tumorigenic after only 5 weeks of treatment with sublethal doses of an alkylating agent, BCNU. Following treatment these subpopulations often show a sharp decrease in mitotic index with long lag periods, but when exponential growth resumes, they are able to grow in soft agar whereas control cultures do not. In contrast, hyperploid cells (3n and 4n chromosome number), although capable of spontaneously generating many new variants during serial passage, appear to be more sensitive to alkylating agents and show increased cell death and failure to grow in soft agar. By passage numbers 15-20, many of these hyperploid subpopulations no longer grow. Karyotypic analysis of these events reveals considerable genotypic remodeling causing a continued evolution of phenotypes. Mechanisms include segregational error, inactivation, induction or mutation of a gene or genes. Since malignant cells do not act independently, cell-cell interactions as well as developmental events may play key roles in the modification of any such phenotype. The goal of this work is no longer one of simply identifying heterogeneity within a system, but rather identifying and isolating those cells which permit the continued progression of the neoplastic state from the multitude of cells that seem to be generated by most malignant tumors.

Rational Basis for Chemotherapy, pages 45–59
© **1983 Alan R. Liss, Inc., 150 Fifth Avenue, New York, NY 10011**

SPECIFIC KARYOTYPIC AND TUMORIGENIC CHANGES IN CLONED SUBPOPULATIONS OF HUMAN GLIOMAS EXPOSED TO SUBLETHAL DOSES OF BCNU[1]

Joan R. Shapiro and William R. Shapiro

George C. Cotzias Laboratory of Neuro-Oncology
and Department of Neurology
Memorial Sloan-Kettering Cancer Center
Department of Neurology
Cornell University Medical College,
New York, NY 10021.

ABSTRACT   Five human gliomas were dissociated into single cells which were karyotyped and cloned.   Clones, cytogenetically identified as part of the original tumor, were expanded and treated with sublethal doses of BCNU.   The control and treated clones were analyzed at passages 2 and 12 to determine retention or loss of specific chromosomes and growth potential in soft agar.   The untreated clones that were near-diploid in chromosome number remained stable in vitro and retained their parental karyotypes without producing new variants, while hyperploid (3n and 4n) clones were unstable, generating many new variant cells.   During serial passage the stable clones lost and/or gained few chromosomes while the unstable clones frequently lost chromosomes 1, 3, 9 and 22, and/or gained chromosome 19.   Only one control clone, JVC-11, grew in soft agar at passage 12.   This clone reduced its chromosome number to a near-diploid range.   Treatment of stable and unstable clones with BCNU (1 µg/ml for one hour) 3 times weekly, for 5 consecutive

[1]This work was supported by Grant CA 25956-03 and CA 18856-07 from the National Cancer Institute and BRSG 3854 and Memorial Sloan-Kettering Cancer Center.

weeks, altered both the chromosomal complement and tumorigenicity of the clones. By passage 12, 6 of 10 treated clones showed a decrease in modal chromosome number. Five of the 8 clones, all of which had near-diploid chromosome numbers, grew in soft agar. Within these 5 clones there was a noted loss of chromosome 22 and a gain of chromosome number 17. The loss and retention of specific chromosomes may identify those important in tumorigenicity and drug resistance.

INTRODUCTION

Cytogenetic analysis of freshly resected human gliomas (anaplastic astrocytomas and glioblastoma multiforme) have identified many subpopulations and isolated cell types (1). Within a single tumor, the size of a subpopulation(s) and the proportion of individual cell types may differ, permitting tumors to have a variable phenotypic expression. Such heterogeneity is also evident when one compares the cells or subpopulations of the same histologically graded tumor in different patients. Here again, the distribution of cell types varies from one patient to another.

Techniques using quantitative autoradiography on animal brain tumor models have shown that in addition to heterogeneous cell types there is the problem of heterogeneous drug delivery. Blood-brain barrier and blood flow differ regionally in such tumors resulting in some cells in one location receiving low doses of a chemotherapeutic agent while those located elsewhere in the tumor receive higher doses (2).

It is this variability that leads to the difficulty in treating human gliomas. Subpopulations identified in tumors that were grown for several passages in vitro showed a differential sensitivity to both BCNU and cis-platinum (3). This intrinsic resistance was small in magnitude but statistically significant. In addition to inherent cellular resistance, cells may also be induced to become resistant through the repeated exposure to a chemotherapeutic agent.

Our laboratory efforts have been directed at trying to isolate from the myriad of cells those that are intrinsically resistant and those that can be induced to acquire resistance.

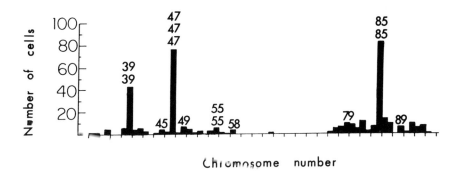

FIGURE 1. The distribution of cells containing chromosome numbers in tumor AN. Chromosome preparations were made on cells mechanically dissociated and grown in suspension culture (karyotyped 6-24 h post resection) or in short-term monolayer culture (karyotyped 48 to 72 h post resection). The chromosome preparations were Q- or G-banded for cytogenetic analysis. Three hundred sixty-nine metaphases were analyzed to determine the probable number of cellular subpopulations present at the time of resection. A subpopulation was designated as a cellular representative of the resected tumor if 5 or more karyotypes with identical deviations were found. The dissociated cells were also dilution-plated and clones were isolated 7-28 days later. The numbers above each of the bars represent clones that were matched to the subpopulations of the tumor. Two clones having 39 chromosomes and identical karyotypic deviations were isolated from different flasks and presumably represent two cells isolated from the same subpopulation. Other cells for which multiple clones were isolated include chromosome numbers 47, 55 and 85.

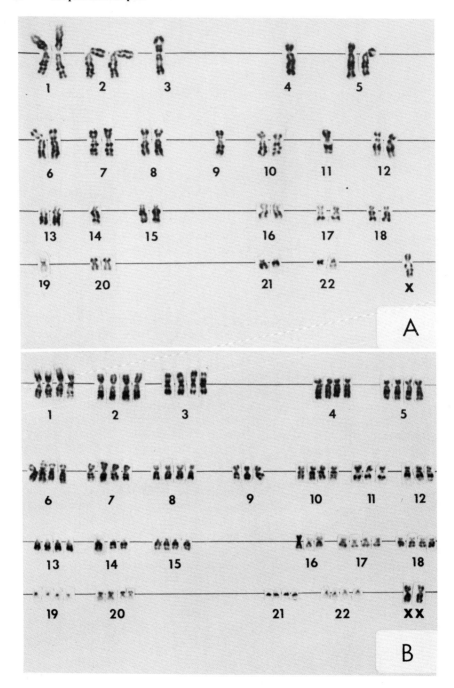

KARYOTYPIC HETEROGENEITY

The histogram of tumor AN is shown in Figure 1. It is representative of the kinds of karyotypic heterogeneity found in glioblastoma multiforme. The chromosome number ranges from hypodiploid cells to hyperploid (3n and 4n) cells. There are usually 1 to 3 clusters of chromosome numbers of which 1 or 2 are generally in the near-diploid range. Even within such clusters, there are often cells with different chromosomal distributions and others of isolated karyotypic deviations (1). Cloning mechanically dissociated cells directly from the tumor permitted the isolation of tumor subpopulations that were identified in the primary cytogenetic analysis of the tumor (1) Fig. 2, A and B). In this manner the cells we investigated were those shown to exist in the tumor at the time of resection rather than variant cells generated in vitro with a selective growth advantage. Clones ANC-2 and ANC-23 were representative of the clonal subpopulations found in our gliomas (Fig 2A and B). The karyotypes demonstrated numerical aberrations in the majority of metaphases analyzed in the primary and short-term analysis. Of the total metaphases analyzed, structural rearrangements were found as isolated cell types in no more than 3% of the cells of the tumors in this experimental group. Karyotypes with extensive chromosomal translocations or rearrangements could not be matched to those of any of the subpopulations. Three tumors AN, MA and RP carried stable marker chromosomes involving chromosomes 3, 10 and 11 (4).

The karyotypic heterogeneity at resection represents a single time point in the evolution of the neoplasm. Following serial passage of the clonal subpopulations, our results indicated two patterns of cellular evolution in vitro (5). Clones that were hypodiploid or near-diploid in chromosome number produced few variant cells; during 12

FIGURE 2. G-banded karyotypes of clones ANC-2 and ANC-23. A second clone, isolated from different flasks (not shown) carried these same numerical karyotypic deviations and presumably represent cells from the same subpopulations.
A) Clone ANC-2 has 39 chromosomes with no apparent structural rearrangement with standard G-banding techniques.
B) Clone ANC-23 has 85 chromosomes all with a normal G-banding pattern.

serial passages they retained their parental karyotypic deviation in 50% or more of the cells analyzed - the stable cell phenotype. Hyperploid cells ranging from 3n and 4n chromosome numbers often generated many new tissue culture variants; the parental karyotypic deviation was lost within 3 or 4 serial passages - the unstable cell phenotype. All five tumors, AN, MS, RP, MA and JV, showed a similar pattern of evolution. Based upon this in vitro behavior, we divided the clonal subpopulations into either stable or unstable groups.

TABLE 1
Clonogenicity of 5 Clonal Subpopulations[a]

Clone Designation	Passage Number 2 Control/Treated	Passage Number 12 Control/Treated
Stable Clones		
ANC-2	ND[b]	ND
MSC-1	0/0	0/203
RPC-2	0/0	0/291
MAC-1	0/0	0/197
JVC-26	0/0	0/107
Unstable Clones		
ANC-10	ND	ND
MSC-8	0/0	0/0
RPC-7	0/0	0/0
MAC-9	0/0	0/0
JVC-11	0/47	18/468

a. Clonal subpopulations isolated directly from 5 glioblastoma multiforme were treated 3x weekly for 1h for 5 consecutive weeks with 1 µg/ml BCNU. At passages 2 and 12, 5 x 10^5 cells/ml were plated in duplicate 6 well dishes. Colony formation was assessed 21-28 days later and each colony scored was not less than 50 µm in diameter.
b. ND = not done.

EFFECTS OF REPEATED ADMINISTRATION OF LOW DOSE BCNU

Our data for intrinsic sensitivity to BCNU and cis-platinum have been reported (3). We found that stable, near-diploid cells differed from unstable, hyperploid cells in their response to BCNU (Table 1).

Following repeated administration of low dose BCNU treatment, stable cells developed marked changes in the distribution and structure of some chromosomes and changed their ability to grow in soft agar. The stable control cultures showed no growth or clonogenicity in soft agar during their 3- to 4-week cultivation and our initial attempts to recover these cells and replate them as a mono-layer culture failed. However, in a second experiment (6), 2 of 5 clones which had not grown in agarose could be recovered and maintained as a monolayer culture. In contrast, the stable treated cultures receiving 1 μg/ml BCNU for 1h, 3x weekly for 5 consecutive weeks all showed growth in soft agar. The unstable clonal populations at passage 2 showed no clonogenicity. By passage 12, JBC-11 of this group grew a number of colonies in soft agar by 3 weeks. Three of the 4 unstable clones treated with BCNU failed to grow in soft agar at passages 2 and 12. JBC-11 was the only clone that produced colonies at passage 2 after treatment and 26-fold more colonies at passage 12. The chromosomes of each subpopulation at passages 2 and 12 were compared (Table 2).

The untreated stable clones did not generate many variants and therefore had few karyotypic changes. The variants from the untreated unstable clones frequently lost chromosomes 1, 3, 9 and 22, and/or gained chromosome number 19. The modal chromosome number of the stable control clones did not change while the unstable controls showed an increase for clone MSC-8, a decrease for clones RPC-7 and JVC-11 and a bimodal distribution for MAC-9. Ninety-seven metaphases from this group at passage 2 were analyzed and 0.003% carried structural rearrangements by standard G-banding. At passage 12, 110 metaphases were analyzed and 0.01% contained structural rearrangements. The treated cultures differed in this respect in that there were many alterations of both chromosome number and structure for both the stable and unstable clones. Eighteen percent of the metaphases in this treated group showed at least one structural rearrangement per metaphase at passage 12. At this same passage number, 6 of 10 clones showed a decrease in modal chromosome number, 3 increased and 1 was bimodal.

Table 2
THE CYTOGENETIC ANALYSIS OF CONTROL AND TREATED SUBPOPULATIONS OF CELLS[a]

CONTROL - STABLE CLONES

Clone Designation[b] (Parental karyotype deviation)	Cell Passage Number	Model Chromosome Number	(Chromosome range)	Karyotypic changes observed[c] in variant cells	
				Loss of Whole Chromosome	Gain of Whole Chromosome
ANC-2 (39, X-3-4-9-11-15-19-X)	2 12	39 39	(34-39) (37-75)	-13	
MSC-1 (45, XX-13)	2 12	45 45	(45-47) (44-49)		
RPC-2 (37, XX del(1p-)-3-5-7-8-9 -9-15-16-16)	2 12	37 37	(37-38) (36-79)		+11+17
MAC-1 (47, Xy +19)	1 12	47 47	(47) (44-58)		+20
JVC-26 (47, Xy +20)	2 12	47 47	(47) (41-101)		+11

Table 2 (Cont.) CONTROL - UNSTABLE CLONES

Clone Designation[b] (Parental karyotype deviation)	Cell Passage Number	Model Chromosome Number	(Chromosome range)	Karyotypic changes observed[c] in variant cells	
				Loss of Whole Chromosome	Gain of Whole Chromosome
ANC-10 (55, XXXX +7+11+11+15+15 +18+19)	2	55	(47-158)	-1-3-X	+19
	12	55	(38-72)	-9-21	+11
MSC-8[d] (74, XXX -1-1-3-7-9-11-11 -13-15-17-18-20-21-22 -22 M₁M₂)	2	74	(49-82)	-4-11	
	12	84	(39-101)	-c-14-22-X	+15
RPC-7[d] (72, XXX -1-2-3-3-5-7-8-9-9 -10-10-12-13-14-14-17-18 +19-20-21-X)	2	72	(69-86)		
	12	69	(44-112)	-1-3-5	+19+20
MAC-9 (64, XXy +2-3+4+7+8+8+10+10 -11+12+13+13+16+17+18+19 +20+21+21+X)	2	64	(56-88)	-1	+19
	12	55&68	(49-93)	-3-11-22	+13+21
JVC-11 (58, Xy +7+9+11+13+15 +15+19+19+21+22+22)	2	58	(49-76)		+17+20+X
	12	43	(47-135)	-3-4-9-10-22	

Table 2 (Cont) TREATED - STABLE CLONES

Clone Designation	Cell Passage Number	Model Chromosome Number	(Chromosome range)	Karyotypic changes observed[c] in variant cells	
				Loss of Whole Chromosome	Gain of Whole Chromosome
ANC-2	2 12	39 42	(39-47) (33-86)	-22	+17+21
MSC-1	2 12	45 47	(41-49) (44-101)	-21	+6+17
RPC-2	2 12	37 43&51	(36-51) (35-99)		+7+17+20
MAC-1	2 12	47 44&47	(47-56) (43-89)	-22	+17
JVC-26	2 12	47 45	(47) (43-162)	-3-11-22	

Table 2 (Cont) TREATED - UNSTABLE CLONES

Clone Designation	Cell Passage Number	Model Chromosome Number	(Chromosome range)	Karyotypic changes observed[c] in variant cells	
				Loss of Whole Chromosome	Gain of Whole Chromosome
ANC-10	2	55	(37-109)	-1-11-X	+17
	12	49&62	(42-111)		
MSC-8	2	74	(35-116)		
	12	65	(47-101)	-5-22	
RPC-7	2	72	(49-96)	-3-X	
	12	63&65	(43-98)	-1-5	+19
MAC-9	2	64	(47-88)	-5	
	12	52&54	(39-104)	-1-2-X	
JVC-11	2	58	(41-86)	-2-22	+17
	12	49	(40-124)	-1-2-7-X	+17+20

JVC-11, which showed the greatest capacity for clonogenicity, had a decrease in the modal chromosome number consistent with the chromosomal numbers of the other clonogenic clones. When the variant cells were analyzed for chromosome loss and gain, it was found that chromosomes 1, 2, 5 and 22 were most often lost and chromosome 17 was gained. When stable treated and untreated clones were separated, 3 of 4 treated stable clones that grew in soft agar became monosomic for chromosome 22 and were diploid, triploid or tetraploid for chromosome 17. Only RPC-2 was diploid for chromosome 22 and trisomic for 17. JVC-11, originally grouped as a hyperploid unstable clone (chromosome number 58), reduced its chromosome number to near-diploid range (chromosome number 49) in which some cells were monosomic for 22 and diploid or trisomic for 17 along with other loses and gains of chromosomes.

We observed that the unstable clones grew very poorly following the sublethal BCNU administration and we continued to passage the 10 treated clones beyond passage 12 (data not shown). At passage 20, all of the stable populations treated with BCNU were growing vigorously as was the unstable clone JBC-11. Clones ANC-10, MSC-8 and RPC-7 failed to grow after serial passage 13, 18 and 19 respectively, and clone MAC-9 terminalized at passage 22. The control clones from these 4 subpopulations as well as the unstable control populations all continued to grow vigorously at passage 25.

TABLE 2:

a. A G-banded cytogenetic analysis was made on all stable and unstable clones in the control and treated divisions at passage 2 and 12.

b. The parental karyotypic deviation is recorded for each clonal subpopulation. Except for RPC-2 with a del of chromosome 1 all other chromosomes had normal banding patterns with standard G-banded analysis.

c. A karyotypic change seen in the variant cells was not recorded unless it was seen 3 or more times. Marker chromosomes are not included in this report.

d. The karyotypic deviation is based on a 4n cell; all other cells are a deviation of a 2n cell.

DISCUSSION

The karyotypic heterogeneity found in primary and short term analysis of freshly resected human gliomas involved primarily numerical aberrations. The chromosome range extended from 35 to 100 chromosomes per cell. Tumor RP and MA carried a common marker chromosome (3)(pter→ p21:). This marker was found in less than 1% of the RP tumor metaphases, but was found as a subpopulation in tumor MA. Tumor RP also contained a 10q+ and an 11p+ chromosome respectively in 5% and 17% of the metaphases. The 11p+ was identified in 3 of 21 subpopulations and represented a very stable marker chromosome. Other structural rearrangements were seen only in isolated cell types. These alterations were very complicated and the number of metaphases carrying all these rearrangements in the primary analysis did not exceed 1% for tumors AN, MA, MS and JV and 2.0% for tumor RP. Several reasons may account for the low incidence of structurally rearranged chromosomes in high grade tumors. Most rearrangements that tumor cells can undergo are not stable and are not suited for cell survival in vivo. Further, such cells may arise in hypoxic or necrotic areas, neither of which provides an environment suitable for cell growth.

Unlike these primary and early passage studies, established glioma lines have been reported as showing numerous chromosomal rearrangements (7-10). Such lines have been in culture for many years and it is uncertain if any of these marker chromosomes occurred in vivo or were selected as the tumor evolved in vitro. In our laboratory, clones in serial passage for 3-6 months all developed marker chromosomes (5). The administration of sublethal doses of BCNU increases the instability of glioma clonal subpopulations causing numerous numerical and structural rearrangements. Because of the possible relationship between chromosomal stability and in vitro evolution we compared stable and unstable clones with respect to clonogenicity (growth in soft agar) following BCNU. Treated, near-diploid clones were more easily induced to grow in soft agar than were the unstable hyperploid clones. Thus, 4 of 4 near-diploid stable clones grew in soft agar after BCNU, while only one hyperploid unstable clone grew after treatment. The latter, JVC-11, decreased its modal chromosome number from 58 to 43 in the control and from 58 to 49 after treatment, thus becoming near-diploid.

Alkylating agents increase segregational errors, predisposing the cells to generate many new combinations of chromosomes in the variants. Some of these variant cells have a growth advantage while in the presence of BCNU and are selected from the myriad of genotypes. We looked for specific chromosomal changes that might have occurred in the evolution of the cells during the sublethal drug administration. A specific pattern of loss and/or gain of chromosomes consistent for every clone was not seen. Few chromosomes were lost in the untreated, stable group while there was a loss in three or more clones for chromosomes 1, 3, 9 and 22 and a gain of chromosome 19 in the unstable group. The treated clones, both stable and unstable, increased the number of chromosomes lost and/or gained. The most notable loss was that of chromosome 22 in 5 of 10 clones and a gain of chromosome 17 in 6 of 10 clones. Changes in these two chromosomes may be of special importance in the evolution of brain tumors since the growth receptor has been provisionally assigned to chromosome 17 (11) and the loss of chromosome 22 has been associated with neurogenic tumors (12-14).

We have drawn several conclusions from these preliminary findings. In a heterogeneous population of cells, near-diploid cells appear to be those most capable of surviving sublethal doses of BCNU. These cells also appeared to evolve to a more malignant state following such treatment as evidenced by their ability to grow in soft agar. While chromosomal changes occur in both treated and untreated cells, there is an increased frequency of loss for chromosome 22 and/or gain of 17 in the treated populations that grow in soft agar. Using this experimental protocol, it may be possible to correlate a specific loss or gain of a chromosome(s) as it relates to tumorigenicity and drug resistance.

REFERENCES

1. Shapiro JR, Yung W-KA, Shapiro WR (1981). Isolation, karyotype and clonal growth of heterogeneous subpopulations of human malignant gliomas. Cancer Res 41:2349.
2. Shapiro WR, Voorhies RM, Basler GA. Blasberg RG (1982). Regional methotrexate entry into experimental rat brain tumors as measured by quantitative autoradiography (QAR). Proc AACR 23:179.

3. Yung W-KA, Shapiro JR, Shapiro WR (1982).
    Heterogeneous chemosensitivities of subpopulations of
    human glioma cells in culture. Cancer Res 42:992.
4. Shapiro JR. The cytogenetic finding of 19 human
    gliomas. (Manuscript in preparation).
5. Shapiro JR, Dato VM, Yung K-WA, Shapiro WR. In vitro
    clonal evolution of human glioma subpopulations.
    (submitted to In vitro).
6. Shapiro JR, Shapiro WR. The effects of sublethal dose
    of BCNU on clonal subpopulations of freshly resected
    human gliomas. (Manuscript in preparation).
7. Mark J (1974). G-Banded analyses of an established
    cell line of a human malignant glioma. Humangenetik
    22:323.
8   Mark J (1974). Origin of the marker chromosomes in an
    established hypotriploid glioma cell line studied with
    G-banded technique. Acta Neuropath. 29:223.
9. Mark J, Anten J, Westermark B (1974). Cytogenetic
    studies with G-band technique of established cell
    lines of human malignant gliomas. Hereditas 78:304.
10. Mark J, Westermark B, Ponten J, Hugosson R (1977).
    Banding patterns in human glioma cell lines.
    Hereditas 87:243.
11. Owerbach D, Rutter WJ, Martial JA, Baster JD, Shows
    TB (1980). Genes for growth hormone, chorionic
    somatomammotropin, and growth hormone-like gene on
    chromosome 17 in humans. Science 209:289.
12. Douglass EC, Poplack DG, Whang-Ring J (1980).
    Involvement of chromosome No. 22 in neuroblastoma.
    Cancer Genet.Cytogenet. 2:287.
13. Yamada K, Kondo T, Yoshioka M, Cami H (1980).
    Cytogenetic studies in twenty human brain tumors:
    association of the No. 22 chromosome abnormalities
    with tumors of the brain. Cancer Genet.Cytogenet.
    2:293.
14. Zang KD, Singer H (1967). Chromosomal constitution of
    meningiomas. Nature 216:84.

Rational Basis for Chemotherapy, pages 61–69
© 1983 Alan R. Liss, Inc., 150 Fifth Avenue, New York, NY 10011

CHEMOTHERAPEUTIC RESPONSE IN XENOGRAFTS:
INTER- AND INTRA-TUMOR HETEROGENEITY

Peter J. Houghton[1] and Janet A. Houghton

Department of Biochemical and Clinical Pharmacology
St. Jude Children's Research Hospital
Memphis, Tennessee 38101

ABSTRACT   Cross resistance between anthracyclines,
actinomycins and Vinca alkaloids is a common phenomenon in both neoplastic cells in culture and in murine
tumors in situ. This study was designed to examine
patterns of intrinsic resistance (de novo) in human
malignancies under conditions of in situ growth. The
sensitivity of 5 lines of rhabdomyosarcoma (RMS) each
derived from a different child, and grown as xenografts in mice, was examined using doxorubicin,
actinomycin D and vincristine as examples of these
classes of cytotoxic agent. The results indicate that
resistance de novo to one agent is not associated
necessarily with cross resistance. Development of
resistance to vincristine in situ was examined. Only
in 2 tumor lines which show slight sensitivity have
resistant lines been derived. These data suggest that
the initial tumor response is determined by subpopulations of cells having different intrinsic sensitivity
to vincristine.

INTRODUCTION

The problem of cross-resistance between anthracycline,
actinomycin and Vinca alkaloid classes of drug has considerable significance to the treatment of many pediatric
neoplasms. In the therapy for rhabdomyosarcoma (RMS), for
example, doxorubicin, actinomycin D and vincristine comprise standard effective therapy (1). Where resistance is
induced in vitro to a Vinca alkaloid (or colchicine), cells

This work was supported by Grants CH-156 and CH-156A from
the American Cancer Society, CA-23099 from the National
Cancer Institute, and by ALSAC.

are usually found to be cross-resistant to doxorubicin and
actinomycin D (2,3,4), although this is not definitive
where resistance is developed in vivo (4,5). Patterns of
cross-resistance in P388 murine leukemic cells selected in
vivo for resistance to either vincristine or doxorubicin
are also different, suggesting that different mechanisms of
resistance are operative (6). Further, the choice of an in
vivo model may prove equally as important. Johnson et al.
(6) stressed that the pattern of cross-resistance displayed
by the sublines of P388 leukemia probably is not evident in
clinical cancer. Recently, it has been demonstrated that
only at high levels of resistance to vincristine is cross-
resistance to other natural products observed, whereas at
lower levels of resistance, mechanisms of resistance may be
specific for a particular drug or class of agent (7).

In the present study, we have examined the intrinsic
sensitivity to doxorubicin, actinomycin D and vincristine
of 5 human rhabdomyosarcomas grown as xenografts in mice in
order to determine whether resistance de novo to agents
from one class was associated with cross-resistance. Data
is presented also on the development of tumor lines resistant to vincristine.

MATERIALS AND METHODS

CBA/CaJ inbred female mice were immune-deprived by the
technique of infant thymectomy (in 4-wk-old mice), followed
3 weeks later by whole-body irradiation (850 rad; Varian 4
MeV linear accelerator). Within 4 hours of irradiation,
each mouse received iv injections of 2.5×10^6 bone marrow
cells derived from thymectomized syngeneic mice (8). Mice
were used for the implantation of neoplastic tissue 2 weeks
after the transplantation of murine bone marrow. In
general, 2- to 4-mm^3 pieces of tumor were implanted. The
incision wound was irrigated with a solution containing
penicillin (20,000 U/ml) and streptomycin (20 mg/ml). All
procedures were done in a type B laminar flow hood. Mice
were caged in an air-conditioned room (26-28°C) lighted for
12 hours each day. Cages, litter, and food (Purina #5010,
autoclavable) were sterilized, and mice were placed in
fresh cages twice weekly.

The growth of tumors was assessed by measuring two
perpendicular diameters at 7-day intervals. As tumor shape
of HxRh12, HxRh14, HxRh18 and RD approximated that of a
sphere, tumor volumes were calculated with the use of the
formula $(\pi/6)xd^3$, where d is the mean diameter (8), whereas
the formula $axb^2/2$ where a is the greater and b the lesser

diameter was used to calculate the volume of HxRh28 xenografts, the shape of which approximated that of a hemielip-
soid. With the exception of HxRh28 tumors, each of the
tumor lines used has been described previously (8-10).
HxRh28 was established from a metastatic lesion in the
axilla of a child with alveolar RMS.

RESULTS

   Data in Figure 1 show dose response curves for HxRh12
and HxRh14 xenografts treated with a single administration

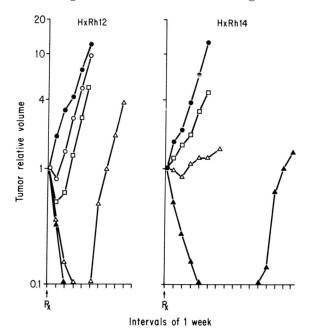

FIGURE 1. Typical dose response curves for HxRh12 and
HxRh14 xenografts. Mice bearing bilateral tumors were given
a single administration of vincristine (ip) at O 0.375 mg,
□ 0.75 mg, △ 1.5 mg, or ▲ 3.0 mg per kg. For HxRh12 tumors
complete regressions (CR) were obtained at 1.5 mg/kg and
"cures" (> 3 months with non-detectable disease) were obtained at 3 mg/kg. No "cures" were obtained in HxRh14 xenografts. The tumor volume relative to that at treatment is
plotted against time. Each curve represents the mean response for 14 individual tumors. ● untreated controls.
   For comparison with data presented in Table 1, responses in HxRh12 xenografts (left panel) would be classi-
fied:O= ±,□= +,△= ++++;▲= +++++.

of vincristine. For HxRh12 tumors, complete regression (CR) of established tumors (0.5-1.0 g) was achieved at 1.5 mg/kg as a single administration, and 'cures' (> 3 months with non-detectable disease) were obtained at 3 mg/kg (approximately an LD_{10} level of dosage). Complete regressions in HxRh14 tumors were achieved at the highest dose level only, with subsequent regrowth of all tumors. 'Cures' were also obtained in HxRh28 tumors treated with vincristine (3 mg/kg).

The sensitivity of each tumor line to doxorubicin and actinomycin D is contrasted to that for vincristine in Table 1. Several points are of interest. Under the experimental conditions used a) resistance de novo to actinomycin D can be separated from resistance to either doxorubicin or vincristine; b) resistance de novo to doxorubicin is not necessarily associated with resistance to vincristine; c) exquisite sensitivity to vincristine (HxRh12, HxRh28 tumors) does not necessarily convey collateral sensitivity to agents of other classes. These data suggest that resistance de novo is mediated by mechanisms

TABLE 1
TUMOR RESPONSE

Tumor Line	Vincristine	Tumor Response[a] Doxorubicin	Actinomycin D
HxRh12	+++++	+++	−
HxRh14	++++	−	−
HxRh18	+++	+++	+++
HxRh28	+++++	+++	+
RD	++	−	−

[a]−, no growth inhibition; +, 1 to 1.5 volume doublings of growth inhibition; ++, 1.5 to 2 volume doublings of growth inhibition; +++, > 2 volume doublings of growth inhibition; ++++, complete regression with subsequent regrowth; +++++, complete volume regressions, apparent "cures." Each agent was administered once only at the maximum tolerated dose level (LD_{10}) to groups of seven mice bearing bilateral tumors.

specific for the mechanism of drug action, rather than a pleiotropic mechanism proposed for highly resistant cell lines in culture. This may be consistent with altered tubulin binding (3) rather than a membrane transport defect for vincristine-resistance de novo.

In an earlier report (9), we developed a stable line of RD resistant to vincristine. In mice treated with vincristine every 7 days (1.5 mg/kg) tumors resumed growth after 6 weeks despite continued treatment. The parent RD tumor line is relatively resistant to vincristine (Table 1), whereas HxRh12 and HxRh14 tumors are very sensitive. It was therefore of interest to examine the rate at which resistant cell populations were selected under in situ conditions. In Figure 2 is presented an ongoing study with HxRh18 xenograft-bearing mice, treated with vincristine.

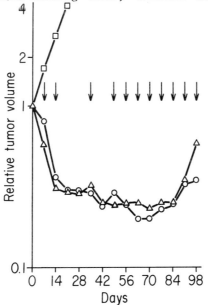

FIGURE 2. Development of resistance in HxRh18 xenograft tumors exposed to chronic administration of vincristine (1.5 mg/kg; arrows). Tumor volume relative to that at the start of therapy is plotted against time. O △ treated, □ control.

Using this schedule, tumors regressed by approximately 70 percent and remained stable for 10 weeks after which tumors progressed despite continued treatment. In contrast, using a maximal tolerated dose of vincristine (3 mg/kg; single administration) a resistant tumor line was selected

rapidly, Figure 3. In this experiment, seven mice bearing
bilateral HxRh18 tumors were treated with a single administration of vincristine. When the tumors reached four-fold
their volume at treatment, one tumor (VCR-2) which

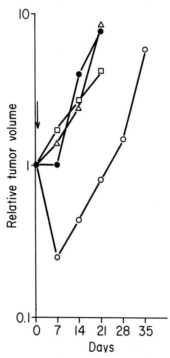

FIGURE 3. Development of a resistant line of HxRh18
tumor after a single administration of vincristine (3
mg/kg). ○ Growth of parent line HxRh18, after vincristine
treatment which upon regrowth tumor was transplanted in 14
mice which were treated with vincristine △ (3 mg/kg)
(VCR-2); one of these tumors was subsequently transplanted
and its sensitivity to vincristine re-evaluated ● (VCR-3);
□ growth of untreated parent line.

exhibited an initial response (> 80% volume regression) was
transplanted into a further seven mice which were subsequently treated with vincristine when the tumors were 0.5
to 1 g. It is apparent that these tumors were resistant to
vincristine, as were tumors taken from this experiment and
treated similarly on the subsequent passage (HxRh18 VCR
3). Attempts to develop resistant lines from the HxRh12 or
HxRh14 xenografts which are iniitally sensitive to vincris-

tine, using either weekly injections or a single administration of vincristine with subsequent transplantation,
have not yet yielded resistant variants.

DISCUSSION

These investigations attempted to examine the patterns
of resistance de novo in xenografts derived from patients
that had not received treatment with either vincristine,
doxorubicin or actinomycin D. The HxRh14 tumor was, however, derived from a child that relapsed over two years
after therapy with these agents had been terminated. It is
clear under the experimental conditions employed that
resistance de novo to either actinomycin D or doxorubicin
is independent of that for resistance to vincristine. Resistance to these agents appears to be based upon the
mechanism of action of each drug rather than the chemical
nature or molecular weight, as had been hypothesized for
CHO cells made highly resistant to actinomycin D (11). Our
data are consistent with the recent observations by Conter
and Beck (7), who have demonstrated that the pattern of
cross-resistance in CCRF-CEM human leukemic cells made
resistant to vincristine was dependent upon the degree of
vincristine resistance. Thus, the mechanisms determined on
cells selected for resistance by subculturing in progressively higher concentrations of cytotoxic agent may not
prove applicable to resistance developed under pharmaco-
logic conditions in situ. Under these conditions resistant
variants from RD and HxRh18 tumors have been derived, but
we have not been successful in developing resistant lines
from HxRh12 and HxRh14 xenografts which are initially more
sensitive to vincristine. Thus resistant lines have been
derived rapidly in tumors which have only slight sensitivity to vincristine. The most plausible explanation
appears to be that the initial response of the tumors is
determined by the sensitivity of both sensitive and resistant cell populations. Thus, the greater the proportion of
cells resistant to therapy, the poorer the initial
response, and the more rapid would be the emergence of a
resistant cell population. Alternatively, for example, if
both HxRh18 and HxRh12 tumors were comprised of homogeneous
cell populations, their response would be determined by the
intrinsic sensitivity of cells to vincristine. Under these
circumstances, although the response to therapy would be
different, development of resistance would be expected to
occur at approximately the same time. Both possibilities

assume that the rate of spontaneous mutation to resistance is similar in each tumor. The data presented suggest that the initial response to vincristine is determined by a heterogeneous population of cells, although both this and the mechanism of resistance require further examination using cell lines derived from these xenografts. In an earlier study a vincristine resistant line of RD xenograft was selected rapidly, and demonstrated an altered karyotype (9). The data in both studies are consistent with the hypothesis that the initial response to therapy is determined by heterogeneous cell populations having different intrinsic sensitivities to vincristine.

REFERENCES

1.   Green DM, Jaffe N (1978). Progress and controvery in the treatment of childhood rhabdomyosarcoma. Cancer Treat Rev 5:7.
2.   Riehm H, Biedler JL (1971). Cellular resistance to daunomycin in chinese hamster cells in vitro. Cancer Res 31:409.
3.   Ling V, Aubin JE, Chase A, Savangi F (1979). Mutants of Chinese Hamster ovary (CHO) cells with altered colcemid-binding affinity. Cell 18:423.
4.   Valeriote F, Medoff C, Dicckman J (1979). Potentiation of anticancer agent cytotoxicity against sensitive and resistant AKR leukemia by amphotericin B. Cancer Res 39:2041.
5.   Schabel FM, Skipper HE, Trader MW, Laster WR, Corbett TH, Griswold DP (1980). Concepts for controlling drug-resistant tumor cells. In Mouridsen HT, Palshof T (eds): "Breast Cancer. Experimental and Clinical Aspects," Oxford: Pergamon Press, p 199–211.
6.   Johnson BK, Chitnis NP, Embrey WM, Gregory EB (1978). In vivo characteristics of resistance and cross resistance of an adriamycin-resistant subline of P388 leukemia. Cancer Treat Rept 62:1535.
7.   Conter V, Beck WT (1982). Cross-resistance (CR) properties of CCRF-CEM cells selected for resistance (R) to vincristine (VCR), adriamycin (ADR) and VM-26. Proc Am Assoc Cancer Res 23:197.
8.   Houghton JA, Houghton PJ, Webber BL (1982). Growth and characterization of childhood rhabdomyosarcomas as xenografts. J Natl Cancer Inst 68:437.

9. Houghton JA, Houghton PJ, Brodeur GM, Green AA (1981). Development of resistance to vincristine in a childhood rhabdomyosarcoma growing in immune-deprived mice. Int J Cancer 28:409.

10. Houghton JA, Houghton PJ, Green DM (1982). Chemotherapy of childhood rhabdomyosarcomas growing as xenografts in immune-deprived mice. Cancer Res 42:535.

11. Biedler JH, Riehm H, Peterson RHF, Spengler BA (1975). Membrane-mediated drug resistance and phenotypic reversion to normal growth behavior of Chinese hamster cells. J Natl Cancer Inst 55:671.

Rational Basis for Chemotherapy, pages 71–92
© 1983 Alan R. Liss, Inc., 150 Fifth Avenue, New York, NY 10011

GENE AMPLIFICATION AND PHENOTYPIC INSTABILITY IN
DRUG-RESISTANT AND REVERTANT CELLS[1]

June L. Biedler, Tien-ding Chang, Robert H.F. Peterson,
Peter W. Melera,[2] Marian B. Meyers, and
Barbara A. Spengler

Laboratories of Cellular and Biochemical Genetics and
RNA Synthesis and Regulation,[2] Sloan-Kettering Institute
for Cancer Research, Rye, New York 10580

ABSTRACT Chinese hamster, mouse, and human cell lines
selected in a stepwise manner for high levels of resistance to antifolates, vincristine, or actinomycin D were
tested for phenotypic stability in absence of drug. Dihydrofolate reductase-overproducing cells characterized
by homogeneously staining metaphase chromosome regions
(HSRs) or double minute chromosomes (DMs) declined in
resistance, level of target enzyme, and size or number
of HSRs or DMs. Such cells are known to contain amplified dihydrofolate reductase genes associated with these
abnormal chromosome structures. In contrast, transport
defective methotrexate-resistant cells were stably resistant when grown in drug-free medium.
     HSR- or DM-containing vincristine-resistant per-
meability mutant cells declined in resistance and HSR
length or DM number in absence of drug. Actinomycin D-
resistant permeability mutant Chinese hamster cells with
no cytological evidence of amplified genes were also
phenotypically unstable. The hamster cells with acquired
resistance to vincristine or actinomycin D are cross-resistant to a wide range of chemically unrelated agents,
have a diminished phenotypic expression of malignancy,
and express a prominent high molecular weight plasma
membrane glycoprotein component designated gp150. The

[1]This work was supported by NIH grants CA-08748, CA-
28595, CA-28679, CA-24635, The Fairchild Foundation New
Frontiers Fund, and the Kleberg Foundation.

predominant glycoprotein species of spontaneously
transformed, tumorigenic control cells has an apparent
molecular weight of 100 KD. Vincristine-resistant cells
oversynthesize, in addition, a low molecular weight,
acidic, cytosol protein designated V19. Revertant cells
show increased drug uptake related to decrease in resistance and accompanying loss, in vincristine-resistant
cell lines, in HSR length or DM number. They also regain morphologic and growth characteristics of malignant
cells, synthesize relatively less gp150 and more of the
100 KD glycopeptide species and, in the case of vincristine-resistant cells, show a decline in synthesis of
V19. Cytological indication of gene amplification in
vincristine-resistant cells and the observed correlations
between phenotypic expression of resistance and synthesis
of gp150 and V19 implicate these molecular species as
candidate products of amplified genes.

INTRODUCTION

The mechanisms by which cancer cells become resistant to
antitumor drugs have been an area of extensive investigation
over the years. Although considerable information has been
gained about biochemical mechanisms of drug action and biochemical mechanisms of drug resistance, many fundamental
questions remain as to how, for specific drugs, cells undergo
the phenotypic alterations associated with development of resistance. Does acquisition of resistance involve genetic
changes, i.e., changes in the DNA, or epigenetic changes,
i.e., changes in gene expression not requiring alteration of
nucleotide sequence? One approach to this problem, initiated
some years ago in a number of laboratories, was to determine
whether there were metaphase chromosome alterations specifically related to development of resistance to a particular
drug, with the notion that a specific karyotypic alteration
would denote a genetic alteration. This cytogenetic approach,
simplistic in retrospect, did provide cytological indication
of amplification of the dihydrofolate reductase gene in antifolate-resistant cells (1); direct evidence of preferential
amplification of this gene in cells selected with methotrexate
and overproducing high levels of the target enzyme was obtained subsequently (2). Thus, acquired resistance to antifolates associated with increased levels of dihydrofolate
reductase may occur as the result of DNA sequence alteration
involving amplification of the structural gene and

accompanying sequences of DNA (1-6).

A second general, but not obligatory, finding has emerged from cytogenetic analysis of dihydrofolate reductase-overproducing cells with acquired resistance to antifolate. In sublines with high levels of resistance, amplified dihydrofolate reductase genes may be manifested either as a poorly banded or nonbanded, homogeneously staining region (HSR) of a chromosome (1,3,5-8) in metaphase cells stained by trypsin-Giemsa banding methods, or as small, paired extrachromosomal bodies known as double minute chromosomes (DMs) and present in variable numbers and sizes (6,9) in cells stained by various methods. Thus, HSRs and DMs are useful cytological indicators of amplified genes in a variety of antifolate-resistant cells.

Recent studies in our laboratories have indicated that cells with high levels of acquired resistance to the cancer chemotherapeutic agent, vincristine, may also display either HSRs or large numbers of DMs (10,11). Although the putative gene product has not yet been identified, we have implicated two candidate proteins which are involved in expression of the drug resistant phenotype. In this report we summarize results of our investigations of these permeability mutant cells as well as of actinomycin D-resistant cells which likewise display reduced drug permeability and broad-ranged cross-resistance to other agents including vincristine. We also describe new results of comparative studies of phenotypic stability of cells resistant to antifolates, vincristine, or actinomycin D and grown in absence of drug, and we raise the question of whether phenotypic instability may, like presence of HSRs and DMs, be a concomitant of gene amplification occurring as a consequence of drug selection pressure.

METHODS

Drug resistance was measured in a growth assay procedure based on relative cell counts in control and drug-treated cultures, and is expressed as the ratio of the 50% inhibitory drug concentration for resistant to control cells (12). Number of DMs per cell was determined after conventional Giemsa staining procedures and presence of HSRs by trypsin-Giemsa banding methods (1). Methods of SDS-PAGE and 2D gel electrophoresis are detailed in the publications cited.

RESULTS

Antifolate-Resistant Cells: Cytogenetic Studies and
Reversion of Resistance.

Several drug-resistant Chinese hamster lung cell lines
selected with methotrexate or methasquin (Table 1) were
studied for stability of the resistant phenotype in absence
of drug.   Cells of the DC-3F/MQ19 and DC-3F/A3 sublines are
characterized by high levels of target enzyme dihydrofolate
reductase overproduction and the presence of an HSR on a
single chromosome 2q homologue (1,8).   When cell clones derived from each of the sublines were grown in absence of
antifolate, resistance gradually declined (8).   As shown in
Figure 1, DC-3F/MQ19 cells maintained in methasquin-free
medium exhibited an early and rapid decline in resistance

TABLE 1
DRUG-RESISTANT CELL LINES

Cell Line	Drug[a]	Maintenance conc. (µg/ml)	Increase in resistance[b]
DC-3F	None		1
DC-3F/MQ19	Methasquin	10	1,583
DC-3F/A3	Methotrexate	50	108,400
DC-3F/VCRd-5	Vincristine	5	500
DC-3F/AD IV	Actinomycin D	1	376
DC-3F/AD X	Actinomycin D	10	2,450
CLM-7	None		1
CLM-7/A XVIII	Methotrexate	50	32,200
MAZ	None		1
MAZ/A/MQ60	Methotrexate	500	52,500
MAZ/VCR	Vincristine	20	2,050
SH-SY5Y	None		1
SH-SY5Y/VCR	Vincristine	10	1,256

[a]Abbreviations are: MQ, methasquin; A, methotrexate
(amethopterin); AD, actinomycin D; VCR, vincristine.
[b]Resistance was determined after 10-15 days of growth
in absence of drug.

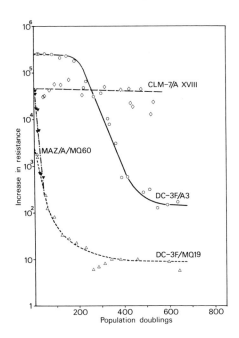

FIGURE 1. Degree of resistance of antifolate-resistant Chinese hamster and mouse sublines grown in drug-free medium.

reaching, after approximately 300 cell population doublings or 10 months, a plateau level 10-fold higher than that of DC-3F control cells. In contrast, resistance of methotrexate-selected DC-3F/A3 cells was initially stable in absence of antifolate and began to decrease rapidly only after approximately 150 population doublings or 5 months in drug-free medium. After about 1.5 years, resistance stabilized at a level that was 200-fold higher than control. For both sublines, decline in resistance was accompanied by a decrease in dihydrofolate reductase activity and in length of the HSR (8). Target enzyme activity and mean HSR length declined in parallel until enzyme activity reached a level that was on average 20-fold higher than control and HSR-containing cells were no longer observed (Figure 2). The structurally rearranged, HSR-bearing chromosome 2 of DC-3F/A3 cells and a cell with a shortened HSR are illustrated in Figures 3a and 3b.

We have demonstrated (4,13) that DC-3F/MQ19 and DC-3F/A3 cells contain amplified dihydrofolate reductase genes and that the amplified genes are preponderently localized to the

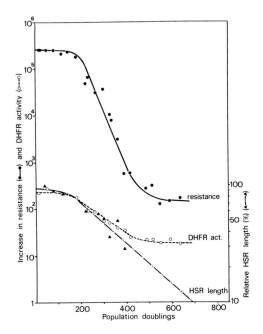

FIGURE 2. Correlation between degree of resistance, level of dihydrofolate reductase (DHFR) activity, and mean length of the HSR of methotrexate-resistant Chinese hamster DC-3F/A3 cells grown in drug-free medium.

HSR (Figure 3c). At the end of the 2-year experimental period of growth in methotrexate-free medium, DC-3F/A3 cells (designated A3-P-U) were devoid of HSRs but had a 7-fold higher dihydrofolate reductase gene copy number than DC-3F cells (4). Retention of a small number of amplified genes may explain the stable 20-fold elevation in target enzyme activity of the revertant subline. Whether the amplified genes are located at a site proximal to that of the HSR deletion site or at a distant chromosomal site(s) is not known.

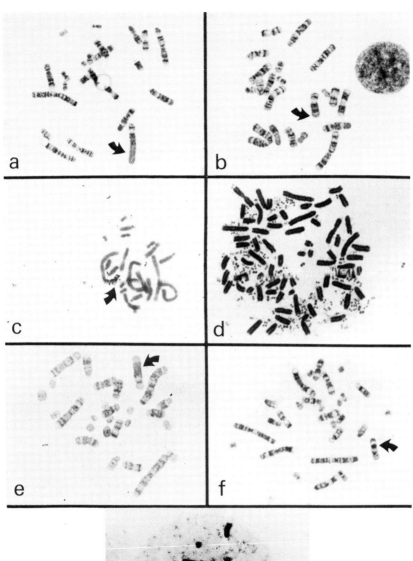

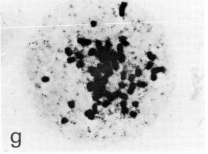

FIGURE 3. HSRs and DMs of drug-resistant sublines. (a)
Long HSR (arrow) on abnormal chromosome 2 of methotrexate-
resistant Chinese hamster DC-3F/A3 subline. (b) Shortened
HSR in a revertant DC-3F/A3 cell after growth in drug-free
medium. (c) Cluster of silver grains over terminal segment
(arrow) corresponding to known HSR location on a chromosome
2q of a methasquin-resistant DC-3F/MQ19 cell hybridized in
situ with nick-translated, ^{125}I-labeled recombinant plasmid
pDHFR6 probe (4,15). (d) Antifolate-resistant MAZ/A/MQ60
mouse cell with several hundred variably sized DMs. (e)
Typical, interstitial HSR (arrow) on a marker chromosome of
vincristine-resistant DC-3F/VCRd-5 cells. (f) Shortened HSR
(arrow) on the marker chromosome of a revertant DC-3F/VCRd-5
cell after growth of subline in drug-free medium. (g) Vincristine-resistant MAZ/VCR mouse tumor cell with hundreds of
very small DMs.

Just as high level amplification of the dihydrofolate
reductase gene is the result of a stepwise drug selection
process, so gene loss in the absence of selection pressure
appears to occur gradually. During the period of reversion
of DC-3F/A3 (Figure 2), the mean length of the HSR decreased
progressively over a 1.5-year period (8). Karyotype analyses
carried out during the reversion period showed that, although
at any one time point HSRs varied in length, cells did not
abruptly lose all or even a large segment of an HSR.
We have also examined the reversion propensity of cells
selected with methotrexate which developed resistance via an
altered drug transport mechanism. The CLM-7/A XVIII subline
(Table 1), selected from a Chinese hamster bone marrow-de-
rived line, CLM-7, exhibits a 32,000-fold increase in resistance and only a 2-fold elevation in dihydrofolate reductase
activity (14). Measurement of intracellular methotrexate
concentration indicated that these cells have an impaired
ability to transport drug. Two clonally-derived sublines of
CLM-7/A XVIII were maintained in drug-free medium for 1.5
years. There was no appreciable loss of resistance during
this period (Figure 1). Although the genetic basis of the
transport alteration has not been elucidated, the observed
stability of the resistant phenotype suggests that this mode
of resistance to antifolate does not prominently involve a
gene amplification mechanism.
In contrast to dihydrofolate reductase-overproducing
antifolate-resistant Chinese hamster cells which usually contain HSRs (1,3,5,8), target enzyme overproducing mouse cell

lines often contain DMs which may likewise carry amplified
dihydrofolate reductase genes (6,9). We have developed and
studied a resistant subline, MAZ/A/MQ60, selected sequentially
with methotrexate and methasquin from the cloned MAZ cells
isolated from a line established in vitro from a hydrocarbon-
induced tumor of a C57BL/6 mouse (Table 1). Control MAZ
cells, like many rodent tumor cell lines described in the
literature, contain variable numbers of DMs whose origin and
possible function are not known (Table 2). MAZ/A/MQ60 cells
exhibit a 361-fold increase in dihydrofolate reductase activity, large increases in amount of protein as demonstrated by
SDS-PAGE and, as shown in Table 2 and Figure 3d, a variable
and very high number of DMs (16). The number of DMs rapidly
decreased when cells were grown in methotrexate-free medium
until at 11 weeks there was a 12-fold reduction in mean number
per cell (Table 2). After almost 10 months in absence of
drug, only a few cells displayed DMs. In fact, the DM number
for the revertant cells was considerably lower than for the
"natural" DM population of the MAZ tumor cells. Loss in resistance was correspondingly rapid (Figure 1). Dihydrofolate reductase activity also declined (16). Whether resistance will decrease to control level is not yet known.

These various experimental results indicate that antifolate resistance occurring as a consequence of dihydrofolate
reductase overproduction is unstable in absence of selective
agent whereas resistance associated with altered drug transport, for the cells under study in our laboratory, is stable.

Some Phenotypic Characteristics of Vincristine- and
Actinomycin D-Resistant Cells.

In a different series of investigations we developed, by
multistep selection procedures, cell lines with very high
levels of acquired resistance to vincristine or actinomycin D
(Table 1). As detailed in previous publications (10,12,17,
18), drug-resistant sublines selected from spontaneously
transformed Chinese hamster cells including the DC-3F line
utilized in studies of antifolate resistance (1,8,14) consistently displayed the following characteristics:
(a) Cross-resistance to a wide variety of cancer chemothera-
     peutic and other agents correlated in general with
     molecular weight.
(b) Reduced permeability to both vincristine and actino-
     mycin D.

TABLE 2
DECREASE IN DMs OF DRUG-RESISTANT MOUSE TUMOR CELLS
WITH TIME IN DRUG-FREE MEDIUM

Days without drug	Frequency (%) of cells with DM nos. of:					Mean no. of DMs/cell ± SD
	0	1-50	51-100	101-200	>200	
MAZ/A/MQ60						
5	0	26	22	16	36	348 ± 502
13	0	26	30	14	30	199 ± 250
76	20	62	10	6	2	30 ± 49
286	98	2	0	0	0	0.02
MAZ/VCR						
0	0	0	34	42	24	183 ± 143
3	0	26	30	26	18	139 ± 136
10	0	17	33	23	27	171 ± 162
24	0	48	34	16	2	59 ± 47
52	4	62	26	8	0	43 ± 49
MAZ						
(control)	35	54	5	5	1	24 ± 46

(c) Cell morphology and in vitro growth behavior associated
     with normal cells in culture (in contrast to drug-
     sensitive, control cells with morphologic and growth
     characteristics associated with malignancy).
(d) Suppression of the tumor phenotype in relation to
     degree of resistance, as indicated by reduced tumori-
     genicity in immunosuppressed hosts.
     Reversion of vincristine- and actinomycin D-resistant
cells toward a more normal phenotype (10,18) is not unique
to the Chinese hamster sublines under investigation in our
laboratory. Wicker et al. (19) studied an actinomycin D-

resistant subline selected from SV40-induced Syrian hamster
tumor cells established in vitro. Maintained at 2 μg/ml of
actinomycin D, resistant cells exhibited a strong reduction
in tumorigenicity and ability to grow in soft agar. To further test the generality of the phenotypic reversion phenomenon, we selected vincristine- and actinomycin D-resistant
sublines from cloned lines including MAZ (Table 1). The
various drug-resistant sublines, among them MAZ/VCR (Table 1),
showed a reduced capacity for uptake of isotopically-labeled
actinomycin D in proportion to degree of resistance as well
as markedly reduced oncogenic potential when tested in syngeneic mice and in several different types of immunosuppressed
host animals (10). Thus, we have found that reduced or non-
expressed malignancy is a general concomitant of high levels
of acquired resistance to both vincristine and actinomycin D.

Since our studies indicated that reduced permeability to
drug was an important determinant of resistance to the two
agents and implicated the plasma membrane as mediator of at
least some of the other observed alterations in cell phenotype as well, we began investigations of plasma membrane composition. SDS-PAGE analysis of plasma membranes isolated
from cells metabolically labeled with ^{3}H-glucosamine demonstrated that spontaneously transformed, tumorigenic Chinese
hamster DC-3F cells expressed a prominent glycoprotein species
with an apparent molecular weight of 100,000 daltons (10,20).
In contrast, actinomycin D-resistant DC-3F/AD IV and DC-3F/AD X
as well as vincristine-resistant DC-3F/VCRd-5 cells (Table 1)
synthesized a 150,000 dalton species as the major glycopeptide
component (10,17). Expression of the high molecular weight
150 KD species, now designated gp150, is correlated with degree of drug resistance (10). Further, when the highly resistant (2450-fold) DC-3F/AD X subline was grown in absence
of drug for over three years, there was a decline in resistance to actinomycin D (18), a relative decrease in synthesis
of gp150 and an increase in the lower molecular weight 100 KD
membrane component (10). Decrease in resistance was accompanied also by an increase in tumorigenicity and a partial
return to malignant cell culture characteristics (18). Decrease in expression of gp150 by revertant DC-3F/AD X cells
substantiated observations of a quantitative relationship
between increase in resistance to actinomycin D and vincristine (and also daunorubicin) and increased synthesis of gp150
(10).

Recent results obtained by 2D gel electrophoretic analysis (Figure 4) confirmed the earlier observations. Both the
2450-fold resistant DC-3F/AD X cells and 2800-fold resistant

³H-GLUCOSAMINE LABELED MEMBRANE GLYCOPROTEINS

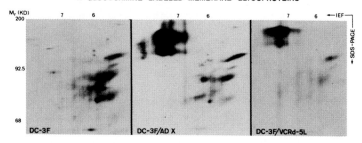

FIGURE 4. Detail of 2D gel electrophoretic analysis of
plasma membrane glycoproteins of DC-3F control, actinomycin
D-resistant DC-3F/AD X and 2800-fold vincristine-resistant
DC-3F/VCRd-5L cells.

DC-3F/VCRd-5L cells (newly selected with 50 μg/ml of vincristine from the 500-fold resistant DC-3F/VCRd-5 subline listed
in Table 1) prominently exhibit gp150, which appears in 2D
gels as a family of glycopeptides in a molecular weight range
of about 135 to 170 KD and within a pI range of about 6.7 to
7.5. The predominant 100 KD glycoprotein species of control
cell membranes are more acidic, with a broad pI range of 4.8
to 5.8 and appear as at least three major groups of spots
within a wide molecular weight range of approximately 70 to
135 KD. This glycopeptide component is also synthesized by
the resistant cells, as is particularly apparent for the
actinomycin D-resistant subline (Figure 4), but to a lesser
degree.
    Observations of enhanced expression of plasma membrane
gp150 in cells exposed to and developing resistance to three
agents (vincristine, actinomycin D, daunorubicin) apparently
unrelated in chemical structure and/or mode of cytotoxic
action suggest that synthesis of the high molecular weight
glycopeptide species is associated with the apparently non-
specific, altered membrane permeability phenotype of these
resistant cells.

Vincristine-Resistant Chinese Hamster, Mouse, and Human Cells
have HSRs or DMs.

    Trypsin-Giemsa banding analysis of actinomycin D-resistant Chinese hamster DC-3F/AD X and vincristine-resistant DC-3F/VCRd-5 cells (Table 1) has demonstrated that the vincristine-resistant cells consistently contain an HSR (10). Unlike the antifolate-resistant DC-3F sublines in which HSRs and also the specific abnormally banding regions characterizing low level dihydrofolate reductase-overproducing sublines are preferentially located on the long arm of chromosome 2 (8,13), the HSR of the vincristine-resistant cells is interstitially located on a rearranged marker chromosome comprising an entire chromosome 8 (new nomenclature) and the distal segment of the late-replicating, X chromosome long arm (Figure 3e). Actinomycin D-resistant DC-3F/AD X chromosomes have no HSR nor putative pre-HSR manifested cytologically as regions with deranged band patterns (8,13).

Vincristine-resistant MAZ/VCR cells (Table 1), selected as were the antifolate-resistant MAZ/A/MQ60 cells from the MAZ tumor cell line (Table 1), likewise show a marked increase in number of DMs (Table 2; Figure 3g). In the presence of vincristine, all MAZ/VCR cells examined had at least 50 DMs per cell with a mean number of 183. In general, the DMs of the vincristine-resistant cells are very small, sometimes just visible microscopically (Figure 3g) whereas those of the MAZ subline maintained in methotrexate are usually larger and more variable in size (Figure 3d).

As described in a preliminary report (21), two vincristine-resistant human neuroblastoma lines were also found to have either DMs or an additional HSR. The 1260-fold resistant SH-SY5Y/VCR subline (Table 1) has DMs in 100% of cells. The DMs are extremely small and generally range in number from 10 to 100; 6% of cells may have several hundred. Most of the human neuroblastoma cell lines established in culture and examined to date have either HSRs or variable and often large numbers of DMs (1,22-24). However, the SK-N-SH line from which the thrice-cloned SH-SY5Y line was derived is one of the few that has never exhibited either HSRs or DMs. Another drug-resistant human neuroblastoma line, MC-IXC/VCR, was selected with 1 µg/ml of vincristine and is 1200-fold more resistant than control MC-IXC cells (21). The resistant cells have a newly-acquired HSR on chromosome 19p in addition to the HSR-like segment on 22p in both resistant and control cells (21).

Low Molecular Weight Acidic Protein, V19, in Vincristine-Resistant Cells.

Since HSRs or DMs were found in four different vincristine-resistant sublines and not in the actinomycin D-resistant cells that we have examined to date, we sought to identify a candidate cell product that might be encoded by amplified genes contained in the aberrant chromosome structures. Results of 2D gel electrophoretic analysis of supernatant and pelleted fractions of ^{35}S-methionine-labeled cells revealed that a 19,000 dalton acidic (pI, 5.7) protein designated V19 is oversynthesized in vincristine-resistant Chinese hamster DC-3F/VCRd-5 and murine MAZ/VCR cells; presumed counterpart species were visualized on 2D gels of the two vincristine-resistant human neuroblastoma lines (11). The peptide was found in the soluble fraction and not detected in the pelleted membraneous fractions. V19 or its human counterpart was present in only very small amounts in control cells and was not oversynthesized in cells of the actinomycin D-resistant DC-3F/AD X subline (11).

Stability of the Vincristine- and Actinomycin D-Resistant Phenotype.

In order to examine the relationship between the HSRs and DMs of the three vincristine-resistant sublines listed in Table 1 and expression of the resistant phenotype, cells were grown in absence of vincristine. As shown in Figure 5, the clonally-derived DC-3F/VCRd-5 Chinese hamster line gradually declined in resistance, reaching, after approximately 550 cell doublings or 1.5 years, a plateau level that was 30-fold higher than the response level of DC-3F control cells. Decline in resistance was accompanied by a gradual decline in length of the interstitially positioned HSR (Figure 3f).

When the vincristine-resistant MAZ/VCR mouse cells were maintained in drug-free medium, resistance declined rapidly (Figure 5). Experiments still in progress showed that after 30 population doublings or 7.5 weeks, there was more than a 4-fold decrease in mean number of DMs per cell (Table 2) and DM-negative cells had begun to appear in the population. DM-containing human neuroblastoma SH-SY5Y/VCR cells declined in resistance at a similar rate (Figure 5). Initially exhibiting a 1250-fold increase in resistance, the subline was 85-fold resistant after about 50 population doublings and 8-fold above control level after 100 doublings or about 8 months in

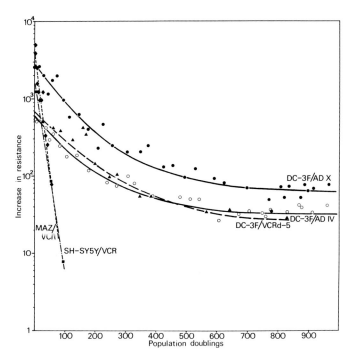

FIGURE 5. Degree of resistance of actinomycin D- and vincristine-resistant Chinese hamster and mouse sublines grown in drug-free medium.

vincristine-free medium. At the latter time point, 16% of cells contained 1-10 DMs per cell and 84% were DM-negative.

The observed correlations between reduction in size or number of HSRs or DMs and decrease in resistance for three vincristine-resistant sublines (Figure 5; Table 2), as well as analogous results with HSR- and DM-containing antifolate-resistant cells (Figures 1 and 2; Table 2) that overproduce dihydrofolate reductase as a consequence of selectively amplified target enzyme-encoding genes, strongly implicate the HSRs and DMs of vincristine-resistant cells as carriers of specifically amplified genes.

Neither HSRs nor DMs have been observed in the actino-mycin D-resistant sublines, DC-3F/AD IV and DC-3F/AD X. Resistance in both lines, however, declined during the three-year growth period in drug-free medium at approximately the same rate as for the HSR-containing DC-3F/VCRd-5 cells and reached plateau levels similar to or slightly higher than the vincristine-resistant cells (Figure 5). This slow pattern of reversion is analogous to that observed in HSR-containing antifolate-resistant Chinese hamster cells as well.

Expression of gp150 and V19 in Revertant Cells.

To further assess the relationship between expression of the drug-resistant phenotype and synthesis of plasma membrane gp150 of vincristine- and actinomycin D-resistant Chinese hamster cells and synthesis of the cytosol protein, V19, of vincristine-resistant hamster and mouse cells, we examined revertant sublines. Analysis by SDS-PAGE of DC-3F/AD X cells grown in absence of actinomycin D for three years and exhibiting a low level of resistance to antibiotic indicated that the revertant cells had regained the 100 KD glycopeptide species highly characteristic of DC-3F control cells as the most prominent membrane species (20). Recent analysis by 2D gel electrophoresis of these revertant cells and of the revertant DC-3F/VCRd-5 cells grown in absence of vincristine has demonstrated that the vincristine-resistant cells likewise synthesize relatively less gp150 and more of the lower molecular weight glycopeptide species (not shown).

Revertant DC-3F/VCRd-5 cells also showed reduced synthesis of V19, which was present in amounts intermediate between that of resistant and control cells (11). The vincristine-resistant MAZ/VCR subline, which rapidly declined in resistance in absence of drug (Figure 5), showed a rapid decline in capacity to synthesize V19. Aliquots containing approximately 5×10^5 cpm of labeled soluble material from MAZ/VCR cells grown without drug for 0, 7, 28, and 35 days were subjected to 2D gel electrophoresis. Spots corresponding to V19 and several reference spots were cut out of gels and solubilized in 30% hydrogen peroxide at 60°C for 16 hours, and incorporation of radioactivity was measured by liquid scintillation spectrometry. There was a progressive decrease in ratio of V19 cpm to total applied cpm; e.g., after 35 days (23 cell doublings) there was a 61% decrease in synthesis of V19.

CONCLUDING DISCUSSION

We have shown that both HSR- and DM-containing anti-folate-resistant cells with directly demonstrated or highly probable increases in dihydrofolate reductase gene copy number are phenotypically unstable in absence of drug. For HSR-containing Chinese hamster lung cells, resistance began to decline either immediately following drug removal or after a 5-month lag period. For DM-containing mouse cells, decline was immediate and somewhat more rapid. Results indicate that both types of aberrant chromosome structures, HSRs and DMs, which may carry the amplified dihydrofolate reductase genes, tend to be lost from cells removed from drug selection pressure. Our findings are incompatible with the notion that HSRs, because they contain chromosomally integrated genes, signify stable amplification in contrast to the rapidly lost, extrachromosomal, gene-carrying DMs of unstably resistant cells (9,25). Nevertheless, our data do indicate that HSRs, and thus the amplified dihydrofolate reductase genes that they encompass, are more stable chromosomal structures than centromere-lacking, segregation-prone DMs and thereby HSRs bestow selective advantage on cells which contain them. From findings reported here and elsewhere (26,27) it appears that HSRs, in comparison to DMs, confer short-term stability and/or a slower rate of dihydrofolate reductase gene loss in cells grown in antifolate-free medium.

Similar results were obtained with HSR- and DM-containing vincristine-resistant cells maintained in absence of the <u>Vinca</u> alkaloid. For the three sublines tested (DC-3F/VCRd-5, MAZ/VCR, and SH-SY5Y/VCR) resistance was unstable and diminished at a greater rate for cells with DMs rather than HSRs.

The striking cytological resemblances between the HSRs and DMs of vincristine- and antifolate-resistant cells and the loss of these structures in revertant cells of both types are strong indications that gene amplification has occurred in the drug-resistant sublines selected with vincristine. HSR-like segments and DMs have also been found in vincristine-resistant Chinese hamster ovary cells (28). Our previous and current investigations of cellular and genetic changes involved in development of resistance to vincristine, and to actinomycin D and daunorubicin as well, have shown that all three types of resistant cells synthesize gp150 as one major plasma membrane glycopeptide species; in contrast, control, drug-sensitive cells display a 100 KD species as the major membrane glycopeptide component (10,20). Vincristine-resistant Chinese hamster, mouse, and human cells also synthesize

increased amounts of V19 or of a counterpart low molecular
weight cytosol protein (11). Both of these proteins, candidate products of amplified genes, are synthesized in progressively lower amounts in revertant cells. Results indicate
that vincristine-resistant cells, at least, may have multiple
genetic changes associated with drug resistance development.
In the actinomycin D- and vincristine-resistant cells which
display multiple phenotypic alterations, e.g., altered permeability to drug, morphological change to a more normal cell
type, reduced oncogenic potential, the specific role of the
plasma membrane gp150 is unclear. This glycoprotein may be
analogous to the 170-190 KD species found on the surface of
vinblastine-resistant human leukemia cells (29) or to the
170 KD species (P-glycoprotein) described for colchicine-
resistant Chinese hamster ovary cells (30). In both of these
instances, synthesis of the plasma membrane glycopeptide
appears to be linked to the altered permeability phenotype
of the resistant cells. It was reported recently that colchicine resistance and expression of P-glycoprotein was conferred
on drug-sensitive mouse cells by DNA-mediated gene transfer
from resistant hamster cells (31). This finding indicates a
genetic basis for expression of the membrane glycopeptide and
implicates it as a mediator of drug resistance. Presence of
HSRs in colchicine-resistant Djungarian hamster and mouse L
cells and loss of HSRs in phenotypically unstable revertant
cells (32) suggest that development of resistance to this
agent may involve selective gene amplification. It is possible that, in our cell system, permeability alteration,
suppression of the tumor phenotype, and synthesis of gp150
are causally linked in some as yet unknown way. Although we
have not observed HSRs or DMs in actinomycin D-resistant
Chinese hamster sublines, Massino et al. (33) reported that
actinomycin D-resistant Djungarian hamster permeability
mutants have HSRs and are phenotypically unstable in absence
of drug. These results and our own observations suggest
that development of resistance to actinomycin D as well as
to vincristine may involve gene amplification mechanisms.
Cytogenetic analyses of additional actinomycin D-resistant
sublines in our laboratory and studies directed toward
identification of products of amplified genes are in progress.

REFERENCES

1. Biedler JL, Spengler BA (1976). Metaphase chromosome anomaly: Association with drug resistance and cell-specific products. Science 191:185.
2. Alt FW, Kellems RE, Bertino JR, Schimke RT (1978). Selective multiplication of dihydrofolate reductase genes in methotrexate-resistant variants of cultured murine cells. J Biol Chem 253:1357.
3. Nunberg JH, Kaufman RJ, Schimke RT, Urlaub G, Chasin LA (1978). Amplified dihydrofolate reductase genes are localized to a homogeneously staining region of a single chromosome in a methotrexate-resistant Chinese hamster ovary cell line. Proc Natl Acad Sci USA 75:5553.
4. Melera PW, Lewis JA, Biedler JL, Hession C (1980). Antifolate resistant Chinese hamster cells: Evidence for dihydrofolate reductase gene amplification among independently derived sublines overproducing different dihydrofolate reductases. J Biol Chem 255:7024.
5. Milbrandt JD, Heintz NH, White WC, Rothman SM, Hamlin JL (1981). Methotrexate-resistant Chinese hamster ovary cells have amplified a 135-kilobase-pair region that includes the dihydrofolate reductase gene. Proc Natl Acad Sci USA 78:6043.
6. Bostock CJ, Tyler-Smith C (1981). Gene amplification in methotrexate-resistant mouse cells. II. Rearrangement and amplification of non-dihydrofolate reductase gene sequences accompany chromosomal changes. J Mol Biol 153:219.
7. Dolnick BJ, Berenson RJ, Bertino JR, Kaufman RJ, Nunberg JH, Schimke RT (1979). Correlation of dihydrofolate reductase elevation with gene amplification in a homogeneously staining chromosomal region in L5178Y cells. J Cell Biol 83:394.
8. Biedler JL, Melera PW, Spengler BA (1980). Specifically altered metaphase chromosomes in antifolate-resistant Chinese hamster cells that overproduce dihydrofolate reductase. Cancer Genet Cytogenet 2:47.
9. Kaufman RJ, Brown PC, Schimke RT (1979) Amplified dihydrofolate reductase genes in unstably methotrexate-resistant cells are associated with double minute chromosomes. Proc Natl Acad Sci USA 76:5669.

10. Biedler JL, Peterson RHF (1981). Altered plasma membrane glycoconjugates of Chinese hamster cells with acquired resistance to actinomycin D, daunorubicin, and vincristine. In Sartorelli AC, Lazo JS, Bertino JR (eds): "Molecular Actions and Targets for Cancer Chemotherapeutic Agents," New York: Academic Press, p 453.

11. Meyers MB, Biedler JL (1981). Increased synthesis of a low molecular weight protein in vincristine-resistant cells. Biochem Biophys Res Commun 99:228.

12. Biedler JL, Riehm H (1970). Cellular resistance to actinomycin D in Chinese hamster cells in vitro: Cross-resistance, radioautographic, and cytogenetic studies. Cancer Res 30:1174.

13. Biedler JL (1982). Evidence for transient or prolonged extrachromosomal existence of amplified DNA sequences in antifolate-resistant, vincristine-resistant, and human neuroblastoma cells. In Schimke RT (ed): "Gene Amplification," New York: Cold Spring Harbor Laboratory, p. 39.

14. Biedler JL, Albrecht AM, Hutchison DJ, Spengler BA (1972). Drug response, dihydrofolate reductase, and cytogenetics of amethopterin-resistant Chinese hamster cells in vitro. Cancer Res 32:153.

15. Lewis JA, Kurtz DT, Melera PW (1981). Molecular cloning of Chinese hamster dihydrofolate reductase-specific cDNA and the identification of multiple dihydrofolate reductase mRNAs in antifolate-resistant Chinese hamster lung fibroblasts. Nucleic Acids Res 9:1311.

16. Biedler JL, Chang TD, Meyers MB, Melera PW, Spengler BA (1980). Diversity of chromosome abnormalities associated with dihydrofolate reductase (DHFR) overproduction in antifolate-resistant mouse tumor cells. Eur J Cell Biol 22:106.

17. Peterson RHF, O'Neil JA, Biedler JL (1974). Some biochemical properties of Chinese hamster cells sensitive and resistant to actinomycin D. J Cell Biol 63:773.

18. Biedler JL, Riehm H, Peterson RHF, Spengler BA (1975). Membrane-mediated drug resistance and phenotypic reversion to normal growth behavior of Chinese hamster cells. J Natl Cancer Inst 55:671.

19. Wicker R, Bourali M-F, Suarez HG, Cassingena R (1972). Propriétés d'une lignée de cellules de hamster transformées par le virus SV40 et résistantes à l'Actinomycine D. Int J Cancer 10:632.

20. Peterson RHF, Biedler JL (1978). Plasma membrane proteins and glycoproteins from Chinese hamster cells sensitive and resistant to actinomycin D. J Supramol Struct 9:289.

21. Meyers MB, Spengler BA, Biedler JL (1981). Vincristine-resistant human neuroblastoma cells have double minutes (DMs) and homogeneously staining regions (HSRs). In Vitro 17:221.

22. Biedler JL, Spengler BA (1976). A novel chromosome abnormality in human neuroblastoma and antifolate-resistant Chinese hamster cell lines in culture. J Natl Cancer Inst 57:683.

23. Balaban-Malenbaum G, Gilbert F (1977). Double-minute chromosomes and the homogeneously staining regions in chromosomes of a human neuroblastoma cell line. Science 198:739.

24. Biedler JL, Ross RA, Shanske S, Spengler BA (1980). Human neuroblastoma cytogenetics: Search for significance of homogeneously staining regions and double minute chromosomes. In Evans AE (ed): "Advances in Neuroblastoma Research," New York: Raven Press, p 81.

25. Schimke RT, Brown PC, Kaufman RJ, McGrogan M, Slate DL (1981). Chromosomal and extrachromosomal localization of amplified dihydrofolate reductase genes in cultured mammalian cells. Cold Spring Harbor Symp Quant Biol 45:785.

26. Tyler-Smith C, Bostock CJ (1981). Gene amplification in methotrexate-resistant mouse cells. III. Inter-relationships between chromosome changes and DNA sequence amplification or loss. J Mol Biol 153:237.

27. Kaufman RJ, Brown PC, Schimke RT (1981). Loss and stabilization of amplified dihydrofolate reductase genes in mouse sarcoma S-180 cell lines. Mol Cell Biol 1:1084.

28. Kuo T, Pathak S, Ramagli L, Rodriguez L, Hsu TC (1982). Vincristine-resistant Chinese hamster ovary cells. In Schimke RT (ed): "Gene Amplification," New York: Cold Spring Harbor Laboratory, p. 53.

29. Beck WT, Mueller TJ, Tanzer LR (1979). Altered surface membrane glycoproteins in Vinca alkaloid-resistant human leukemic lymphoblasts. Cancer Res 39:2070.

30. Juliano RL, Ling V (1976). A surface glycoprotein modulating drug permeability in Chinese hamster ovary cells. Biochim Biophys Acta 455:900.

31. Debenham PG, Kartner N, Siminovitch L, Riordan JR,
     Ling V (1982). DNA-mediated transfer of multi-drug
     resistance and P-glycoprotein expression. J Cell Mol
     Biol (In press).
32. Kopnin BP (1981). Specific karyotypic alterations in
     colchicine-resistant cells. Cytogenet Cell Genet 30:11.
33. Massino JS, Kakpakova ES, Kopnin BP, Pogosiantz EE
     (1981). Association of resistance to actinomycin D of
     mammalian cells with karyotype alterations and the
     decrease of plasma membrane permeability. Genetika
     17:1253.

Rational Basis for Chemotherapy, pages 93–105
© 1983 Alan R. Liss, Inc., 150 Fifth Avenue, New York, NY 10011

EFFECT OF METHOTREXATE ON THE DNA-DIRECTED CYTOTOXICITY PRODUCED BY EQUITOXIC DOSES OF 5-FLUOROURACIL AND 5-FLUORODEOXYURIDINE IN MURINE LEUKEMIA CELLS

Robert Heimer and Ed Cadman

Departments of Medicine and Pharmacology, Yale School of Medicine, New Haven, CT. 06510

ABSTRACT When the fluoropyrimidines, 5-fluorouracil and 5-fluoro-2'-deoxyuridine were administered at equitoxic doses, their cytotoxicity occurred via different routes. Fluorodeoxyuridine was DNA-directed, that is, it inhibited thymidylate synthetase. Its effect was reversed by thymidine and antagonized by methotrexate, which deprived the cells of the folate cofactor needed for the active metabolite, 5-fluorodeoxyuridylate, to bind covalently to thymidylate synthetase. This antagonism was associated with lowered amounts of covalent binding, and greater retention of thymidylate synthetase activity. Fluorouracil was primarily RNA-directed. Its cytotoxicity was partially reversed by uridine at concentrations high enough to compete against the incorporation of FUTP into RNA; thymidine was ineffective at reversing this toxicity. In sequence, methotrexate and fluorouracil were synergistic. This is despite the fact that the DNA-directed effects of fluoropyrimidines were reduced. Less fluorodeoxyuridylate was bound to thymidylate synthetase after methotrexate and the enzyme, tested in vitro after separation from unbound fluorodeoxyuridylate, retained greater activity. We have concluded that the synergy is not a result of enhanced inhibition of thymidylate synthetase but probably resulted from the fourfold augmentation of FUTP incorporation into L1210 RNA.

INTRODUCTION

The work of our laboratory has investigated the action of the frequently used combination of methotrexate (MTX) and 5-fluorouracil (FUra). The starting points were the observations that while these drugs ought to be antagonistic (1,2), if MTX preceded FUra then they acted better than additively against the tumors L1210 (3) and S180 (4) in tumor bearing mice. Our work has confirmed the synergic action of the sequence, demonstrated a biochemical mechanism, and suggested that the events of biological consequence involved augmented incorporation of FUra residues into RNA (5,6).

There has been considerable controversy lately over the cytotoxic action of FUra. The traditional view has held that it is a consequence of the metabolims of FUra to fluorodeoxyuridylate (FdUMP), which inhibits thymidylate synthetase (7) by forming a covalent ternary complex with the enzyme and the folate cofactor N5, N10-methylenetetrahydrofolate (CH_2FAH_4) (8). We have investigated FdUMP formation and the role of ternary complex formation under conditions in which MTX and FUra display synergy. For comparison, we have also studied the combination of MTX and fluorodeoxyuridine (FdUrd). FdUrd is metabolized directly to FdUMP and very little is broken down by L1210 cells in culture to FUra. Therefore comparison of FdUrd and FUra will allow us to separate the RNA-directed from the thymidylate synthetase-directed actions of FUra.

METHODS

L1210 were maintained by thrice weekly passages in Fischer's medium supplemented with 10% horse serum. Cell populations used experimentally were always between 80,000 and 150,000 cells/ml. Equitoxic doses of FUra and FdUrd were determined by cloning L1210 cells in drug free soft agar medium after 1 hr exposure to either drug. This procedure has been previously described (9).

Protection of treated cells was determined by growth in suspension culture. The effects of uridine and thymidine were compared in cells treated with FUra and FdUrd. Cells were counted daily using a Model ZBI Coulter Counter

(Coulter Electronics, Hialeah, FL).

Levels of intracellular FdUMP were quantified by an HPLC method using a BA-X4 anion exchange column (James B. Benson, Co., Reno, NV) (10). To assure that all FdUMP, free and bound to thymidylate synthetase, was counted together, FdUMP was cleaved from ternary complex by incubation of the cell extract at 65° for 20 min (11). Recoveries of FdUMP were >95%.

Thymidylate synthetase ternary complex was quantified using [6-^{3}H]-FdUrd (18Ci/mmol) or [6-^{3}H]-FUra (18Ci/mmol) purchased from Moravek (Brea, CA). A modification of a technique using HPLC and a Toyo Soda G2000SW gel exclusion column was used (12). Cell lysates were prepared in 20mM NaH$_2$PO$_4$ pH 7.3, 10mM β-mercaptoethanol by sonication. RNase (Sigma, St. Louis, MO) was added @ 0.1 mg/ml of extract for 10 min at 19°C. RNase at this mild temperature for the short period cleaved the RNA by >95% while less than 5% of the FdUMP bound to the enzyme was removed. Lysates were spun at 8,700xg for 1 min in a Beckman microfuge. Aliquots were injected onto the G2000SW column and eluted with 100mM NaH$_2$PO$_4$, 10mM β-mercaptoethanol pH 7.1 at 1 ml/min. [^{3}H]-FdUMP bound to the enzyme eluted in a peak with an estimated molecular weight of 34,500 daltons which was clearly separated from unbound FdUMP and other fluoropyrimidine nucleotides and nucleosides. A more detailed account of this method has been recently published (12).

The activity of thymidylate synthetase was measured by a modification of the procedure of Roberts (13) by Armstrong and Diasio (14). Cells were incubated in unlabelled FUra or FdUrd before lysis. The RNase step was excluded. Thymidylate synthetase activity was tested in the appropriate fractions from the G2000SW column. Activities in treated samples were compared to controls.

RESULTS

Cytotoxicity of FdUrd and FUra

L1210 cells were treated for 1 hr with varying doses of FdUrd and FUra. 0.1μM FdUrd and 10μM FUra achieved the same cell kill: approximately 55%. These doses were used throughout this investigation. We attempted to protect cells from the lethal effects of fluoropyrimidine treatment using 10μM thymidine and 0.6mM uridine. The dose of uridine was chosen to insure that elevated levels of UTP would at least partially compete with FUTP incorporation into RNA. (Unfortunately, doses of uridine which decreased the rate of FUra incorporation by more than 50% -- greater than 1mM -- were themselves cytostatic). FUra or FdUrd was coincubated with 0.6mM uridine, which decreased FUra incorporation by 35%, for 4 hr before drugs were removed. Following the removal of drug-containing medium the cells were counted daily. Uridine did not protect cells from FdUrd and afforded only partial protection from FUra,a 31.8% reversal of toxicity (Table 1). Thymidine in the same regimen, in place of uridine, did not protect cells from FUra but completely prevented the cytotoxic action of FdUrd. When uridine and thymidine were combined, only a slight increase in protection from FUra was noticed. Hence, the cytotoxic effect of FdUrd was probably mediated by thymidylate synthetase inhibition and was circumvented by the addition of thymidine. The cytotoxic effects of FUra were more complicated. In fact, thymidine was virtually inactive in preventing cytotoxicity despite the fact that it completely reversed the FUra-induced inhibition of DNA synthesis (Table 2). In contrast, uridine reversed the inhibition of DNA synthesis by only 40%.

Formation of FdUMP and Thymidylate Synthetase Ternary Complex

The equitoxic doses of FUra and FdUrd produced not very different levels of total intracellular FdUMP after 1 hr; 1052 fmoles/10^6 cells from 10μM FUra; 807 fmoles/10^6 cells from 0.1μM FdUrd. However, the rates of formation were very different. Transport and phosphorylation of FdUrd were essentially complete within 5 min while transport of FUra and formation of FdUMP were linear for at least 90 min.

The consequence of the different rates can be seen in the time course of formation of thymidylate synthetase ternary complex. Appearance of enzyme-bound FdUMP from [^{3}H]-FdUrd was maximal within 20 min and the levels of ternary complex was about the same as the total FdUMP formed (Figure 1). This level represented saturation of the thymidylate synthetase. This was shown in two ways. Extracts

TABLE 1

Reversal of FdUrd Toxicity by Uridine and Thymidine

	-FdUrd		+FdUrd		
	Doubling Time in Hrs	Rate Log Pop HR	Doubling Time in Hrs	Rate Log Pop HR	%Reversal*
No rescue	13.9	.0216	19.7	.0153	
+dThd	13.7	.0220	13.7	.0220	100
+Urd	13.8	.0218	16.4	.0184	46.5
+dThd,Urd	13.9	.0216	13.1	.0230	>100

Reversal of FUra Toxicity by Uridine and Thymidine

	-FUra		+FUra		
	Doubling Time in Hours	Rate Log Pop HR	Doubling Time in Hours	Rate Log Pop HR	%Reversal*
No rescue	12.02	.0250	58.71	.0051	
+dThd	12.08	.0248	50.23	.0060	4.8
+Urd	13.60	.0221	29.62	.0101	31.8
+dThd,Urd	14.15	.0212	23.95	.0125	48.4

$$*\%\text{Reversal} = \frac{\left(\dfrac{\text{Rate (Drug + Rescue)}}{\text{Rate (Rescue alone)}}\right) - \left(\dfrac{\text{Rate (Drug alone)}}{\text{Rate (control)}}\right)}{1 - \left(\dfrac{\text{Rate (Drug alone)}}{\text{Rate (control)}}\right)} \times 100$$

10µM thymidine 0.6mM uridine, and 10µM FUra or 0.1µM FdUrd were administered for 4 hr before cells were washed once with medium free from drug and resuspended in fresh Fischer's medium + 10% horse serum.

TABLE 2

EFFECTS OF FURA AND ATTEMPTED RESCUE WITH THYMIDINE AND URIDINE
ON [^{3}H]-DEOXYADENOSINE AND [^{14}C]-DEOXYGUANOSINE INCORPORATION*

CONDITION	CONCENTRATION	DURATION IN HRS	[^{3}H]-DADO		[^{14}C]-DGUO	
			%CONTROL	%REVERSAL+	%CONTROL	%REVERSAL
CONTROL			100		100	
THD	10uM	3	93.1±12.9		100	
URD	0.6mM	3	101.8±10.3		101	
FURA	10uM	3	60.7±13.2		75.8±1.7	
FURA THD	10uM 10uM	3 3	93.7±14.2	101.6	100	100
FURA URD	10uM 0.6mM	3 3	82.2±2.6	51.0	84.1	30.9

*Two forms of controls demonstrate that these labels are found specifically in DNA in L1210 Cells:

    1. Lability to DNase but not RNase
    2. Co-sedimentation with DNA but not RNA on CsCl isopycnic gradients.

$$+ \text{\% reversal} = \frac{\left(\dfrac{\text{\% drug + rescue}}{\text{\% rescue agent}}\right) - \left(\dfrac{\text{\% drug}}{\text{\% control}}\right)}{1 - \left(\dfrac{\text{\% drug}}{\text{\% control}}\right)} \times 100$$

FIGURE 1

TMP Synthetase Ternary Complex Formation
From 0.1 μM FdUrd

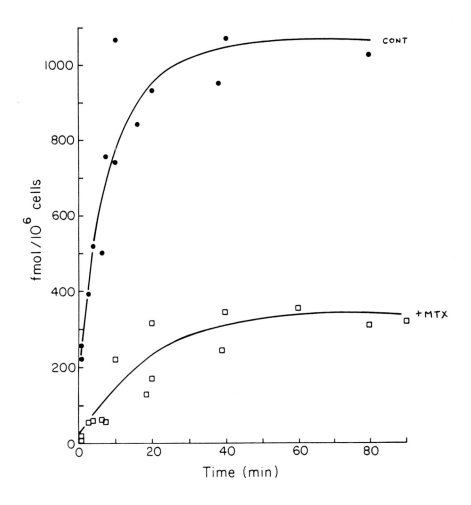

from cells pretreated with $0.1\mu M$ unlabelled FdUrd for 1 hr
neither bound [3H]-FdUMP even in the presence of $30\mu M$
CH_2FAH_4 nor displayed >5% of the enzyme activity of the
control. By contrast, appearance of enzyme-bound FdUMP
from [3H]-FUra was negligible for 0.5 hr and after 2 hr
it was only three quarters of the maximum achievable (Figure
2). After 1 hr, when FdUMP levels were at approximately
1 pmole/10^6 cells, only 57% the FdUMP was bound. Cells
were pretreated with unlabelled FUra at $10\mu M$ for 1 hr and
enzyme activity was assayed. The activity of thymidylate
synthetase was 55% of control. When just more than half
the enzyme is inhibited, the enzyme was just more than
half as active.

Effect of MTX Pretreatment on FdUMP Levels and Ternary
Complex Formation

    In all the experiments described below, MTX was admin-
istered for 3 hr at $1\mu M$ before the addition of fluoropyrimidine. This dose has been shown satisfactory to inhibit
de novo purine biosynthesis (6), to increase 5-phosphori-
bosyl-1-pyrophosphate levels (5), and to enhance the accumulation of FUra. It also inhibited the incorporation of
[3H]-deoxyuridine into the DNA of L1210 cells by >98%.

    This MTX pretreatment had little effect on the accumu-
lation of total cellular FdUMP from FUra or FdUrd. Previous
work had demonstrated increased amounts of free FdUMP from
FUra after MTX pretreatment (5). Here, we heated our lysates as described to allow measurement of total cellular,
rather than just free FdUMP. Under these conditions, there
was little change in total FdUMP: after MTX, FdUMP was increased on the average only 3% to 1080 ± 56.6 fmoles/10^6
cells. FdUMP levels after administration of [3H]-FdUrd was
increased only 10%, from 807 to 889 fmoles/10^6 cells.

    The reason for the increase in free FdUMP that we had
seen was the decrease in FdUMP bound to thymidylate synthetase. Binding of FdUMP from $0.1\mu M$ [3H]-FdUrd to the enzyme after MTX pretreatment was decreased 75% at maximum
values (Figure 1). Instead of rapid saturation seen in
controls, FdUMP binding was linear for at least 45 min. MTX
decreased the binding from $10\mu M$ [3H]-FUra by 80%, although
binding was linear for at least 4 hr (Figure 2). These
decreases in binding of FdUMP were related to increased

FIGURE 2

TMP Synthetase Ternary Complex Formation From FUra

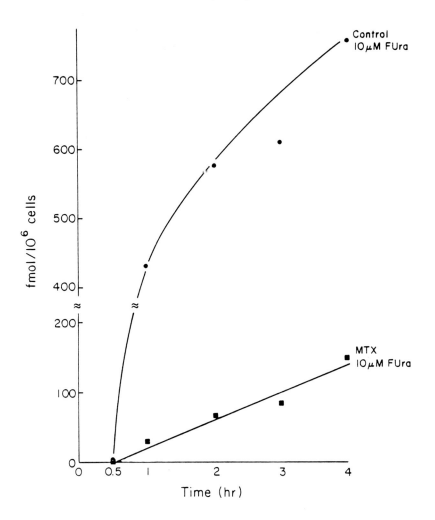

activity of thymidylate synthetase that remained in cell
extracts. After 3 hr of MTX pretreatment, cells were given
unlabelled 10μM FUra or 0.1μM FdUrd for 1 hr. Cell lysates
were injected onto the G2000SW column and the enzyme containing fractions were collected and pooled. Activity of
thymidylate synthetase was increased from 4.5 to 62.5% of
control when MTX preceded FdUrd and from 55% to 84% of
control when MTX preceded FUra.

Cloning of L1210 Cells After MTX and Fluoropyrimidines

FUra and FdUrd doses and times were chosen to be equitoxic. A 1 hr treatment of FUra at 10μM and of FdUrd at
0.1μM killed 55% of the cells (Figure 3). MTX for 4 hr at
10μM resulted in only 7% survival. If the MTX followed by
the fluoropyrimidine acted additively, survival should have
been 3.8% (0.07 x .55). The data summarized in Figure 3
demonstrated that the sequential combination of MTX and
FUra is synergistic while MTX and FdUrd is antagonistic.
This has been shown true throughout wide concentration
ranges of MTX (1 to 100μM), FUra (1-300μM), and FdUrd (0.1
to 3μM).

FIGURE 3

CYTOTOXICITY OF SEQUENTIAL MTX - FdUrd AND MTX - FUra
IN L1210 CELLS

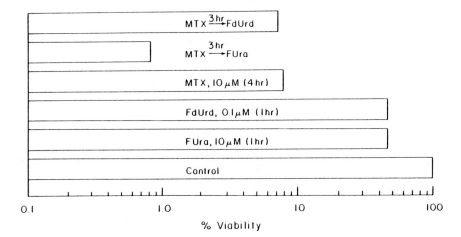

% Viability

DISCUSSION

It is clear that FdUrd, but not FUra, is acting as an inhibitor of L1210 cells growth in culture primarily by inhibiting thymidylate synthesis. At 0.1µM, and even at 1µM, FdUrd is not substantially incorporated into L1210 RNA (12) or DNA (15). MTX prevents the reduction to active tetrahydrofolates of the dihydrofolate generated in the synthesis of thymidylate. A consequence of this is the decrease in the binding of FdUMP to thymidylate synthetase, a binding that requires CH_2FAH_4. Since this is the major route by which FdUrd is cytotoxic, it is not surprising that MTX and FdUrd are, in fact, antagonistic.

However, the situation with 10µM FUra is quite different. Its primary effect in our cells seems not to involve the inhibition of thymidylate synthetase. Its cytotoxicity is not reversed by thymidine, even though the addition of thymidine restores normal DNA synthesis. It does not form FdUMP rapidly enough to completely inhibit thymidylate synthetase. Our lab has shown this in three ways. First, the enzyme is not saturated with the inhibitor; FdUMP. Second, the enzyme has not been completely inhibited: it retains activity assayed in vitro. Third, the incorporation of [^{3}H]-dUrd is inhibited by only 80% after 1 hr (16).

When MTX precedes FUra, the binding of FdUMP to thymidylate synthetase is dramatically reduced despite little change in total FdUMP levels. The enzyme itself is even less inhibited, although [^{3}H]-dUrd incorporation is unchanged because MTX decreases [^{3}H]-dUrd incorporation. Yet, the sequential combination of MTX and FUra is quite better than additive. We believe this is due to the enhanced rate of FUTP incorporation in RNA.

ACKNOWLEDGEMENTS

We would like to thank Robert N. Dreyer for excellent technical help in developing the HPLC methods, Barbara Stanley for tissue culture, Arlene Cashmore for the figures, and Hillary Raeffer for typing the manuscript. Supported in part by grant CH-145 from the American Cancer Society, and the following grants from the National Cancer Institute, CA-27130 and CA-08341. Dr. Cadman is a recipient of a faculty research award from the American Cancer Society.

REFERENCES

1) Ullman B, Lee M, Martin DW Jr, Santi DV (1978). Cyto-totoxicity of 5-fluoro-2'-deoxyuridine: Requirement for reduced folate cofactors and antagonism by methotrexate. Proc Natl Acad Sci USA 75: 980.

2) Bowen D, White JC, Goldman ID (1978). A basis for fluoro-pyrimidine-induced antagonism to methotrexate in Ehrlich ascites tumor cells in vitro. Cancer Res 38: 219.

3) Kline I, Venditti JM, Mead JAR, Tyrer DD, Goldin A (1966). The anti-leukemic effectiveness of 5-fluoroura-cil and methotrexate in the combination chemotherapy of advanced leukemic L1210 in mice. Cancer Res 26: 848.

4) Bertino JR, Sawicki WL, Lindquist CA, Gupta VS (1977). Schedule-dependent antitumor effects of methotrexate and 5-fluorouracil. Cancer Res 37: 327.

5) Cadman E, Heimer R, Davis L (1979). Enhanced 5-fluoro-uracil nucleotide formation after methotrexate admin-istration: Explanation for drug synergism. Science 205: 1135.

6) Cadman E, Heimer R, Benz C (1981). The influence of methotrexate pretreatment on 5-fluorouracil metabolism in L1210 cells. J Biol Chem 256: 1695.

7) Heidelberger C (1965). Fluorinated pyrimidines. Prog Nucl Acid Res Molec Biol 4: 1.

8) Santi DW, McIlenry CS (1972). 5-Fluoro-2'-deoxyuridylate: Covalent complex with thymidylate synthetase. Proc Natl Acad Sci USA 69: 1855.

9) Cadman E, Eiferman F, Heimer R, Davis L (1978). Pyra-zofurin enhancement of 5-azacytidine antitumor activity in L5178Y and human leukemia cells. Cancer Res 38: 4610.

10) Dreyer R, Cadman E (1981). Use of periodate and methyl-amine for the quantification of intracellular 5-fluoro-2'-deoxyuridine-5'-monophosphate by high-performance liquid chromatography. J Chromatog 219: 273.

11) Washtien WL, Santi DV (1979). Assay of intracellular free and macromolecular-bound metabolites of 5-fluoro-deoxyuridine and 5-fluorouracil. Cancer Res 39: 3397.

12) Heimer R, Cadman E (1981). Analysis of thymidylate syn-thetase ternary complex by high-performance liquid steric exclusion chromatography. Anal Biochem 118: 322.

13) Roberts D (1966). An isotopic assay for thymidylate synthetase. Biochemistry 5: 3546.

14) Armstrong RD, Diasio RB (1982). Improved measurement of thymidylate synthetase activity by modified tritium-release assay. J Bioch Biop Methods 6: in press.

15) Ingraham HA, Tseng BY, Goulian M (1982). Nucleotide
    levels and incorporation of 5-fluorouracil and uracil
    into DNA of cells treated with 5-fluorodeoxyuridine.
    Molec Pharmacol 21: 211.
16) Danhauser L, Heimer R, Cadman E (1982). Effect of leu-
    covorin on the activity of 5-fluorouracil in cultured
    L1210 cells pretreated with methotrexate. Proc Amer
    Assoc Cancer Res 23: 741.

Rational Basis for Chemotherapy, pages 107–118
© 1983 Alan R. Liss, Inc., 150 Fifth Avenue, New York, NY 10011

DEVELOPMENT OF A DRUG-SENSITIVITY ASSAY FOR HETEROGENEOUS
TUMORS BASED ON GROWTH IN 3-DIMENSIONAL COLLAGEN GELS[1]

B.E. Miller, F.R. Miller, and G.H. Heppner

Department of Immunology, Michigan Cancer Foundation
Detroit, Michigan 48201

An assay is described in which antineoplastic drugs
may be tested for their ability to inhibit the
3-dimensional growth of tumor cell colonies embedded
in collagen gel. The method allows for sequential,
nondestructive measurement of colony size to assess
growth rates. The assay permit the assessment of
growth of mixtures of cells and thus allows drug
testing to take place in the presence of intracellular
interactions which occur in heterogeneous tumors. The
method has been tested on tumor cells suspended and
embedded in collagen as a bolus, and on small pieces
($<1mm^3$) of tumor embedded without dissociation.

INTRODUCTION

Intra-tumor heterogeneity has been demonstrated in a
substantial number of human and animal cancers (reviewed in
1 and 2). Tumor cell subpopulations from single neoplasms
have been found to differ in many biologically and clinically important characteristics. We have developed a model
system to study the biological implications and therapeutic
consequences of tumor heterogeneity (3-6). This system
consists of a series of tumor subpopulations from a single
strain BALB/cfC3H mouse mammary cancer. These subpopulations differ among themselves in morphology, karyotype, in
vitro growth parameters, sensitivity to therapeutic agents,
antigenicity, and immunogenicity. They also differ in
tumor latency period, TD_{50}, growth rate, and ability to
metastasize spontaneously from a s.c. implant. We have

[1]This work was supported by Public Health Service
Grant CA-27437.

shown that certain of the subpopulations interact to influence each other's growth (7), immunogenicity (8), and sensitivity to chemotherapy (9). The basis for these interactions includes both host and tumor factors. We now have
begun to use the concepts learned from our model system to
develop a new in vitro method to assess the sensitivity of
tumors to chemotherapeutic agents and to evaluate the
influence of heterogeneity on therapeutic regimens.

The current assay of choice for assessing drug sensitivity of tumors in vitro is the soft agar method of
Salmon, et al. (10). This assay appears to be accurate in
detecting drugs to which the patient's tumor will not
respond, but is less successful in predicting effective
chemotherapy (10). Tumor heterogeneity seems to be one
factor in this failure. The soft agar method is highly
selective; only a few tumor cells actually form clones.
Although it is likely that clonogenic cells are tumorigenic, self-renewing cells, all tumorigenic cells do not
clone in soft agar. Thus, cloning in soft agar differentially selects tumor cell subpopulations; those subpopulations unable to grow in the assay system are lost.
Furthermore, we have shown that cells of different subpopulations (only some of which are clonogenic) influence each
other's response to drugs (9). The procedure of placing
cells in suspension and cloning them must modify these
interactions. Another problem inherent in cloning is
illustrated by the recent work of Poste, et al. (11)
showing that tumor cell phenotypes relevant to metastasis
are more stable in mixed population than in cloned lines of
B16 melanoma. Whether a similar consideration holds for
drug sensitivity is not known, but cloning may induce variation that could greatly complicate the results of clonogenic assays. Finally, many of the most common types of
cancer, such as breast cancer, are notoriously difficult to
clone.

What we report here is an attempt to develop an in
vitro assay using the concepts of tumor heterogeneity to
improve test design. Such an assay must meet the following
criteria:

  It must maintain tumor cell interactions. Cloning is
  therefore not desirable.
  It must be as non-selective as possible for growth of
  all elements in the tumor.

It must incorporate procedures to control for zonal
heterogeneity (see below).
It must allow for testing a reasonable number of
drugs.
An additional criterion which we feel to be important
is maintenance of tissue architecture. The failure of
monolayer cultures to provide an adequate assay of drug
sensitivity may be taken as evidence of this (4). Three-
dimensional architecture can also influence sensitivity to
therapeutic agents (12). Whether this is due to some
interactions between stromal and tumor cells, to parameters
of drug delivery, or to unknown factors, it seems prudent
to attempt to mimic, as closely as possible, the in vivo
situation in an in vitro assay.

To establish the basic parameters of the assay we are
using our tumor subpopulations and spontaneous mouse
mammary tumors.

DRUG SENSITIVITY ASSAY

Recently human and mouse breast cancers (and normal
tissue) have been shown to grow at high frequency in
collagen cultures (13). In our laboratory, we are using a
modification of this technique in which cells are embedded
between two layers of collagen. Under these conditions an
array of morphologically different outgrowths occurs,
including "duct-like" tubes, branching tubes, discs and un-
organized cells. Cells of our different subpopulations
produce distinctive and different outgrowth patterns.
Tumors grown from 68H cells, a variant-producing line (14),
produce a variety of patterns. This suggests that outgrowth in collagen can be used to detect different variants. Furthermore, it appears to be the least selective
method available for growing mammary cancer, both animal
and human.

We have used a modification of the method of Yang et
el. (13) in preparing our collagen culture system. Collagen stock solutions are prepared from rat tail fibers,
which are sterilized in 70% ethanol, than dissolved in
dilute acetic acid. Cold collagen stock is mixed with concentrated Dulbecco's modified eagle medium (DME) and NaOH
to bring the pH to 7.4. This dilute gelatin mixture will
not gel if kept on ice. For embedding, 0.5 ml of the cold

gelation mixture is allowed to gel at room temperature in a
well of a Multiwell tissue culture plate. Pieces from
tumors grown in vivo or 10^5 cultured cells in 1 μl of cold
gelation mixture are placed on the surface, then overlaid
with 0.3 ml of cold gelation mixture. Cultures are fed
twice a week with 0.8 ml of DME, supplemented with serum
and antibiotics.

Outgrowth of cells from the embedded bolus or tumor
piece is readily determined by observation with an inverted
microscope. An image of the colony is projected onto paper
with a camera lucida (Leitz Wetzlar, Germany) and sketched
by hand. The area of the projected magnified image is
measured with a compensating polar planimeter (Keuffel and
Esser Co., Morristown, N.J.). An example of data obtained
by this method is shown in Figure 1.

Preliminary experiments are necessary to see whether
optional drug exposure will be by addition to the fluid
phase above the gel or by incubation of tumor pieces in
drug containing medium prior to plating. It may be
necessary to add different drugs in different ways. The
effect of length of time of incubation will also be
established empirically. In experiments to date, we have
chosen to add drug to the fluid bathing the gel, and to
treat continuously during the entire period of colony
growth. Experiments with ^{14}C-hypoxanthine indicate that
small molecules are readily washed out of collagen gels by
changing the media so that it is possible to remove drugs
from the cultures.

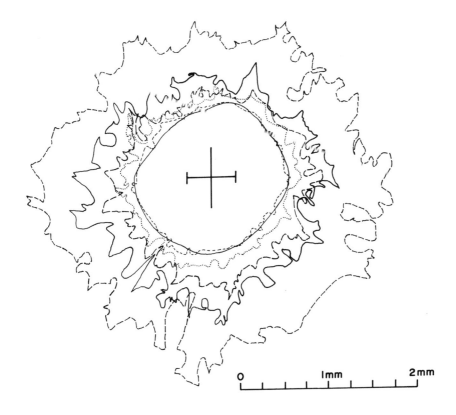

Figure 1.   Growth of embedded bolus of line 410.4 cells, no drug treatment. The projected colony area was sketched on day 0, 1, 2, 3, 4, and 7 after embedding.

Shown in Figure 2 is the effect of continuous exposure to methotrexate (MTX) on colony expansion of an embedded bolus of cells of mammary tumor subpopulation 410.4. As can be seen, little effect of MTX is seen at concentrations less than 10^{-6}M. This is far in excess of the concentration of MTX needed to inhibit monolayer growth of cultures of the same cell line (Table 1). This decreased sensitivity to MTX in cultures grown on collagen was also seen with line 67, a related cell line (Table 1). We have not yet determined the reason for this decreased sensitivity to MTX. In contrast, concentration-response curves for 5-fluorouracil (5-FU) and thioguanine are similar in collagen cultures vs. cells grown on plastic.

TABLE 1

EFFECT OF SUPPORT MATRIX ON METHOTREXATE RESPONSE OF TWO CELL LINES[a]

Cell Line	Matrix	Percent inhibition of growth[b] at MTX concentration:			
		10^{-8}M	10^{-7}M	10^{-6}M	10^{-5}M
67	Plastic	3	97	107	107
	Collagen	10	14	45	70
410.4	Plastic	62	104	102	103
	Collagen	0	9	39	57

[a]Both cell lines were originally isolated from the same mouse mammary tumor. Line 67 is 2X less sensitive than 410.4 when grown on plastic (9).
[b]Cultured cells were either plated at 8 X 10^3 cells/cm^2 (1.6 X 10^4 cells/well) onto the plastic bottom of multiwell plates, for which growth was determined by trypsinizing and counting cells, or embedded as a bolus of 10^5 cells, for which growth was determined as described in Text. In both cases, treated wells were compared to control wells after 4 days continuous exposure to drug.

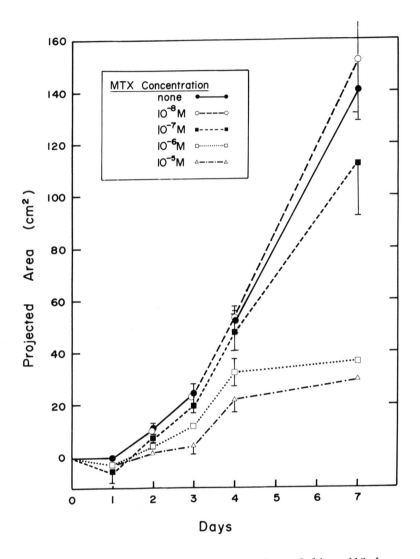

Figure 2. Growth of embedded bolus of line 410.4 cells treated with MTX. Bars represent the range of values determined with three different colonies in one experiment.

APPLICATION OF THE ASSAY TO HETEROGENEOUS TUMORS

In our experiments so far, we have used cell populations which are as homogenous as possible in order to refine the collagen assay. Our goal, however, is to develop an assay useful for determining drug sensitivity in heterogeneous tumors. We plan to use the collagen gel assay for testing both spontaneously arising mouse mammary tumors and transplanted tumors consisting of mixtures of cells of different drug sensitivities. The results of these in vitro assays will be compared to in vivo assays by transplanting and testing these same tumors in mice.

Solid tumors (at least 10mm X 10mm) will be surgically removed under sterile conditions and grossly necrotic areas trimmed. Initially, the tumor will be cut into 1 mm^3 pieces and each piece embedded into collagen in a single well of a multiwell plate. This sampling procedure allows for expression of zonal heterogeneity in drug sensitivity (see below) and further maintains opportunity for cellular interaction. A 1mm^3 size allows for adequate diffusion of nutrients into the tissue (15). The pieces will be cut according to a standard plan and each piece will be numbered so that its position relative to the others in the tumor will be known.

Drugs (A, B, C, etc. up to 5 drugs) and some or all of their combinations (AB, AC, ABC ...) will be added to the wells of each replicate plate in a randomized fashion. Preliminary experiments indicate the need for at least 6 replicates for each single drug. Growth will be determined by planimeter on days 5, 10, and 15.

Growth curves will be fit using regression analysis for each drug, drug combination, and for the no drug controls. Various response indices will be calculated to determine which are the most predictive for drug sensitivity in vivo.

Our assay scheme depends upon a zonal (i.e. non-random) distribution of cells with differential sensitivity to drugs. Zonal tumor heterogeneity for drug sensitivity has been demonstrated by Siracky (16) and by Hakanssen and Trope (17,18). Zonal distribution of heterogeneous populations within tumors has also been shown by Prehn (19) and Fidler and Hart (20).

We are able to reproducibly grow 1mm^3 pieces of transplantable mammary tumors in collagen culture. So far, we
have only tested a few tumors with two drugs, MTX and 5-FU.
We have found far more heterogeneity in growth rates of
both drug-treated and control tumor pieces than of embedded
boluses of cultured cells. The amount of heterogeneity in
growth of untreated pieces seems characteristic of the
tumor line. 5-FU inhibits growth of tumor pieces in our
assay, but the dose required may be more than that required
to inhibit growth of the embedded tumor cell line. Interestingly, we have found low doses of MTX (10^{-7}M) continuously present in medium to be very stimulatory to tumor
pieces from lines which do not grow well in collagen (for
example, we embedded a 68H tumor in which only 20% of untreated pieces grew as compared to 90% of pieces treated
with MTX). The stimulation of growth of some tumor pieces
by MTX in the subrenal capsule assay was reported by Reich
et al. (21).

DISCUSSION

That a wide variety of solid tumors are composed of
heterogeneous "subpopulations" of tumor cells is a well-
established fact. Certainly it has been long appreciated
that cells of individual tumors vary at any one time in
many morphological and cell cycle criteria. It is also
known that tumor populations are not static, but undergo
progression, defined as the acquisition of new, generally
more malignant, characteristics. Since the mechanism of
progression is thought to involve the development and
selection of variant tumor cells, a process which requires
time, it is certain that tumor cells differing in be-
havioral characteristics must co-exist in the same tumor.
We have shown that tumor subpopulations isolated from a
single mouse mammary tumor differ in many respects and are
capable of interacting to influence each other's growth,
immunological characteristics, and sensitivity to chemotherapeutic drugs. The concept of the tumor which emerges
from our work is that of a dynamic, interactive ecosystem.
We know that the mechanisms of interaction are multiple and
involve both tumor and host factors. Our conviction that
the principles we have already learned can be extended into
clinically important areas has led us to a new approach to

in vitro drug testing in which we are incorporating the concepts of tumor heterogeneity into the test design.

ACKNOWLEDGMENTS

We wish to thank the E. Walter Albachten bequest and the United Foundation of Greater Detroit for their continuing support of our work. We also thank Ms. Clare Rogers and Ms. Jennifer Kimball for excellent technical assistance.

REFERENCES

1. Fidler IJ (1978). Tumor heterogeneity and the biology of cancer invasion and metastasis. Cancer Res 38:2651.
2. Heppner GH, Shapiro WR, Rankin JC (1981). Tumor heterogeneity. In Humphrey GB, (ed): "Pediatric Oncology," Vol 1, The Hague: Martinus Nijhoff Publishers NV, p 91.
3. Dexter DL, Kowalski HM, Blazar BA, Fligiel Z, Vogel R, Heppner GH (1978). Heterogeneity of tumor cells from a single mouse mammary tumor. Cancer Res 38:3174.
4. Heppner GH, Dexter DL, DeNucci T, Miller FR, Calabresi P. (1978). Heterogeneity in drug sensitivity among tumor cell subpopulations of a single mammary tumor. Cancer Res 38:3758.
5. Miller FR, Heppner GH (1979). Immunologic heterogeneity of tumor cell subpopulations from a single mouse mammary tumor. J Natl Cancer Inst 63:1457.
6. Blazar BA, Laing CA, Miller FR, Heppner GH (1980). Activity of lymphoid cells separated from mammary tumors in blastogenesis and Winn assays. J Natl Cancer Inst 65:405.
7. Miller BE, Miller FR, Leith J, Heppner GH (1980). Growth interaction in vivo between tumor subpopulations derived from a single mouse mammary tumor. Cancer Res 40:3977.
8. Miller FR, Heppner GH (1980). Intratumor immunologic interactions. Proc AACR 21:201a.

9. Miller BE, Miller FR, Heppner GH (1981). Interactions between tumor subpopulations affecting their sensitivity to the antineoplastic agents cyclophosphamide and methotrexate. Cancer Res 41:4378.

10. Salmon SE, Hamburger AW, Soehnlen B, Durie BG, Alberts DS, Moon TE (1978). Quantitation of differential sensitivity of human-tumor stem cells to anticancer drugs. N Engl J Med 298:1321.

11. Poste G, Doll J, Fidler IJ (1981). Interactions among clonal subpopulations affect stability of the metastatic phenotype in polyclonal populations of B16 melanoma cells. Proc Nat Acad Sci USA 78:6226.

12. Wibe E (1980). Resistance to vincristine of human cells grown as multicellular spheroids. Br J Cancer 42:937.

13. Yang J, Richards J, Bowman P, Guzman R, Enami J, McCormick K, Hamamoto S, Pitelta D, Nandi S (1979). Sustained growth and three-dimensional organization of primary mammary tumor epithelial cells embedded in collagen gels. Proc Natl Acad Sci (USA) 76:3401.

14. Hager JC, Fligiel S, Stanley W, Richardson AM, Heppner GH (1981). Characterization of a variant-producing tumor cell line from a heterogeneous strain BALB/cfC$_3$H mouse mammary tumor. Cancer Res 41:1293.

15. Bogden AE, Cobb WR, Lepage DJ, Haskell PM, Gulkin TA, Ward A, Kelton DE, Esber HJ (1981). Chemotherapy responsiveness of human tumors as first transplant generation xenografts in the normal mouse: Six day subrenal capsule assay. Cancer 48:10.

16. Siracky J (1979). An approach to the problem of heterogeneity of human tumor-cell populations. BR J Cancer 39:570.

17. Hakansson L, Trope C (1974). On the presence within tumors of clones that differ in sensitivity to cytostatic drugs. Acta Path Microbiol Scand Section A 82:35.

18. Hakansson L, Trope C (1974). Cell clones with different sensitivity to cytostatic drugs in methylcholanthrene induced mouse sarcomas. Acta Path Microbiol Scand Section A 82:41.

19. Prehn RT (1970). Analysis of antigenic heterogeneity within individual 3-methylcholanthrene-induced mouse sarcomas. J Natl Cancer Inst 45:1039.

20. Fidler IJ, Hart IR (1981). Biological and experimental consequences of the zonal composition of solid tumors. Cancer Res 41:3266.
21. Reich SD, Griffin TW, Cote TH, Bogden AE (1981). Stimulation of tumor growth by anticancer agents in the subrenal capsule assay. Breast Cancer Res and Treatment 1:164a.

Rational Basis for Chemotherapy, pages 119–136
© 1983 Alan R. Liss, Inc., 150 Fifth Avenue, New York, NY 10011

CHEMOTHERAPEUTIC DRUG SENSITIVITY
OF CULTURED HUMAN MAMMARY EPITHELIAL CELLS [1,2]

Helene S. Smith,[3,4] Edward M. Acton,[5]

and Adeline J. Hackett,[3,4]

[3] Peralta Cancer Research Institute
3023 Summit Street
San Francisco, California

[4] Donner Laboratory
Lawrence Berkeley Laboratory
Berkeley, California   94720

[5] SRI International
333 Ravenswood Avenue
Menlo Park, California   94025

ABSTRACT   Epithelial cells were isolated and cultured from a number of human mammary specimens of both malignant and nonmalignant origin.   At second passage, single cells were plated onto irradiated fibroblasts to form a highly efficient

[1]We wish to thank Mr. Alan J. Hiller for excellent technical assistance. This work was supported by the Peralta Hospital Association and National Cancer Institute grants, CA32158, CA25418, CA33303.

[2]Address correspondence to Dr. Helene S. Smith, Peralta Cancer Research Institute, 3023 Summit Street, Oakland, CA 94609.

clonogenic assay suitable for measuring chemotherapeutic drug dose response curves. Dose response curves for adriamycin were generated using a number of different cultures of tumor and nonmalignant tissue. Among cultures tested, the adriamycin concentrations required to kill 50% of the cells varied approximately 30 fold (from 2.5 ng/ml to 78 ng/ml). No consistant differences were observed between cultures derived from nonmalignant and malignant tissues. Heterogeneity in drug response was also detected among subpopulations within a single culture. This heterogeneity was manifested as biphasic dose response curves and also by a reduced range in drug concentrations required to kill 99% of the cells. The sensitivity of one tumor derived culture to two experimental adriamycin analogues was also evaluated. On a molar basis, both analogues were more efficient than adriamycin for killing approximately 50% of the cells; however, adriamycin was more efficient for killing the remaining resistant subpopulation.

INTRODUCTION

Techniques have been developed to evaluate chemotherapeutic drug sensitivity of dissociated cancer cells in agar suspension (1,2). Recent studies indicate that this assay correlates with patient response (3-7). One technical difficulty with the agar assay is that the plating efficiency is often lower than one colony per 10^4 cells plated. This low plating efficiency makes it impossible to evaluate heterogeneity in drug sensitivity of subpopulations within a single tumor specimen.

In order to amplify the number of mammary tumor cells available for drug sensitivity testing, we developed techniques for isolating and readily culturing human mammary epithelial cells (both normal and malignant) in mass culture (8,9) and as a highly efficient clonogenic assay suitable for testing drug sensitivity (10). We previously found variability in adriamycin sensitivity among cultures derived from both malignant(11) and nonmalignant (Smith, H.S., Stampfer, M.R., Hackett, A.J., Manuscript submitted for publication) specimens . Because the techniques that we developed result in plating efficiencies as high as 1 to 40 percent, we are also able to detect the presence of small resistant subpopulations within a given specimen. In this report, we review both the techniques resulting in the highly efficient clonogenic assay for mammary cells and our studies on adriamycin sensitivity; we also extend our drug senstivity studies to explore the possibility of utilizing this system to evaluate new drug analogues.

MATERIALS AND METHODS

Tissue Collection and Preparation

Tissue was obtained as discard material from reduction mammoplasties, mastectomies or metastases. Processing of tissue for separation of epithelial from stromal components was as described previously (8). For the reduction mammoplasties, skin and grossly fatty areas were removed. The remaining mammoplasty as well as carcinomatous tissue was gently lacerated. The material was then digested with collagenase and hyaluronidase to digest stroma and basement membranes. Because of the junctional complexes connecting the epithelial cells, they remained as clumps or organoids after the treatment and were separated from the dissociated stromal cells by filtration with polyester screen filters. The organoids were either plated directly or stored frozen in multiple ampoules in liquid nitrogen. Depending upon the amount of tissue obtained, and the epithelial content of that tissue, 10 to 70 ampoules containing approximately 100 to 250 organoids each could be stored frozen from each reduction mammoplasty, while 1 to 6 ampoules could be stored from each carcinoma.

Culturing of Organoids

To initiate experiments, an ampoule was quickly thawed and the organoids plated into multiple T-25 flasks (Corning) in an enriched medium (termed MM) which was a modification of the enriched medium previously designed for human mammary epithelial cells (8) and which consisted of the following: 30% Dulbecco's Modified Eagles medium

(DME), 30% Ham's F-12, 15% conditioned medium from human fetal intestine epithelial cells, 74Int (12,13), 15% conditioned medium from human bladder epithelial cell line 767B1 (12,13), 9.5% conditioned medium from human myoepithelial cell line 578 Bst (14), 0.5% fresh newborn or fetal calf serum, 10 ug/ml insulin (Sigma, St. Louis, MO), 5 ng/ml epidermal growth factor (Collaborative Research), 10^{-8}M triiodothyronine (Sigma), 1 ng/ml cholera toxin (Schwartz Mann), penicillin and streptomycin.

Within 24-48 hours, epithelial cells migrate from the organoids and begin extensive proliferation. By 6-8 days after plating, the combined effect of cell migration and extensive proliferation was a wide area of epithelial cells with extensive mitotic activity surrounding each clump. By briefly treating with trypsin at this stage many of the cells peripheral to the organoid were dissociated leaving the central organoid and some peripheral cells remaining on the dish. The dish was then refed and the process repeated from three to eight times.

Clonal Assay for Drug Sensitivity

The clonal assay was performed as described previously (10,11). Briefly, human skin fibroblasts were trypsinized and irradiated in suspension for 6 seconds at 24 inches from an ultraviolet germicidal light (General Electric #30T8, 30 watts). The irradiated fibroblasts were seeded at 1.5×10^4 cells onto 35 mm tissue culture dishes. The next morning, cells dissociated from the organoid cultures were dispersed to a single cell suspension, counted with a hemocytometer and plated onto the irradiated fibroblasts at either 350, 10^3 or 3500 cells/dish with MM medium. As previously discussed in detail (10), great care was taken to insure that only single cells were plated. Dissociated cells were examined with an inverted microscope during trypsinization and were plated only when a single cell suspension was observed. For each experiment, randomly selected dishes were observed twenty four hours post seeding. If any clumps were seen, all of the dishes were examined and those containing clumps were discarded. This situation occurred only rarely; for most experiments, no clumps were observed. Sixteen to nineteen hours after seeding the epithelial cells, the media was removed and MM medium with the desired drug concentration was added to each dish. Four dishes were used for each drug dose. For lower drug concentrations, two dishes were seeded with 10^5 cells and two dishes with 3.5×10^4 cells; for higher drug concentrations, two dishes were seeded with 3.5×10^5 cells and two with 10^5 cells. The dishes were incubated with various drug concentrations at 37 C; four hours later, the medium was removed, and the dishes washed one time with basal salts. Each dish was then refed with MM medium containing an additional 10^4 freshly trypsinized and irradiated fibroblasts. Dishes were refed twice weekly until readily visualized colonies were present (usually within 5 to 10 days). Dishes were rinsed with phosphate buffered saline, fixed with methanol, and stained with May Grunwald-Giemsa.

Preparation of Drugs

Adriamycin (doxorubicin) in lyophilized powder (Adria Laboratories, Inc.) was diluted with sterile physiologic saline at 1 mg/ml, aliquoted and frozen at -20 C. For each experiment, a new ampoule was used.

Adriamycin analogues were dissolved in absolute methanol at concentrations of 1 mg/ml, aliquoted, dried with nitrogen gas, and stored in the dark at room temperature. The analogues were reconstituted in methanol; unused portions were redried with nitrogen and reused up to 5 times.

RESULTS

We have examined the sensitivity to adriamycin of mammary epithelial cells cultured from a number of different specimens of both malignant and nonmalignant origin. Table 1 summarizes the patients' histories.

Table 1

History of Patient Donors

Specimen	Age of Donor	Tissue Pathology
Nonmalignant Tissue		
a. reduction mammoplasties		
H59E	23	Normal
H161E	17	Normal
H184E	21	Normal
H191E	56	Slight Fibrocystic
H208E	45	Mild duct ectasia, focal apocrine metaplasia
b. tissue peripheral to carcinomas		
H200P	68	Fibrocystic; focal areas of sclerosing adenosis
Primary Carcinoma		
H66T	55	Invasive ductal carcinoma (lobular pattern)
H72T	71	Invasive ductal carcinoma
H82T	49	Infiltrating carcinoma (comedo pattern)
H192T	42	Infiltrating lobular carcinoma
H200T	68	Infiltrating ductal carcinoma
PH326T	59	Infiltrating ductal carcinoma
PH328T	42	Poorly differentiated infiltrating ductal carcinoma
PH329T	64	Infiltrating ductal carcinoma
PH331T	58	Infiltrating ductal; areas of in situ and lobular carcinoma
Metastatic Carcinoma		
PH303T	68	To vagina
PH313T	unknown	To hypodermis
PH325T	54	To hypodermis

Figure 1 illustrates the dose response curves to adriamycin, plotted semilogarithmically, of typical tumor derived specimens. For one primary carcinoma specimen, H66T (fig. 1) the dose response curve indicated a rather sensitive population since the slope of the curve was quite steep and there was no evidence of a shoulder. The curve was also biphasic with the initial slope of the curve being more steep than the slope of the curve at drug concentrations greater than approximately 0.01 ugm/ml. The fact that the dose response curve had two phases indicated that the tumor specimen was heterogeneous and contained two populations with different sensitivities to adriamycin. The lower section of the curve extrapolated to approximately 45% on the y axis indicating that 45% of the cells in the specimen had the more resistant phenotype. At the other extreme, the dose response curve for metastatic specimen PH303T (fig. 1) indicated marked resistance since there was a broad shoulder on the curve and it took approximately twenty-fold more drug to kill 50% of PH303T cells than an equivalent number of 66T cells. At the drug concentrations tested, there was no indication of heterogeneity for specimen PH303T. At 0.25 ug/ml of drug, there were no surviving colonies of PH303T among 9×10^3 cells plated (data not shown); however, survival was not tested at drug concentrations between 0.1 and 0.25 ug/ml. The dose response curve for metastatic specimen PH313T (fig. 1) was intermediate in sensitivity between H66T and PH303T. Like H66T, it had a biphasic dose response curve. The second phase of the curve extrapolated to the y axis at approximately 80% survival indicating that 80% of the population was more resistant while 20% of the population was even more sensitive than specimen H66T.

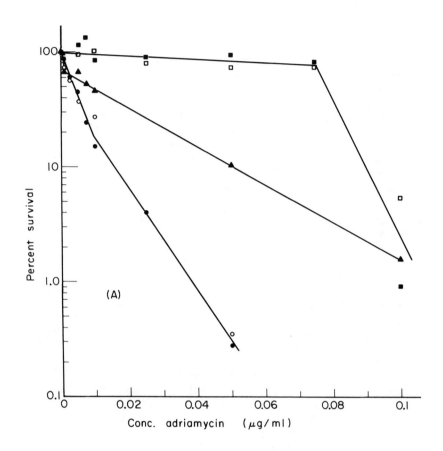

<u>Figure 1</u>   Response to adriamycin by different
tumor derived cultures.

●,○ two different assays for carcinoma
H66T; ▲ hypodermal metastasis PH313T;
■,□ two different assays for hypodermal
metastasis PH303T

We also examined the adriamycin sensitivity of
nonmalignant specimens derived from reduction mammoplasties

and uninvolved mastectomy tissue peripheral to carcinomas. Figure 2 illustrates the dose response curves for two reduction mammoplasties. Specimen H161E is similar to metastatic specimen PH303T in that the dose response curve had a broad shoulder with a steep drop indicating a homogeneously resistant population. In contrast, specimen H184E had a dose response curve which could be extrapolated to 100% survival with no shoulder indicating a homogeneous sensitive culture.

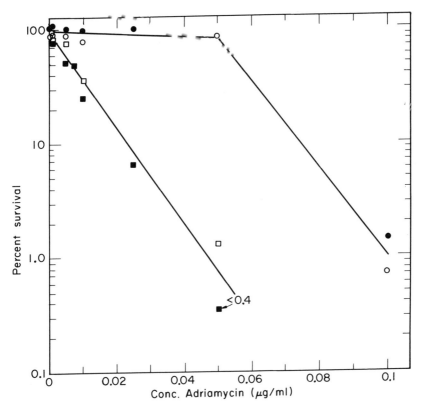

Figure 2   Response to adriamycin by different reduction mammoplasty specimens.

        □, ■   two different assays for specimen H184E; ○, ● two different assays for specimen H161E.

Figure 3 illustrates a composite of all the dose response curves to adriamycin that we have accumulated on malignant specimens. The specimens seem to fall into three distinct categories; sensitive, intermediate, and resistant. Within many of the sensitive specimens, there also appear to be subpopulations of the intermediate type. Figure 4 shows a similar composite for the nonmalignant specimens. Of the seven specimens tested to date, three had biphasic curves indicating heterogeneity in response to adriamycin. One of the three with biphasic curves was obtained with cells derived from tissue peripheral to a carcinoma (192P) while the others, H59E and H208E, were derived from reduction mammoplasties.

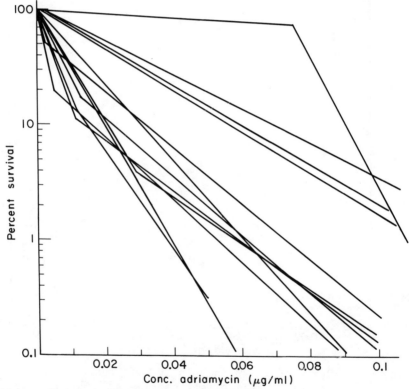

Figure 3   Composite of adriamycin dose
response curves for malignant
specimens.

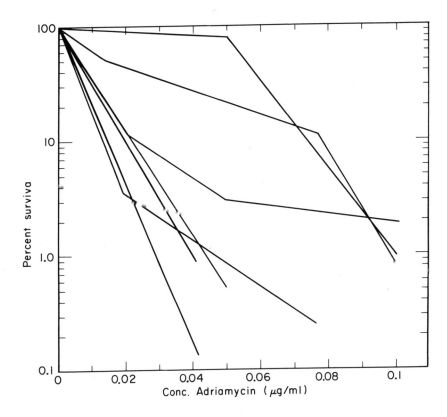

Figure 4   Composite of adriamycin dose response curves
for nonmalignant specimens.

        We have also used this system to evaluate the
sensitivity to two experimental adriamycin analogues,
bis(daunorubicin)   succinhydrazone   (NSC266210)   and
2-Iminodaunorubicin (NSC254681). Figure 5 illustrates the
data for one tumor specimen. When the data are plotted on
a linear scale, (Figure 5A), it is clear, on a molar basis,
that both the bis compound and the imino compound are more
efficient than adriamycin for killing approximately 50% of
the cells.   However,   when   the   data   are   plotted
logrithmically,   so   that   the   effect   on   resistant
subpopulations are emphasized, adriamycin is a more
effective agent than either analogue (Figure 5B).

Table 2

Summary of Data for Adriamycin Sensitivity Response

Specimen	Drug conc. (ng/ml) resulting in[1]	
	50% Survival	1% Survival
Nonmalignant Tissue		
a. reduction mammoplasties		
H59E	3.7	46
H161E	56	100
H184E	7	45
H191E	15	102
H208	6	130
b. tissue peripheral to carcinomas		
H200P	4.5	29
Primary Carcinomas		
H66T	3.0	39
H72T	3.5	60
H82T	12	82
H192T	6.4	59
H200T	5.0	63
PH326T	2.5	53
PH328T	9	61
PH329T	17.5	119
PH331T	20.5	138
Metastatic Carcinomas		
PH303T	78	104
PH313T	8.6	110
PH325T	14	110

[a]Where more than one assay was performed, the mean value from all assays is indicated.

Table 2 summarizes the data on adriamycin sensitivity of all specimens tested to date. The concentrations required to produce 50% survival varied among the specimens over a 31-fold range from 2.5 ng/ml to 78 ng/ml. In contrast, there was only a 5-fold range in drug concentrations required to reach 1% survival among various specimens.

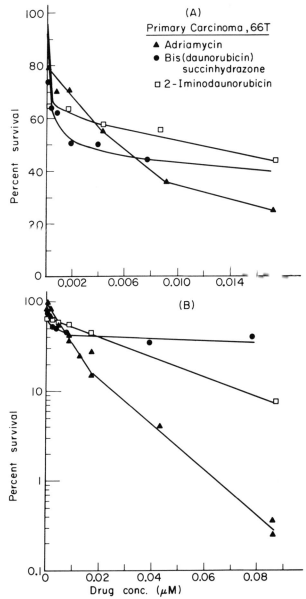

Figure 5: Response to adriamycin analogues by a primary carcinoma specimen (H66T)
A. Data plotted on a linear scale.
B. Same data plotted on a logarithmic scale.

DISCUSSION

This assay has potentially high relevance to the human chemotherapy of breast tumors, both for selection of existing drugs for treatment and for development of better new drugs. In this report we examined the sensitivity of a number of human mammary epithelial cell cultures at second passage to a drug currently in use against breast tumors. We have also begun comparisons with several new adriamycin analogues. Previous reports have described the generally high rate of success and high efficiency of cloning (1-40%) with this assay (10,11). Because the assay was so efficient most tumors produced a biphasic dose-response curve that indicated the presence of subpopulations of varying drug sensitivity or resistance. This is consistent with the clinical experience that patient relapse often follows an initial response to chemotherapy and may be due to the presence of a highly resistant form of the tumor. The ability in the present assay to detect resistant subpopulations in primary untreated specimens can have important application. Various experimental parameters that can be used in comparisons and correlations are obtainable (figures 1-5) from the dose-response curves. These include the concentrations required for a threshold effect on cell survival, the concentrations at the breakpoint in a biphasic curve, the slopes of the curves, and the concentrations required for nearly total cell kill. In this study, we have compared only the concentrations that resulted in 50% and in 1% survival of the cells.

For the 18 tissue specimens (Table 2) that were treated with adriamycin, no consistent differences were observed between cultures derived from malignant and those from nonmalignant tissues.

Overall, there was a thirty-fold range in adriamycin concentrations required to kill 50% of the cells. On the other hand, there was only a four-fold range in drug concentration required for 1% survival. This decreased range was from the resistant subpopulations in the cultures that evidently require higher concentrations of drug for cell kill. The wide variation in senstivity seems to be with the subpopulations that are more responsive to drug treatment.

The capacity to test and compare both malignant and nonmalignant tissues is an advantage for this assay that is unprecedented. If a sufficient number of malignant and nonmalignant specimens are compared, it should be possible to predict selectivity of the drug for tumor and the relative absence of cytotoxic side effects. To define the number of specimens required for a valid comparison requires further study and analysis. The fact that nonmalignant specimens as well as tumors varied in adriamycin sensitivity raises the question as to whether these differences are common to all cell types from a given donor or whether they arise as a result of mammary gland differentiation. Further studies with fibroblasts from the same donors will help answer this question. The capacity to compare a tumor specimen with nonmalignant tissue from the same donor is of very great utility, especially for designing patient treatment but also for new drug development. In the one example so far (Table 2), tumor specimen H200T and tissue peripheral to this carcinoma (H200P) showed similar dose responses to adriamycin. It will be important to obtain and accumulate clinical results for comparison with such assay data on a patient-by-patient basis.

A difficulty in obtaining the needed clinical correlations is that breast cancer patients are usually treated with combinations of drugs. A possible but less satisfactory alternative would be to compare drug sensitivities using both this assay and tha agar clonogenic assay. Since good single drug clinical correlations are available for some tumors using the agar clonogenic assay (3-7) it would be encouraging if both assays made the same predictions concerning sensitivity of a specimen. Preliminary comparisons already show some interesting differences that require explanation. For the agar clonogenic assay, the concentrations of adriamycin required to kill cells in culture were much higher (3) than those required in the mammary cell assay described here. One possibility is that the difference between the two assays is the result of differences in media components. For example, lowered serum levels in MM media might bind less adriamycin thus making more of it available for cell uptake. Alternately, the fact that we first allow cells to enter into a proliferative phase may affect drug sensitivity. Further studies to distinguish among these alternatives are in progress.

The importance of the studies--few so far--of new adriamycin analogues must not be underestimated. It is the objective of drug development studies to rank new analogues against the parent drug. Before this assay can be used systematically for that purpose, further studies must be done, but even the very first tests are useful in showing that the new analogues possess activity against human tumor cells and are therefore worth examination by other criteria. The use of assays involving human tumor cells at second passage will be a major advance in drug development. Up to now most assays for antitumor activity rely on mouse tumors. Such assays have the advantages of an in vivo test and the use of established homogeneous cell lines, but their predictiveness is uncertain. Results with mouse tumors seem to predict for clinical activity only in the most general way, and not for spectrum of activity or quantitatively for rate of response. Prediction of spectrum of activity is not improved by increasing the number and type of mouse tumors. The NCI has recently found (oral report to the Board of Scientific Counselors, Division of Cancer Treatment, NCI, June 4, 1982) that most of the active compounds detected by a panel of 8 mouse tumors could be predicted by only 3 of the tumors. The issue of predictiveness is quite different with a clonogenic assay using human specimens in culture. The major question for the development of new drugs and predicting their clinical activity is how to generalize from individual human specimens. Presumably this can be accomplished by statistically defining the minimum number of random specimens that give a significant overall correlation in the clinic, and by recognizing the role that in vivo drug delivery and pharmacokinetics can play.

In conclusion, we have demonstrated the existence of a useful new clonogenic assay for both malignant and nonmalignant human mammary specimens. Most specimens have been successfully cultured with high (1-40%) plating efficiency. Treatment of the cultures with adriamycin and several of its analogues over a range of concentrations produced dose-response curves that in many cases were biphasic indicating the presence of subpopulations with varying sensitivity. These curves can yield numerous parameters for comparing the activity of drugs and the sensitivity of human tumors.

REFERENCES

1. Courtenay, V.I., Selby, P.J., Smith, I.F., Miller, J., Peckham, M.J. Growth of Human Tumor Cell Colonies from Biopsies Using Two Soft-agar Techniques. Br. J. Cancer 38:77-82, 1978.
2. Hamburger, A.W., Salmon, S.E. Primary Bioassay of Human Tumor Stem Cells. Science 197:461-463, 1977.
3. Salmon, S.E., Hamburger, A.W., Soehnlen, B., Durie, B.G.M., Alberts, D.S., and Moon, T.E. Quantitation of Differential Sensitivity of Human Tumor Stem Cells To Anticancer Drugs. The New England Journal of Medicine 298:1321-1327 1978.
4 Salmon, S.E., Alberts, D.S., Meyskens, F.L., Durie, B.G.M., Alberts, D.S., and Moon, T.E. Quantitation of Differential Sensitivity of Human Tumor Stem Cells. Salmon, S.E., ed. Alan Liss, Inc., New York 223:245, 1980.
5. MacIntosh, F.R., Evans, T.L., and Sikic, B.I. Methodologic Problems In Clonogenic Assays of Spontaneous Human Tumors. Cancer Chemotherapy and Pharmacology 6:205-210, 1981.
6. Alberts, D.S., Salmon, S.E., Chen, H.S.G, Surwit, E.A., Soehnlen, B., Young, L., and Moon, T.E. Predictive Chemotherapy of Ovarian Cancer Using An In Vitro Clonogenic Assay. Lancet II. 340-342, 1980.
7. Von Hoff, D.D., Cowen, J., Harris, G., Reisdorf, G. Human Tumor Cloning: Feasibility and Clinical Correlations. Cancer Chemotherapy and Pharmacology 6:265-272, 1981.
8. Stampfer, M.R., Hallowes, R.C., Hackett, A.J. Growth of Normal Human Mammary Cells In Culture. In Vitro 16:415-425, 1980.
9. Stampfer, M.R. Cholera Toxin Stimulation of Human Mammary Epithelial Cells in Culture. In Vitro, In Press.
10. Smith, H.S., Lan, S., Ceriani, R., Hackett, A.J., and Stampfer, M.R. Clonal Proliferation of Cultured Nonmalignant and Malignant Human Breast Epithelia. Cancer Research 41:4637-4643, 1981
11. Smith, H.S., Hackett, A.J., Lan, S., Stampfer, M.R. Use of An Efficient Method For Culturing Human Mammary

Epithelial Cells To Study Adriamycin Sensitivity.
Cancer Chemotherapy and Pharmacology 6:237-244, 1981.

12. Smith, H.S., Hackett, A.J., Riggs, J.L., Mosesson,
M.L., Walton, J.R., Stampfer, M.R. Properties of
Epithelial Cells Cultured from Human Carcinomas and
Nonmalignant Tissues. Journal of Supramolecular
Structure 11:147-166, 1979.

13. Owens, R.B., Smith, H.S., Nelson-Rees, W.A., and
Springer, E.L. Epithelial Cell Cultures From Normal
and Cancerous Tissues. J. Natl. Cancer Inst.
56:843-849, 1976.

14. Hackett, A.J., Smith, H.S., Springer, W.L., Owens,
R.B., Nelson-Rees, W.A., Riggs, J.L., and Gardner, M.
Two Syngeneic Cell Lines From Human Breast Tissue: One
Aneuploid Mammary Epithelial (Hs578T) and One Diploid
Myoepithelial (Hs578Bst). J. Natl. Cancer Inst.,
58:1795-1806, 1977.

Rational Basis for Chemotherapy, pages 137–151
© 1983 Alan R. Liss, Inc., 150 Fifth Avenue, New York, NY 10011

THE ANDROGEN RESISTANCE SYNDROMES

James E. Griffin

Department of Internal Medicine
The University of Texas Southwestern Medical School
Dallas, Texas 75235

ABSTRACT   Hereditary defects in androgen action
cause resistance to the hormone both during
embryogenesis and in later life and hence usually
cause developmental defects of the male urogenital
tract.   In genetic males such defects produce a
phenotypic spectrum ranging from infertile but
otherwise normal men to individuals with varying
degrees of ambiguous genitalia to phenotypic
women.   These disorders can be classified on the
basis of the step in androgen action that is
affected by the individual mutations.   5α-Reduc-
tase deficiency is an autosomal recessive enzyme
defect that impairs the conversion of testosterone
to dihydrotestosterone. The internal male genital
tract virilizes normally, but the external genitalia are predominantly female in character.   The
syndrome is the result of one of several mutations
that impair the function of the 5α-reductase
enzyme.   A variety of disorders influence the
androgen receptor that mediates the action of both
testosterone and dihydrotestosterone.   At least
four phenotypic variants can be distinguished --
complete testicular feminization, incomplete
testicular feminization, the Reifenstein syndrome, and the infertile male syndrome, each of
which is inherited as an X-linked trait.   Absence
of receptor binding is found commonly in complete
testicular feminization, but qualitative and/or
less severe quantitative defects in receptor function can be associated with all four variants.   A
third type of disorder -- receptor positive resistance -- also causes variable defects in male

development and is associated with normal 5α-reductase activity and normal androgen receptor. The underlying defect is presumed to lie at the intranuclear site or sites of action of the hormone-receptor complex.

INTRODUCTION

Resistance to the action of a hormone was first described as a mechanism of endocrine disease when it was recognized that pseudohypoparathyroidism is due to resistance to the action of parathyroid hormone. The next endocrinopathy recognized to result from hormone resistance was the syndrome testicular feminization, which is due to resistance to androgen action (1). Subsequently, additional syndromes of androgen resistance have been delineated, so that the phenotypic spectrum ranges from normal-appearing women with testicular feminization to otherwise normal men with infertility. This review will describe the mechanisms by which androgens normally act to virilize the male embryo and maintain normal masculinization in the adult and summarize current concepts of the androgen resistance syndromes. The types of spontaneous mutations in androgen action occurring in the androgen resistance syndromes may serve as models for mechanisms of resistance to the action of other steroid hormones.

PERIPHERAL METABOLISM OF ANDROGENS

Testosterone, formed in the testes under control of luteinizing hormone (LH) from the pituitary, is the principal androgen in the circulation of the male. It serves as the prohormone for the formation in peripheral tissues of two types of active metabolites: 5α-dihydrotestosterone and 17β-estradiol (2). Dihydrotestosterone, formed from testosterone by the 5α-reductase enzyme, mediates androgen action in many target tissues and in most systems is more potent than testosterone. Estradiol, formed from testosterone by the aromatase enzyme complex, acts in some instances in concert with androgens and in others has independent or opposite effects to those of androgens. The formation of each of these testosterone metabolites is physiologically irreversible, and dihydrotestosterone cannot be converted to estradiol. The 5α-reduced metabolites are formed primarily in androgen target tissues (e.g., the prostate), and in the case of estradiol adipose tissue is also a major site for extraglandular estrogen formation. Estradiol and dihydrotestosterone may either act in the tissue in which they are formed (paracrine function) or enter the circulation and act as circulating hormones. In normal men about 85% of the estradiol formed each day is the result of extraglandular aromatization of androgen and only about 15% of estradiol production is directly secreted by the testis (1). However, when plasma LH concentration is increased, direct secretion of estradiol by the testes increases.

MECHANISMS OF ANDROGEN ACTION

Testosterone enters cells primarily by passive diffusion. Inside the cell testosterone can be converted to dihydrotestosterone by the 5α-reductase enzyme. The two hormones bind to the same high affinity androgen receptor in the cytosol. The hormone-receptor complexes diffuse into the nuclei and interact with presumed specific sites on the chromosomes to result in the generation of new messenger RNA and ultimately new protein synthesis in the cytoplasm of the cell. The final result can be viewed as effecting the major functions of androgen in males: regulation of gonadotropin secretion by the hypothalamic-pituitary system, initiation and maintenance of spermatogenesis, formation of the male phenotype during sexual differentiation, and promotion of sexual maturation at puberty. The testosterone receptor complex is thought to mediate gonadotropin regulation, spermatogenesis, and the wolffian stimulation component of sexual differentiation; the dihydrotestosterone-receptor complex is thought to mediate external virilization during sexual differentiation and most aspects of pubertal virilization (3). The reason that dihydrotestosterone formation is required for some androgen actions is not entirely clear. The mechanisms by which estrogens act to augment or block androgen action are also unclear. In prostatic hyperplasia estrogens appear to enhance androgen action by increasing the levels of androgen receptor (4), whereas in the male breast estrogens and androgens appear to be antagonists (5).

THE CONTROL OF MALE PHENOTYPIC DEVELOPMENT

Normal sexual development consists of three sequential processes (6). Chromosomal sex is established at the time of fertilization, the 46,XY complement being male and the 46,XX complement female. Normally chromosomal sex determines gonadal sex, i.e., the Y chromosome carries genetic determinants that induce the indifferent gonad to become a testis. In the absence of this influence of the Y chromosome (as in the normal female) the indifferent gonad becomes an ovary.

Likewise, gonadal sex normally determines phenotypic sex. The internal genital tracts in the two sexes are derived from separate anlagen, the mullerian and wolffian ducts, which are present along with the indifferent gonad in early embryos of both sexes. In the male the wolffian ducts give rise to the epididymides, vas deferentia, and seminal vesicles, and the mullerian ducts regress. In the female the mullerian ducts give rise to the fallopian tubes, uterus, and upper vagina, and the wolffian ducts regress. In contrast to the internal genitalia, the urethra and external genitalia in the two sexes are derived from common anlagen. The urogenital sinus gives rise in the male to the prostate and the prostatic urethra and in the female to the urethra and lower portion of the vagina. The genital tubercle becomes the glans penis in the male and the clitoris in the female. The genital swellings become the scrotum or labia majora, and the urethral fold and groove either fuse and elongate to become the shaft of the penis or form the labia minora.

In the absence of the testis phenotypic development is female (6). Male development is induced by three hormones from the fetal testis. Mullerian inhibiting substance is a peptide hormone secreted by the fetal testis that causes regression of the mullerian ducts, thus preventing the development of the uterus and fallopian tubes in normal males. As discussed above testosterone secreted by the fetal testis stimulates development of the wolffian ducts, whereas dihydrotestosterone formed at its site of action in the embryonic tissues causes development of the prostate and external genitalia.

DISORDERS OF SEXUAL DEVELOPMENT

Disorders of sexual development can be classified in terms of the initial developmental stage influenced; i.e., disorders of chromosomal sex, disorders of gonadal sex, and disorders of phenotypic sex. The androgen resistance syndromes comprise one category of disorders of phenotypic sex in which 46,XY males (normal chromosomal sex) with bilateral testes (normal gonadal sex) fail to develop as completely normal men (so called male pseudohermaphroditism). Although testosterone synthesis is normal in approximately three-fourths of patients with male pseudohermaphroditism (7, 8), the possibility of an abnormality in testosterone synthesis must be considered in the differential diagnosis of all patients suspected of having androgen resistance. Plasma testosterone is usually low in adults with disorders of testosterone formation, but as a result of increased gonadotropin levels some subjects with partial defects in testosterone synthesis may have an elevation in the plasma levels of the biochemical precursor that accumulates prior to the enzyme block (9).

The androgen resistance syndromes, the focus of this review, are disorders in which mullerian regression and testosterone synthesis are normal but in which affected persons are resistant to the hormone because of a defect in some aspect of androgen action. These abnormalities were originally delineated by studying patients with male pseudohermaphroditism. Subsequently, men with infertility alone as the clinical manifestation of androgen resistance have been identified, extending the clinical spectrum recognized. The molecular defects responsible for androgen resistance may occur at any one of the three major sites in the pathway of androgen action: abnormalities in 5α-reductase, defects in the androgen receptor, or abnormalities in the subsequent phases of androgen action. The latter category has been termed receptor-positive resistance (10).

THE ANDROGEN RESISTANCE SYNDROMES

5α-Reductase Deficiency.

5α-reductase deficiency, a distinct disorder on genetic, phenotypic, and endocrine grounds, was originally described as an autosomal recessive form of male pseudohermaphroditism termed pseudovaginal perineoscrotal hypospadias (11). This entity is now recognized to result from deficient conversion of testosterone to dihydrotestosterone and is termed 5α-reductase deficiency instead of the original anatomic designation (12, 13). The characteristic clinical feature is that of normal male development of wolffian structures that terminate in the vagina but predominantly female development of structures of the urogenital sinus and external genitalia so that the external phenotype is that of a female. Some degree of clitoromegaly is frequently present at birth, and at the time of expected puberty there is variable virilization of the external genitalia and development of normal axillary and pubic hair. Breasts remain infantile (male) in structure. Affected men have less facial and body hair and less temporal hair recession than their unaffected male relatives. No prostatic tissue is palpable or detectable on cystoscopy.

The endocrinology of 5α-reductase deficiency is characterized by normal male plasma levels of testosterone and low plasma levels of dihydrotestosterone in adults, elevated plasma ratios of testosterone to dihydrotestosterone after chorionic gonadotropin stimulation in prepubertal subjects, elevated ratios of urinary 5β- to 5α-reduced steroid metabolites, decreased <u>in</u> <u>vivo</u> conversion of testosterone to dihydrotestosterone, decreased 5α-reductase activity in tissue biopsy specimens, and deficient or abnormal 5α-reductase activity in fibroblasts cultured from genital skin (14-16). Although plasma LH levels are slightly elevated, the levels are lower than in patients with disorders of the androgen receptor. The relatively normal plasma LH levels probably explains why estrogen production is within the normal range for men and why gynecomastia is absent.

The molecular features of the mutation have been studied in fibroblasts cultured from biopsies of genital skin from affected males (14-16). Fibroblasts from the majority of families have very low levels of 5α-reductase activity, as measured under optimal conditions, and appear to form an enzyme with reduced affinity for the testosterone substrate. However, at least one family appears to have a different mutation in which enzyme activity in cultured cells is in the low normal range in spite of a similar <u>in</u> <u>vivo</u> defect to that observed in families with deficient enzyme (17). Whereas the affinity of 5α-reductase for testosterone was normal, the enzyme in cells from this family has a reduced affinity for nicotinamide adenine dinucleotide phosphate (NADPH), the cofactor for the reaction, and is unstable (15). Other families with the disorder appear to have an enzyme with abnormal affinity for both testosterone and NADPH (16). Studies of 15 families with 5α-reductase deficiency have revealed 12 families with very low levels of enzyme activity, two with a combined alteration in affinity for substrate and cofactor, and only the single family with the isolated abnormality in cofactor affinity.

A major unresolved issue is why the external genitalia of patients with 5α-reductase deficiency virilize more at puberty than during embryogenesis. The late virilization may be due to the presence of higher testosterone levels at puberty than during embryogenesis, to the accumulation of some dihydrotestosterone in plasma as a result of the residual 5α-reductase demonstrable in all patients, or to some unidentified change in responsiveness with age. The degree of masculinization at the time of expected puberty varies; furthermore, in some subjects who are untreated until later life a reversal of gender role occurs at the time of pubertal virilization (18). Because of the extreme defect in the external genitalia, most affected persons are raised as females. In such instances castration should be performed before the expected time of puberty to prevent the disfiguring effects of virilization. In persons who are raised as males or who undergo apparent reversal of gender role prior to ascertainment appropriate repair of the hypospadias and any coexisting cryptorchidism should be performed.

Receptor Disorders.

Disorders of the androgen receptor may result in several distinct phenotypes. Despite differences in clinical presentation and molecular pathology these disorders are similar in regard to endocrinology, genetics, and basic pathophysiology. The major clinical features of each of the four disorders will be considered first and followed by a discussion of the endocrine features and pathophysiology.

Complete testicular feminization. Complete testicular feminization is an X-linked recessive disorder characterized by a uniform clinical presentation (1). The phenotype is that of a normal female except for decreased or absent axillary and pubic hair. Breast development and distribution of body fat are truly feminine. The external genitalia are unambiguously female, and the clitoris is normal. The vagina is short and blind-ending. Internal genitalia are absent (neither wolffian nor mullerian derivatives can be identified in most) except for the testes which may be in the abdomen, in the inguinal canal, or in the labia majora.

Histology of the testis invariably reveals incomplete or absent spermatogenesis and normal or hyperplastic Leydig cells. Patients either come to medical attention because of an inguinal hernia or primary amenorrhea. There is often a positive family history of similarly affected family members, but about a third of patients have negative family histories and are presumed to represent new mutations.

Incomplete testicular feminization. Incomplete testicular feminization is about a tenth as common as the complete form and resembles it except that there is some ambiguity of the external genitalia, normal pubic hair, and some virilization as well as feminization at the time of expected puberty (19). There is usually partial fusion of the labioscrotal folds and some degree of clitoromegaly. The vagina is short and blind-ending. In contrast to the complete form of the disorder the wolffian-duct derivatives are usually present but not completely normal. The family history in most cases is uninformative. However, in several instances multiple family members are affected, and in at least one family the pattern of inheritance is compatible with X-linkage.

The management of patients with the two disorders differs. Because tumors of the undescended testes are a potential complication in both the complete and incomplete forms of the disorder, castration is indicated in all patients. Since the risk of tumor formation is minimal prior to adolescence and since patients with the complete form of the disorder undergo successful endogenous feminization at the time of expected puberty, castration can usually be delayed until after the adolescent growth spurt and feminization in these patients. Since patients with the incomplete disorder virilize at the time of expected puberty, prepubertal patients with clitoromegaly or posterior labial fusion should have gonadectomy before adolescence.

Reifenstein syndrome. Reifenstein syndrome is the term now applied to a variety of forms of incomplete male pseudohermaphroditism initially described by Reifenstein, Rosewater, Gilbert-Dreyfus, and Lubs and their colleagues (20). Each of these disorders was originally assumed to be a distinct entity and was designated by a separate eponym. Several pedigrees compatible with X-linkage have now been described in which affected members of the same family exhibit variable phenotypes that span the defects described by these authors, it is now believed that these syndromes probably constitute variable manifestations of a single mutation. The predominant phenotype is male, and the spectrum of defective virilization ranges from gynecomastia and azoospermia to more severe defects such as hypospadias and even to the presence of a pseudovagina. The most common phenotype is that of men with perineoscrotal hypospadias and gynecomastia. Axillary and pubic hair is normal, but chest and facial hair is minimal. Cryptorchidism is common, and the testes are often smaller than normal. Spermatogenesis is usually incomplete. Some subjects have defects in wolffian-duct derivatives such as absence or hypoplasia of the vas deferens. The psychological development in most subjects is unequivocally male. The hypospadias and crypt-orchidism should be corrected surgically. The only success-ful form of treatment of the gynecomastia is surgical removal.

Infertile male syndrome. The infertile male syndrome is the most recently recognized form of androgen resistance and in contrast to the other disorders is not a form of male pseudohermaphroditism (21). Although some of the least severely affected patients in families with Reifenstein syndrome were noted to have azoospermia alone as a manifes-tation of a receptor abnormality, it was not anticipated that individuals with negative family histories and appar-ently idiopathic infertility might have androgen resistance. However, evaluation of men with normal external genitalia, apparently normal wolffian-duct structures, and infertility due to azoospermia or severe oligospermia has suggested that a receptor disorder may be present in a fourth or more (22). As in the other receptor disorders, there is no effective therapy for the infertility.

The endocrine pattern is similar in all forms of androgen receptor disorders but has been best characterized in complete testicular feminization. Plasma testosterone levels and rates of production by the testes are those of normal men (or higher). The elevated rate of testosterone production is secondary to a high mean plasma level of LH, which in turn is the consequence of defective feedback regulation caused by resistance to the action of androgen at the hypothalamic-pituitary level. Elevations in LH are also responsible for the increased estrogen secretion by the testes (1). Thus, variable degrees of androgen resistance coupled with enhanced production of estradiol results in both varying degrees of defective virilization and variable feminization in the four clinical syndromes. In complete testicular feminization the defective virilization is most severe and the full feminizing effect of the increased estrogen is expressed. In incomplete testicular feminization an almost complete feminizing effect of estrogen is expressed together with slight virilization. Estrogen production in Reifenstein syndrome is increased to a similar or greater extent to that in testicular feminization. However, a less severe androgen resistance results in a predominantly male phenotype and less pronounced feminization. Only a few men with the infertile male syndrome have had evaluation of androgen-estrogen dynamics. The hormonal changes seem to be similar to those in the other receptor disorders but less marked, e.g. some men do not have an elevation of plasma LH, at least when assessed by single plasma samples (22).

An abnormality of the androgen receptor in fibroblasts cultured from patients with complete testicular feminization was first demonstrated by Keenan and coworkers (23). The initial patients were shown to have a near absence of high affinity dihydrotestosterone binding. In subsequent studies the pattern has become much more complex. Approximately a third of individuals with the phenotype complete testicular feminization have a qualitative defect in the androgen receptor, in addition patients with incomplete testicular feminization, Reifenstein syndrome, and the infertile male syndrome have been found to have either a decreased amount of an apparently normal receptor or a qualitatively abnormal androgen receptor. In making these distinctions, two methods have been used to identify a qualitatively abnormal receptor: thermolability of dihydrotestosterone binding in fibroblast monolayers (24) and failure of stabilization of the cytosol receptor to ultracentrifugation on sucrose gradients by sodium molybdate (25).

The characteristics of the androgen receptor in genital skin fibroblasts from individuals from 35 families with androgen resistance and putative disorders of the receptor have been studied in our laboratory (25). Absent or near absent binding appears to be primarily associated with complete testicular feminization and was present in 9 families. A qualitatively abnormal receptor was detected in some families with each of the four clinical disorders and was the most common receptor abnormality identified (14 of the 35 families). A decreased amount of an apparently normal receptor was present in 8 families and was primarily associated with the two syndromes with a predominately male phenotype. In four families no receptor abnormality could be identified in spite of a similar clinical and endocrinological picture. In these families as well as in those with fibroblasts having a decreased amount of binding it is not clear whether a more subtle qualitative receptor defect may be present. If, in fact, there is no abnormality of the receptor, the mutation in the four families with normal receptor levels may reside distal to the androgen receptor (see below). Except for the absent binding in complete testicular feminization there is no consistent correlation of the receptor abnormality with the clinical severity of the androgen resistance since the finding of a qualitative abnormality does not indicate the degree of functional impairment of the receptor.

Receptor Positive Resistance.

A category of androgen resistance that does not appear to involve either the 5α-reductase or the androgen receptor was first identified by Amrhein et al (26) in a family with the syndrome of testicular feminization. Subsequent patients have been described with a variety of phenotypes ranging from incomplete testicular feminization to findings similar to those in the Reifenstein syndrome. We have studied individuals from four such families with varying clinical syndromes in whom a receptor abnormality in fibroblasts could not be identified. The hormonal profile is similar to that seen in the receptor disorders. The site of the molecular abnormality in these patients is unclear. If the defect is truly distal to the receptor, there could be failure of generation of specific messenger RNA or an abnormality of its processing. Indeed, it is not established that a uniform defect is present, and the disorder may represent a heterogeneous group of molecular abnormalities. Management depends on the phenotype.

THE NATURE OF ANDROGEN RESISTANCE

Hormone resistance was originally defined as a lack of response to endogenous and exogenous hormone. In the case of androgen resistance, it was assumed that the degree of resistance to the hormone is equal in all tissues at all times of life and that the phenotypic expression of such a disorder was inevitably male pseudohermaphroditism. However, the spectrum of the manifestations of androgen resistance has expanded beyond the original formulations. At the clinical level androgen resistance can be documented in some but not all tissues of the same affected subject.

Therefore, we have adopted a more complex classification of androgen resistance that is dependent on a combination of molecular, genetic, phenotypic, and endocrine characteristics.

Subjects with 5α-reductase deficiency have a special type of androgen resistance -- in these individuals certain target tissues that are resistant to the action of endogenous androgen (testosterone) presumably would have responded normally to the missing end-product (dihydrotestosterone) if it had been administered at the appropriate time during embryogenesis. In contrast, persons with androgen-receptor abnormalities and those with receptor-positive resistance appear to be equally unresponsive to all androgens.

The use of fibroblasts cultured from genital skin has been useful in defining the defects that underlie these various disorders and in the classification of specific entities. In disorders such as 5α-reductase deficiency and testicular feminization, the cultured fibroblast symbolizes the whole body in that the molecular defect present in vivo in all androgen-target tissues is also expressed in fibroblasts cultured from genital skin. The clinical manifestations of these disorders are consistent within families, and the molecular defects are uniform among tissues. The identification of qualitative abnormalities in the 5α-reductase and in the androgen receptor in fibroblasts cultured from some affected families provides additional support for the concept that the defect expressed in the fibroblast is, indeed, the primary genetic defect in the disorders.

For other conditions (e.g., the Reifenstein syndrome and the infertile male syndrome) the relation between the receptor defect and the resulting phenotype is less certain. Even within the same family the phenotypic expression of androgen resistance in these disorders varies from subject to subject and from tissue to tissue despite the fact that affected individuals from a given family have the same abnormality in fibroblasts. Disorders of the androgen receptor are always associated with defective spermatogenesis, whereas the phenotypic abnormalities and degree of sexual maturation at puberty are variable. Unidentified factors must modify hormone action in vivo. In addition, different amounts of androgen receptor may be required for different in vivo actions of the hormone; therefore, a partial defect in the receptor could cause more complete manifestations of androgen resistance in some tissues than in others. The fact that qualitative defects in the androgen receptor have been identified in some families with Reifenstein syndrome and the infertile male syndrome indicates that the fundamental mutation in these disorders does involve the androgen receptor primarily. Thus, the receptor abnormality and the resulting androgen resistance probably cause the disorders, regardless of the mechanism of the incomplete expression of the hormone resistance among tissues and among individuals.

REFERENCES

1. Wilson JD, Griffin JE, Leshin M, MacDonald PC (1982). The androgen resistance syndromes: 5α-reductase deficiency, testicular feminization, and related disorders. In Stanbury JB, Wyngaarden JB, Goldstein JL, Brown MS, Fredrickson DS (eds): "Metabolic Basis of Inherited Disease," New York: McGraw-Hill, in press.
2. Wilson JD (1975). Metabolism of testicular androgens. In Greep RO, Astwood EB (eds): "Handbook of Physiology," Section 7 Vol. 5, Washington DC: American Physiological Society, p. 491.
3. Wilson JD (1978). Sexual differentiation. Annu Rev Physiol 40:279.
4. Moore RJ, Gazak JM, Wilson JD (1979). Regulation of cytoplasmic dihydrotestosterone binding in dog prostate by 17β-estradiol. J Clin Invest 63:351.
5. Wilson JD, Aiman JE, MacDonald PC (1980). The pathogenesis of gynecomastia. Adv Intern Med 25:1.
6. Jost A (1972). A new look at the mechanisms controlling sex differentiation in mammals. Johns Hopkins Med J 130:38.
7. Savage MO, Chaussain JL, Evain D, Roger M, Canlorbe P, Job JD (1978). Endocrine studies in male pseudohermaphroditism in childhood and adolescence. Clin Endocrinol 8:219.
8. Campo S, Moteagudo C, Nicolau G, Pellizzari E, Belgorosky A, Stivel M, Rivarola M (1981). Testicular function in prepubertal male pseudohermaphroditism. Clin Endocrinol 14:11.
9. Griffin JE, Wilson JD (1978). Hereditary male pseudohermaphroditism. Clin Obstet Gynaecol 5:457.
10. Griffin JE, Wilson JD (1980). The syndromes of androgen resistance. N Engl J Med 302:198.
11. Nowakowski H, Lenz W (1961). Genetic aspects in male hypogonadism. Recent Prog Horm Res 17:53.

12. Walsh PC, Madden JD, Harrod MJ, Goldstein JL, MacDonald PC (1974). Familial incomplete male pseudohermaphroditism, type 2: decreased dihydrotestosterone formation in pseudovaginal perineoscrotal hypospadias. N Engl J Med 291:944.

13. Peterson RE, Imperato-McGinley J, Gautier T, Sturla E (1977). Male pseudohermaphroditism due to steroid 5α-reductase deficiency. Am J Med 62:170.

14. Moore RJ, Griffin JE, Wilson JD (1975). Diminished 5α-reductase activity in extracts of fibroblasts cultured from patients with familial incomplete male pseudohermaphroditism, type 2. J Biol Chem 250:7168.

15. Leshin M, Griffin JE, Wilson JD (1978). Hereditary male pseudohermaphroditism associated with an unstable form of 5α-reductase. J Clin Invest 62:685.

16. Imperato-McGinley J, Peterson RE, Leshin M, Griffin JE, Cooper G, Draghi S, Berenyi M, Wilson JD (1980). Steroid 5α-reductase deficiency in a 65-year-old male pseudohermaphroditism: the natural history, ultrastructure of the testes, and evidence for inherited enzyme heterogeneity. J Clin Endocrinol Metab 50:15.

17. Fisher LK, Kogut MD, Moore RJ, Goebelsmann U, Weitzman JJ, Isaacs H Jr, Griffin JE, Wilson JD (1978). Clinical, endocrinological, and enzymatic characterization of two patients with 5α-reductase deficiency: evidence that a single enzyme is responsible for the 5α-reduction of cortisol and testosterone. J Clin Endocrinol Metab 47:653.

18. Imperato-McGinley J, Peterson RE, Gautier T, Sturla E (1979). Androgens and the evolution of male-gender identity among male pseudohermaphrodites with 5α-reductase deficiency. N Engl J Med 300:1233.

19. Madden JD, Walsh PC, MacDonald PC, Wilson JD (1975). Clinical and endocrinologic characterization of a patient with the syndrome of incomplete testicular feminization. J Clin Endocrinol Metab 41:751.

20. Wilson JD, Harrod MJ, Goldstein JL, Hemsell DL, MacDonald PC (1974). Familial incomplete male pseudohermaphroditism, type 1: evidence for androgen resistance and variable clinical manifestations in a family with the Reifenstein syndrome. N Engl J Med 290:1097.

21. Aiman J, Griffin JE, Gazak JM, Wilson JD, MacDonald PC (1979). Androgen insensitivity as a cause of infertility in otherwise normal men. N Engl J Med 300:223.

22. Aiman J, Griffin JE (1982). The frequency of androgen receptor deficiency in infertile men. J Clin Endocrinol Metab 54:725.

23. Keenan BS, Meyer WJ III, Hadjian AD, Jones HW, Migeon CJ (1974). Syndrome of androgen insensitivity in man: absence of 5α-dihydrotestosterone binding protein in skin fibroblasts. J Clin Endocrinol Metab 38:1143.

24. Griffin JE (1979). Testicular feminization associated with a thermolabile androgen receptor in cultured human fibroblasts. J Clin Invest 64:1624.

25. Griffin JE, Durrant JL. Qualitative receptor defects in families with androgen resistance: failure of stabilization of the fibroblast cytosol androgen receptor. J Clin Endocrinol Metab, in press.

26. Amrhein JA, Meyer WJ III, Jones HW Jr, Migeon CJ (1976). Androgen insensitivity in man: evidence for genetic heterogeneity. Proc Natl Acad Sci USA 73:891.

Rational Basis for Chemotherapy, pages 153–176
© 1983 Alan R. Liss, Inc., 150 Fifth Avenue, New York, NY 10011

DETERMINANTS OF GLUCOCORTICOID RESISTANCE
IN LYMPHOID CELL LINES[1]

Judith C. Gasson and Suzanne Bourgeois

Regulatory Biology Laboratory, The Salk Institute
San Diego, California 92138

ABSTRACT This paper presents evidence for two bases
for glucocorticoid resistance in murine T cell lines:
resistance can result either from defects in the
glucocorticoid receptor or in a "lysis" function. All
glucocorticoid resistant variants derived from the
glucocorticoid sensitive cell lines, S49 and W7, have
receptor defects. This can be understood in the case
of the S49, because of the functional hemizygosity of
this line at the locus, r, encoding the receptor.
However, the diploidy of the W7 line at the receptor
locus (r^+/r^+) might have been expected to prevent the
high incidence of receptor defects. Still, approximately 300 W7 glucocorticoid resistant variants
induced by a variety of mutagens have defective
receptor. In view of the difficulties in obtaining
new types of variants by selection in vitro, another
cell line was examined, SAK, which had acquired
glucocorticoid resistance in vivo.
SAK cells contain 30,000 glucocorticoid receptors
per cell with normal nuclear transfer. These receptors are functional since they complement a receptor
defect in W7 cells: hybrids produced by fusion
between SAK cells and receptor deficient W7 cells are
glucocorticoid sensitive. Therefore, the resistance

[1]This work was supported by grant GM20868 from the
National Institute of General Medical Sciences and by a
grant from the Whitehall Foundation to S.B. J.C.G. is recipient of fellowship AM06179 from the National Institute
of Arthritis, Metabolic and Digestive Diseases.

of the SAK line must result from a defect in another
locus, called "ℓ" for lysis. The lysis defect in SAK
cells is recessive, as shown by fusion of SAK cells
with glucocorticoid sensitive W7 cells. Treatment of
SAK cells by 5-azacytidine activates the defective
"lysis" function and renders those cells glucocorticoid sensitive. These results indicate that the
origin of glucocorticoid resistance in the SAK line
is epigenetic, resulting probably from differentiation.
    SAK cells, although resistant to glucocorticoid-
induced cytolysis, show a reduction of cloning efficiency in the presence of glucocorticoids. High cloning efficiency can be restored by the addition of
culture supernatants, containing growth factors, to the
medium. This observation suggests a model to account
for the fact that all glucocorticoid resistant variants
isolated so far from the W7 line have defects in the
receptor, and a possible approach to that problem is
proposed.

INTRODUCTION

    The cytolytic effect of glucocorticoids on T-lymphoid
cells is mediated by cytoplasmic receptors which, after
binding of the hormone, undergo activation and translocation to the nucleus. The step beyond nuclear translocation
and the mechanism of the steroid-induced lysis are entirely
obscure. The availability of cloned T-cell lines derived
from both human (1) and mouse (2,3) tumors allows a genetic
analysis of the cytolytic response and of the bases for
glucocorticoid resistance. Variants resistant to glucocorticoid-induced killing can be isolated from glucocorticoid-
sensitive cell lines; such variants can be characterized
biochemically by receptor assays, and genetically by con-
struction of cell hybrids for complementation and dominance
analyses. Moreover, somatic cell genetic analysis can also
be carried out on T-cell lines that are glucocorticoid
resistant as the result of normal differentiation.
    The results presented in this paper reveal that two
distinct elements are required for the cytolytic response
in murine T-cell lines: the glucocorticoid receptor, and
another function encoded by a "lysis" locus. Two glucocorticoid sensitive cell lines, S49 and W7, have been used
for these studies (4,5). This paper summarizes the evidence that all glucocorticoid-resistant variants selected

from the S49 and W7 lines result from defects in the receptor. These defects appear to be of genetic origin and can
affect receptor quantity or quality. Recent results obtained
with another T-cell line, SAK8, demonstrate that glucocorticoid resistance in this line is due to a defect in the
"lysis" function. This "lysis" defect appears to be of
epigenetic origin, i.e., to result from normal differentiation.

The existence of the "lysis" function raises the question of why no resistant variant defective in "lysis" function was ever selected from a glucocorticoid sensitive line
such as W7. Our results suggest a plausible explanation for
the absence of "lysis" defective W7 variants, and a possible
approach to obtain genetic variants resulting from defects
in the "lysis" function or in other nonreceptor functions
involved in the lytic response.

METHODS

The glucocorticoid-sensitive lines, S49 and W7, have
been described elsewhere (5). Briefly, S49 was cloned from
a thymus-derived lymphoma induced by mineral oil in a
BALB/c mouse. The W7 (WEHI-7) line was cloned from a
thymoma which arose in a BALB/c mouse after X-irradiation
(3). The glucocorticoid-resistant SAK line, of which SAK8
is a subclone, was derived from a spontaneous T-lymphoma in
an AKR/J mouse and cloned by Dr. Robert Hyman (Salk Institute). Derivatives of the S49 and W7 lines that are resistant to 6-thioguanine and 5-bromo-2'-deoxyuridine were isolated as described elsewhere (5).

Cells were grown in suspension in Dulbecco's modified
Eagle's medium containing 10% fetal calf serum (5). Growth
was monitored by counting "living" cells, defined as those
cells which exclude trypan blue. Dexamethasone dose-response curves were obtained by measuring the turbidity of
cultures at 660 nm after 6 or 7 days incubation with
steroid, expressing the results as percentages of the
turbidity reached in the control without dexamethasone (5).

Mutagenic treatments, determinations of the percentage
of survival, and selection for variants resistant to dexamethasone have been described elsewhere (6,7).

Cell hybrids were obtained by polyethylene glycol-
induced cell fusions (8). Both the W7 lines used in fusions
carried a thioguanine or bromodeoxyuridine resistance
marker as well as resistance to 1 to 5 mM ouabain. Hybrids

were selected in medium containing hypoxanthine-aminopterin-thymidine (9) and 1 mM ouabain.

Steroid binding assay, performed on whole cells using [^{3}H]-dexamethasone, and nuclear transfer of the receptor-hormone complex were as described by Pfahl et al. (10).

RESULTS

RESISTANCE RESULTING FROM DEFECTS IN THE GLUCOCORTICOID RECEPTOR

Spontaneous Receptor Defects

Resistance to dexamethasone arises spontaneously in the S49 line at frequencies on the order of 10^{-5} to 10^{-6} (5,11), which is surprisingly high for a genetic event in a pseudodiploid somatic cell. In contrast, the frequency of spontaneous appearance of glucocorticoid-resistant variants of the W7 line is <1.2 x 10^{-10}, i.e., no resistant variant was found when a population of 8.1 x 10^9 W7 cells was examined (5,7). These results prompted us to compare other relevant properties of the S49 and W7 lines, namely their dexamethasone-dose response curves and their glucocorticoid receptor content.

Figure 1 shows the sensitivity of the W7 and S49 lines in the range of 5 to 10 x 10^{-9} M dexamethasone. The cultures were inoculated at a density of 2 x 10^4 cells/ml and exposed to the steroid for a period of time (6 to 7 days) corresponding to approximately eight doublings of the control without hormone. The cellular material present in the culture was measured by turbidity at 660 nm and expressed as percentage of the control. The W7 line is clearly more sensitive to the cytolytic effect of glucocorticoids than the S49 line which displays a sensitivity intermediate between that of the W7 line and that of a fully resistant derivative of W7, clone MS1-R. This difference in sensitivity between the two lines, observed in the range of 5 to 10 x 10^{-9} M dexamethasone, is not obvious if both cell lines are exposed to high concentrations of the steroid, in the range of 10^{-6} to 10^{-5} M, for a long period of time because, in those conditions, the cells of both lines would all eventually lyse.

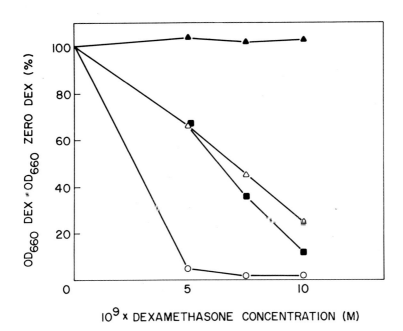

FIGURE 1. Sensitivity to dexamethasone of the S49 and W7 lines. (O-O) W7; (■-■) S49; (△-△) MS1, a derivative of W7 selected in 5 x 10^{-9} M dexamethasone; (▲-▲) MS1-R, a fully resistant derivative of W7-MS1 selected in 10^{-5}M dexamethasone. From Bourgeois, S., "Steroid Receptors and the Management of Cancer," E.B. Thompson and M.E. Lippman, eds., CRC Press, Inc., Boca Raton, Florida, Vol. II, 99, 1979.

The glucocorticoid receptor content of these lines was measured by Scatchard analysis of [^{3}H]-dexamethasone binding data obtained with whole cells (10). While the S49 line contains 15,000 $\pm$ 1,500 dexamethasone binding sites per cell, the W7 line contains 30,000 $\pm$ 3,000 binding sites per cell (5). The receptors from both lines have the same affinity for dexamethasone, K_a = 1.3 $\pm$ 0.3 x 10^8M^{-1}, and in both lines the extent of nuclear translocation of the

receptor hormone complex is on the order of 70% in the
conditions of our nuclear transfer assay (10,12).

The presence of half as much receptor in the S49 line
as in the W7 line led us to postulate that the S49 line is
functionally hemizygous for the gene (r^+) encoding the
glucocorticoid receptor. The amount of receptor would,
then, reflect the activity of two r^+ alleles in the W7 line
(r^+/r^+) and of only one allele in the S49 line (r^+/r^-).
This interpretation also accounts for the high spontaneous
frequency of glucocorticoid resistant variants in the S49
line, and suggests that acquisition of glucocorticoid resistance in the W7 line could proceed in two steps, as
shown in Table 1.

TABLE 1

TWO STEP MODEL OF ACQUISITION OF RESISTANCE

$$r^{+/+} \xrightarrow{\sim 10^{-6}} r^{+/-} \xrightarrow{\sim 10^{-6}} r^{-/-}$$

Cell line	W7	S49	Dex^R
Frequency of Dex^R	$\sim 10^{-12}$	$\sim 10^{-6}$	
Sites per cell	30,000	15,000	0 or altered
Dex 10^{-9} to 10^{-8}M	S	R	R
Dex 10^{-6} to 10^{-5}M	S	S	R

Each step, occurring at a frequency of 10^{-6} to 10^{-5},
corresponds to the inactivation of one functional r^+ allele.
Therefore, the frequency of resistant variants in the W7
line would be in the range of 10^{-12} to 10^{-10}, in good
agreement with our estimate of $<1.2 \times 10^{-10}$ (7). This
interpretation was confirmed by selecting derivatives of
W7 resistant to 5×10^{-9}M dexamethasone, a concentration at
which the S49 line exhibits considerable resistance (see
Fig. 1). If this partial resistance of S49 is due to its
reduced receptor content, then selection for W7 variants
resistant to such low concentrations should yield W7 hemizygotes (r^+/r^-) similar to the S49 line. Such variants
were isolated and characterized (5). The sensitivity of
one such variant, MS1, as shown in Figure 1 is similar to
that of S49. Moreover, such partially resistant W7 variants
contained $15,000 \pm 1,500$ receptors per cell and, like S49,
yielded fully resistant variant at a high frequency on the
order of 10^{-6} (5).

These results have several important implications.
They indicate that the level of glucocorticoid receptors

limits the biological response in these cells. This sytem
was used to demonstrate a tight correlation between receptor level and glucocorticoid sensitivity (13). The fact
that hemizygous variants (r^+/r^-) are present in cell populations at a frequency of 10^{-6} to 10^{-5} and are resistant to
low concentrations of glucocorticoids suggests that physiological concentrations of glucocorticoids in vivo could
selectively enrich the lymphocyte population for these
partially resistant cells. This could have clinical relevance since these hemizygotes give rise to fully resistant
variants at high frequency. If it were not for this two-
step mode of acquisition of resistance, full resistance to
glucocorticoids would only be observed at extremely low
frequencies.

The hemizygosity of the S49 line at the r locus has
recently been confirmed by karyotypic analysis which assigned
the gene encoding the glucocorticoid receptor to chromosome
18 of the mouse (14). The origin of that hemizygosity is
unknown: the tumor from which the S49 line was derived could
have been hemizygous in the animal, or the r^+/r^- derivative
could have been selected by prolonged passage of the S49
line in tissue culture containing serum with low levels of
glucocorticoids. In any event, our results account for the
fact that all of the approximately 500 glucocorticoid resistant variants derived from S49 result from defects in the
receptor (11,12). Some of the S49 variants described by
Sibley and Tomkins (11) as having normal receptor appear to
have receptor defects as well (for a discussion, see ref.
15). The most important conclusion of our results, in terms
of the genetic analysis of glucocorticoid resistance, is
that the S49 line should not be used to attempt to generate
defects in functions other than the receptor because its
hemizygousity at the r locus greatly favors the appearance
of receptor defects. Therefore, we have pursued our studies
of glucocorticoid resistance with the W7 line in which the
diploidy of the r^+ allele should be expected to protect
against the high incidence of receptor defects.

Mutagen-Induced Receptor Defects

Because of the low spontaneous frequency of glucocorticoid resistant variants in the W7 line ($<1.2 \times 10^{-10}$), mutagens were used to induce such variants. Three classical
mutagens were first utilized: N-methyl-N'-nitro-N-
nitrosoguanidine (MNNG), ethyl methanesulfonate (EMS) and
UV irradiation. As shown in Table 2, these mutagens increase

TABLE 2

INDUCTION OF DEXAMETHASONE-RESISTANT VARIANTS OF THE W7 LINE BY VARIOUS MUTAGENS[a]

	Mutagen µg/ml	Number of cells in sample	Percentage of survival	Number of variants in sample	Frequency
	none	8.1×10^9	–	0	$<1.2 \times 10^{-10}$
MNNG	1.25	2.6×10^8	5 – 10	136	5.2×10^{-7}
EMS	530	1.7×10^8	5 – 10	42	2.5×10^{-7}
UV	–	6.0×10^8	10 – 40	30	5.0×10^{-8}
Mitomycin	1	7.4×10^8	5	77	1.0×10^{-7}
Bleomycin	47	1.4×10^{10}	10 – 15	49	3.5×10^{-9}
Streptonigrin	0.1	3.2×10^8	2	4	1.2×10^{-8}
Ellipticine	0.03	4.3×10^9	3 – 10	8	1.8×10^{-9}
Colcemid	0.01	5.6×10^9	40	6	1.0×10^{-9}

[a]Summary of results published elsewhere (6,7).

the frequency of W7 glucocorticoid resistant variants to values ranging from 5×10^{-8} to 5×10^{-7}. Increased frequencies of dexamethasone-resistant variants by mutagens were also observed in the S49 line (4,12). These results suggest that in both lines, the acquisition of glucocorticoid resistance has a genetic origin and results from mutations in the r locus. This view is confirmed by the observation that, although some of these variants contain no detectable dexamethasone binding activity, some of them contain receptor protein with altered properties such as decreased or increased nuclear translocation or altered behavior on DNA cellulose (11,12,16).

Because all W7 variants induced by classical mutagens resulted from receptor defects, we turned to treatments by antitumor drugs known to induce large deletions and chromosome rearrangements or elimination (7). The induction of extensive deletions or monosomy could increase the probability of inactivating an as yet unknown function involved in the cytolytic response. The drugs used were mitomycin C, bleomycin, streptonigrin, ellipticine and colcemid. Except for mitomycin, these drugs had never been tested for mutagenicity on animal cells. As shown in Table 2, all of these antitumor drugs increase the frequency of W7 glucocorticoid resistant variants to values ranging between 10^{-9} and 10^{-8}. However, all the variants induced by these drugs turned out to be of the same type as those induced by classical mutagens, namely defective in glucocorticoid receptor, although the nature of the receptor defects varied with the treatment used (7).

These results suggest the possibility that, in combination therapies, glucocorticoid resistant variants could be induced by the antitumor drug and selected by the presence of the hormone. Another question raised by these results is that of possible cross-resistance. Since these glucocorticoid-resistant variants were selected amongst populations of cells which had survived treatment by highly toxic drugs, the possibility that these variants were also resistant to the drug used as a mutagen was tested. Figure 2 shows that glucocorticoid resistant variants induced by bleomycin (panel b) or by mitomycin (panel c) have retained their sensitivity to the drug used as a mutagen. The absence of cross-resistance between drug and hormone is expected since these variants result from glucocorticoid receptor defects which should not alter their sensitivity to bleomycin or mitomycin C.

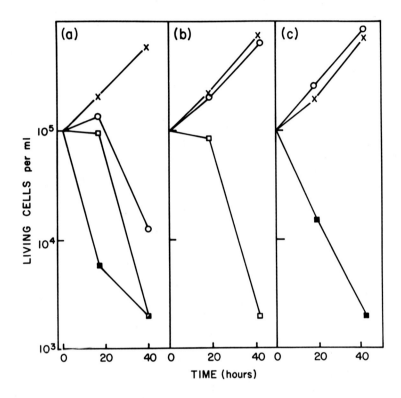

FIGURE 2. Tests of cross-resistance between dexamethasone and cytotoxic drugs. (a) W7 parental line; (b) glucocorticoid-resistant variant induced by bleomycin; (c) glucocorticoid resistant variant induced by mitomycin C. (X-X)
control; (O-O) 10^{-6} M dexamethasone; ($\square$-$\square$) 47 µg/ml
bleomycin; ($\blacksquare$-$\blacksquare$) 1 µg/ml mitomycin C. From Huet-Minkowski,
M. et al., "Drug and Hormone Resistance in Neoplasia," N.
Bruchovsky and J.H. Goldie, eds., CRC Press, Inc., Boca
Raton, Florida, in press, 1982.

The absence of W7 variants containing normal receptor
amongst approximately 300 variants induced by a variety of
mutagenic treatments appears highly significant. Since
this cell line appears functionally diploid for the receptor
locus (r^+/r^+) the fact that all variants obtained result

from receptor defects cannot be attributed to hemizygosity
at that locus, as was the case in S49 cells. Several possible explanations, discussed elsewhere (15), could account
for this result and lead one to conclude that the isolation
in vitro of new types of glucocorticoid-resistant variants
from sensitive lines such as W7 may not be possible. Therefore, we turned to another approach, namely the screening
of a collection of murine T-cell lines for glucocorticoid
resistance that could have a different basis because it was
acquired in vivo.

RESISTANCE RESULTING FROM A DEFECT
IN THE "LYSIS" FUNCTION

Response of the SAK8 Line to Glucocorticoids

Amongst a collection of murine T-cell lines tested,
one line, SAK, derived from a spontaneous T-lymphoma in an
AKR/J mouse, appeared resistant to the lytic effect of glucocorticoids while having normal glucocorticoid receptor.
The effect of dexamethasone on the growth of the SAK line,
as compared to the effect of the steroid on the W7 line and
on a W7 receptor deficient variant, is shown in Figure 3.
While the W7 line undergoes lysis (panel a) and the W7
receptor deficient variant is unaffected by dexamethasone
(panel b), the SAK line displays a partial growth inhibition
in the presence of the steroid (panel c). However, examina-
of the SAK cells in the microscope did not reveal any lysing
cells in the presence of dexamethasone, therefore, the
steroid appears to have only a minor effect on the growth
rate without killing the cells. To ensure that this behavior
did not result from a mixed population of cells, some fully
resistant and some growth inhibited, the SAK line was subcloned. All 20 subclones tested behaved in the presence of
dexamethasone exactly as the parental SAK line, and subclone
SAK8 was used in some of the subsequent experiments.

Dexamethasone binding assays (data not shown) measured
approximately 30,000 binding sites per SAK cell with a K_a
of $10^8 M^{-1}$ for dexamethasone and approximately 65% nuclear
translocation. These values, similar to those obtained for
the W7 line and for a glucocorticoid-sensitive AKR/J T-
lymphoma line, indicate that the receptor of SAK cells is
normal. Moreover, SAK cells do respond to dexamethasone by
the formation of cell aggregates accompanied by a 2- to 3-
fold induction of murine leukemia viral protein, gp70, and
accumulation of leukemia virus mRNA (17,18). Thus, the

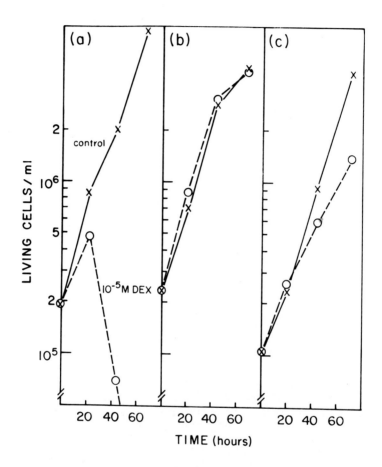

FIGURE 3.   Effect of dexamethasone on the growth of three cell lines.   (X-X) no dexamethasone; (O-O) 10^{-5}M dexamethasone.   Panel (a) W7 line; panel (b) W7 receptor deficient variant; panel (c) SAK line.

presence of apparently normal receptors and an identifiable response indicate that the SAK line is glucocorticoid responsive but resistant to the lytic effect of the hormone because of a defect in a function other than the receptor. This function was named the "lysis" function, encoded by a genetic locus designated as "ℓ", the SAK line being "lysis

defective" ($\mathcal{L}/\mathcal{R}^-$). However, these results have to be
interpreted with caution because binding assay could fail
to reveal a subtle alteration in the receptor. Moreover,
the capacity of a receptor to trigger one type of response
(such as cell aggregation and induction of MuLV) does not
necessarily imply the capacity to induce another response
(such as lysis). Therefore, it was necessary to obtain a
formal genetic proof that the SAK receptor can be functional
in inducing the lytic response.

Complementation Between Receptor and Lysis Defects

The genetic test performed consisted in showing complementation between the "lysis" defect of SAK cells and the
receptor defect of a glucocorticoid-resistant W7 variant.
The principle and result of that complementation test are
shown in Table 3.

TABLE 3

COMPLEMENTATION BETWEEN DEX^r VARIANTS

Fusion:	SAK	X	W7 ——▶	Hybrid
Genotype:	$2r^+/2\ \mathcal{L}^-$		$2r^-/2\ \mathcal{L}^+$	$2r^+/2\ \mathcal{L}^+$
Receptors per cell:	$30,700\pm2,800$		none	$27,000\pm1,800$
Phenotype:	Dex^r		Dex^r	Dex^s

Assuming that the SAK line is normally diploid at the receptor locus but defective at both lysis loci ($2r^+/2\ \mathcal{L}^-$), fusion
with a receptor deficient W7 variant which should have two
normal lysis genes ($2r^-/2\ \mathcal{L}^+$) should yield a hybrid cell containing two normal receptor alleles and 2 normal lysis
alleles ($2r^+/2\ \mathcal{L}^+$). Therefore, this fusion between two glucocorticoid resistant lines should yield glucocorticoid
sensitive hybrids. Several hybrid clones were obtained
after polyethylene glycol induced fusion. All hybrids
tested were shown to contain the approximately 30,000
glucocorticoid receptors contributed by the SAK parent,
and all hybrids were lysed by dexamethasone (19,20). This
result demonstrates that the receptors of the SAK line are
capable of inducing the lytic response and, therefore, that
SAK cells are resistant because of a defect in another
function necessary for lysis to occur, the "$\mathcal{L}$" function.

Dominance and Segregation of the Lysis Function

Fusion between the SAK line and the glucocorticoid sensitive parental W7 line ($2r^+/2 \ell^+$) established dominance of the normal ℓ^+ allele and demonstrated that the lytic function could be lost by chromosome segregation. The principle and results of that fusion are shown in Table 4.

TABLE 4

DOMINANCE AND SEGREGATION OF THE ℓ^+ FUNCTION

$$\text{SAK} \quad \text{X} \quad \text{W7} \longrightarrow \text{Hybrid} \xrightarrow[10^{-6}\text{M Dex}]{\text{selection}} \text{Hybrid}$$

SAK	W7	Hybrid	Hybrid
$2r^+/2\ \ell^-$	$2r^+/2\ \ell^+$	$4r^+/2\ \ell^+$	$4r^+$
$30,700\pm2,700$	$35,000\pm3,000$	$50,900\pm3,600$	$50,900\pm4,300$
Dex^r	Dex^s	Dex^s	Dex^r

Chromosome numbers: 80   78

The hybrids obtained were shown to contain approximately the expected sum of the receptors present in the SAK and the W7 lines. All hybrids tested were lysed by glucocorticoids, confirming the hypothesis that the absence of lytic response in the SAK line is due to a recessive defect. This makes it unlikely that the SAK line produces a substance that "protects" cells from lysis since such a model would predict the resistant phenotype of SAK to be dominant.

The receptor content of the hybrids reflects the presence of four r^+ alleles, while only two active ℓ^+ alleles, contributed by the W7 cells, are expected to be present in these cells. It has been demonstrated (13) that glucocorticoid sensitive hybrids obtained by fusion between W7 lines give rise to glucocorticoid resistant derivatives at high frequency by loss of chromosomes bearing the r^+ allele. The glucocorticoid sensitive hybrids generated by the fusion shown in Table 4 give rise, upon selection in the presence of 10^{-6}M dexamethasone, to glucocorticoid resistant variants at a frequency on the order of 2.5×10^{-5}. In this situation, the hybrids are expected to result from the segregation of the chromosomes bearing the ℓ^+ alleles, present only in two copies, rather than the four chromosomes carrying the r^+ alleles. Dexamethasone binding assays showed that these glucocorticoid resistant hybrid derivatives indeed contained the same amount of receptors ($50,900 \pm 4,300$) as the sensitive hybrids (see Table 4). Moreover, karyotypic analysis of both a dexamethasone sensitive and resistant hybrid showed that the modal number of chromosomes in the sensitive hybrid is 80, while in the resistant hybrid the modal number of chromosomes had shifted to a value of 78. These results are consistent with the idea that the dexamethasone sensitive hybrid has acquired resistance by segregation of the two chromosomes containing the ℓ^+ alleles. This approach could allow the assignment of the ℓ^+ locus to a mouse chromosome.

Altogether, this genetic analysis of the basis for the resistance of the SAK line to glucocorticoid-induced lysis provides strong evidence for the existence of the "lysis" function encoded by a locus, "ℓ", distinct from the locus, r, encoding the receptor. Moreover, the recessivity of this resistant phenotype indicates that the ℓ locus of SAK cells is defective rather than encoding a "protective" substance. However, this analysis does not give information about the origin of the resistance of SAK cells, which could be due either to a mutation in the ℓ gene or to the absence of expression of the ℓ gene through a process such as differentiation. If the ℓ gene is intact but silent, one might be able to activate its expression by DNA demethylation, since increasing evidence points to a correlation between hypo methylation of DNA and gene expression (reviewed in ref. 21). Recovery of the lytic response in SAK cells by activation of expression of the ℓ locus would eliminate the possibility of a genetic mutation in that locus as the origin of the resistant phenotype.

ACTIVATION OF THE "LYSIS" LOCUS BY TREATMENT WITH 5-AZACYTIDINE

The drug 5-azacytidine has recently been shown to cause DNA hypomethylation resulting in heritable changes in the phenotype of a variety of cell lines (see e.g.,ref. 22). Therefore, SAK8 cells were treated by 5-azacytidine as shown in Figure 4. Exponentially growing SAK8 cells were treated with 3 μM 5-azacytidine for 13 hours, extensively washed, and allowed to recover in fresh medium until exponential growth had resumed. After 48 hrs recovery, corresponding to two cell divisions, the treated cells were subcloned and individual clones were tested for dexamethasone sensitivity. Figure 5 shows the growth response to dexamethasone of representative SAK8 clones treated with 5-azacytidine. The untreated SAK8 cells (Figure 5, first column) grow in the presence of 10^{-8} or 10^{-7}M dexamethasone, although the number of SAK8 cells growing in the presence of the hormone appears slightly lower than in the control because of the small growth inhibition and of the aggregation response mentioned

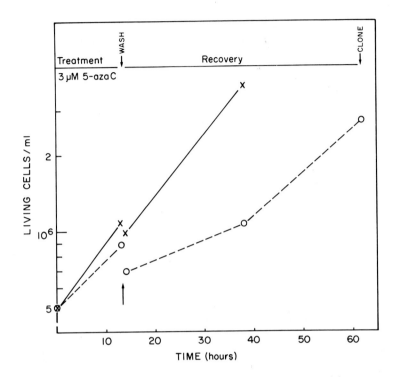

FIGURE 4.   Treatment of SAK8 cells with 5-azacytidine.
(X-X) untreated cells; (O-O) 5-azacytidine treated cells.

earlier.   The 5-azacytidine treated clones shown in Figure
5, rows a and b, are highly sensitive to dexamethasone,
while the clones shown in rows c and d are partially sensitive to the hormone.   Clone e is as resistant to dexamethasone as the untreated SAK8 line.   Growth curves in the
presence of dexamethasone (data not shown) confirmed that
sensitive clones resulting from 5-azacytidine treatment
were in fact lysed by the hormone, rather than growth
inhibited.   Approximately 10 to 20% of the 5-azacytidine-
treated clones displayed sensitivity to dexamethasone.
Some of these clones, however, appear unstable in that they
eventually revert to dexamethasone resistance.   The basis
for this instability is currently under investigation.

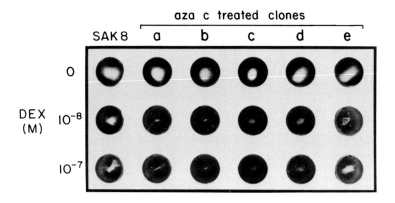

FIGURE 5. Glucocorticoid sensitivity of SAK8 clones after 5-azacytidine treatment. SAK8 cells or 5-azacytidine treated subclones were inoculated into a tissue culture tray at a titer of 5 x 10^4 cells/ml. The concentration of dexamethasone is shown on the left. The cells were allowed to grow for 5 days before the tray was photographed.

These results confirm the idea that the origin of gluco-corticoid resistance in the SAK8 line is epigenetic, i.e., results from a phenotypic change in gene expression rather than from a mutation in the ℓ locus.

EFFECT OF DEXAMETHASONE ON THE CLONING EFFICIENCY OF THE SAK8 LINE

Although SAK cells do not respond to glucocorticoids by lysis, these cells, as mentioned earlier, exhibit three other responses to dexamethasone, namely: (1) cell aggre-gation, (2) induction of leukemia virus proteins and mRNA; and (3) partial growth inhibition. As shown in Figure 1, a culture inoculated with 10^5 cells/ml reaches a lower cell density after 60 hrs in the presence of 10^{-5}M dexamethasone than the control without steroid, although no dead cells are seen in such a culture. However, when single cells are inoculated to determine cloning efficiency, the number of SAK8 clones observed is considerably reduced in the pre-sence of 10^{-6}M dexamethasone. Table 5 shows the results obtained by inoculating 96 tissue culture wells with one cell per well, and counting the wells which show no growth after 20 to 25 days using the Poisson distribution to determine the cloning efficiency. The results of three experiments illustrate that the cloning efficiency of SAK cells in the usual culture conditions (Dulbecco's modified Eagle's medium (DME) containing 10% fetal calf serum (FCS)) is reduced by 10^{-6}M dexamethasone to values of 50% (Exp. I, line 1), 30% (Exp. II, line 4) or 20% (Exp. III, line 6), of the control without steroid. Although these values vary from 20% to 50% in separate experiments, a considerable reduction in cloning efficiency is consistently observed in the presence of dexamethasone. Moreover, the clones obtained are very small and appear only after 3 weeks of incubation.

TABLE 5

CLONING EFFICIENCY OF SAK8 IN 10^{-6}M DEXAMETHASONE

Expt. #		Medium	% FCS Serum	Supernatant	Cloning efficiency[a]
				Cloning conditions	
I	1	DME	10	–	50%
	2	DME	20	–	70%
	3	50% DME+ 50% HAMS	10	–	60%
II	4	DME	10	–	30%
	5	DME	20	–	100%
III	6	DME	10	–	20%
	7	DME	10	23% EL4.El	86%
	8	DME	10	8% EL4.El	44%
	9	DME	10	23% spleen	57%
	10	DME	10	8% spleen	22%

[a]Cloning efficiencies expressed as percentage of a control without dexamethasone in which the cloning efficiency is 100% in all culture conditions tested.

One possible interpretation of this response is that glucocorticoids inhibit the production of T-cell growth factor (interleukin 2, Il 2) or other growth factor(s) necessary for clonal expansion of these cells. In cultures inoculated at high cell density, such as shown in Figure 1, the SAK cells might produce enough growth factor(s) to continue to proliferate in the presence of dexamethasone. This hypothesis is based on the work of Gillis et al. (23) who showed that glucocorticoids inhibit mitogen-induced

Il 2 production and T cell proliferation, and that the addition of Il 2 restores the proliferation of mitogen-stimulated T cells in the presence of dexamethasone. Therefore, we tested the effect of different culture supplements on the cloning response of SAK8 cells to dexamethasone. As shown in Table 5 (lines 2 and 5), increasing FCS from 10 to 20% restores the cloning efficiency of SAK8 cells from 50 to 70% in experiment I and from 30 to 100% in experiment II. Enriching the medium in nutrients by addition of HAMS F-12 medium (line 3) had little effect on the cloning efficiency. We also tested the effect of two culture supernatants from EL4.El cells (24) and from ConA stimulated mouse spleen cells (25). As shown in Table 5, both these supernatants increase the cloning efficiency of SAK8 cells in dexamethasone (lines 7 and 10). These culture supernatants as well as serum contain a variety of factors any of which could be responsible for restoring the high cloning efficiency of SAK8 cells in the presence of dexamethasone. Although it is not clear yet whether the factor(s) necessary for the growth of SAK8 cells is Il 2 or is different from Il 2, these preliminary results support the idea that glucocorticoids reduce the cloning efficiency of these cells by inhibiting the production of a factor which is both produced by SAK8 cells and required for their growth. This observation could have important implications, as discussed below, in terms of the effect of the culture medium on the types of glucocorticoid resistant variants that can be selected from glucocorticoid-sensitive lines.

DISCUSSION

This paper presents evidence for the existence of two bases for glucocorticoid resistance in murine lymphoid T cell lines: resistance can result either from defects in the glucocorticoid receptor or from a defect in expression of the "lysis" function. Defects in the receptor can result in a reduction in receptor quantity, or can alter receptor quality such as in "nuclear transfer defective" receptor variants. The receptor defects observed in glucocorticoid resistant variants derived from the sensitive S49 and W7 lines appear to be of genetic origin because their frequency of appearance is low, dependent on the ploidy of the r^+ allele, and increased by various mutagens. In contrast, the "lysis" defect observed in SAK cells appears to be of epigenetic origin, because the expression of the "lysis" function can be activated at high frequency by treatment with 5-azacytidine. Therefore, this "lysis" defect cannot be due to a mutation that has altered the base sequence of the gene but appears to involve an inheritable DNA modification, probably methylation. Since DNA methylation has been implicated in differentiation (see, e.g., 22) it is possible that SAK cells represent a T-cell type in a glucocorticoid-resistant state of differentiation.

Glucocorticoids have multiple effects on T-cells, some stimulatory and some inhibitory. Some of these effects, all mediated by the glucocorticoid receptor, are schematically represented in the following diagram:

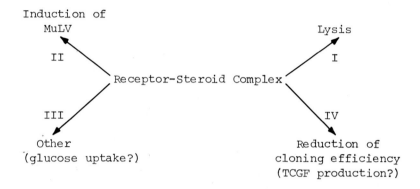

While the lysis pathway (I) is specifically blocked in SAK cells, glucocorticoids are still capable of inducing murine leukemia virus (pathway II). Moreover, glucocorticoids also modulate glucose metabolism in T cells (pathway III). The fact that, through a process which appears to be differentiation, SAK cells become lysis defective while retaining normal receptor allows these cells to still display the other T-cell responses to glucocorticoids. Among these, the reduction of cloning efficiency (pathway IV) is of special interest because, in the absence of the necessary growth factor(s), this response can be lethal, like the lytic response. However, these two pathways are clearly distinct because only pathway IV can be reversed by addition of factors to SAK8 cells (see Table 5) while the lytic pathway I is insensitive to the addition of factors in W7 cells (data not shown).

These considerations suggest a plausible explanation to a dilemma raised by our results, namely, in view of the existence of the "lytic" function why was a genetic variant

defective by mutation at the "ℓ" locus never found amongst
the 300 W7 variants isolated? Because the glucocorticoid-
sensitive W7 parental line undergoes lysis in the presence
of glucocorticoids (pathway I) the reduction of cloning
efficiency by these steroids (pathway IV) cannot be seen.
However, it is known that W7 cells produce Il 2 (26), and
therefore it is tempting to speculate that glucocorticoids
block Il 2 production in these cells as well. If this is
the case, W7 variants defective along the lytic pathway (I)
may not form clones in the culture medium (DME + 10% FCS)
routinely used. From our experience with SAK cells, it is
also likely that clones of W7 "lysis" variants, if they were
able to grow at all, could easily be missed because they
would appear very small and after long incubation while
receptor defective W7 variants appear, after only one week,
as large clones that outgrow the wells of microtiter plates.
The addition of the necessary factors, such as Il 2, should
overcome this problem, and allow W7 variants blocked in the
"lysis" function to form clones in the presence of dexamethasone. Such experiments which should yield new types of
glucocorticoid resistant W7 variants containing normal
receptors, are currently in progress in our laboratory.
This approach should allow further genetic analysis of the
steps involved in the lytic pathway and induced by glucocorticoids after nuclear translocation of the receptor-
hormone complex. It is worth pointing out that the lytic
pathway may involve several steps and, therefore, several
"lysis" functions. A defect in any one of these would be
sufficient to confer glucocorticoid resistance. The nature
of the specific "lysis" function defective in SAK cells is
unknown, but our results allow the conclusion that this
function is unlikely to be a vital housekeeping function or
structural element because its absence in SAK cells would
then be lethal. This "ℓ" function appears to be facultative
to the cell and specifically induced, either directly or
indirectly, by glucocorticoids.

Finally, our results with murine lymphoid cell lines
raise some questions that could be of clinical relevance.
It would be of obvious interest to know whether the same
two bases for glucocorticoid resistance exist in human
lymphoid cells. Work with the glucocorticoid sensitive
human leukemic CEM-C7 cells (27) has established that
resistance can result from receptor defects. The spontaneous frequency of glucocorticoid resistant receptor defective variants of the CEM-C7 line is on the order of 10^{-5}
and increased by mutagens. No evidence for a "lysis" defect

similar to that observed in SAK cells has not yet been obtained with human cell lines. If such a defect exists in glucocorticoid resistant human lymphoid cells, treatment by 5-azacytidine could activate a function rendering those cells glucocorticoid sensitive. If this were the case, 5-azacytidine could be viewed not only as a useful cytotoxic drug when used alone, but also as a drug that could, even transiently, make some glucocorticoid resistant lymphoid malignancies sensitive to glucocorticoids.

ACKNOWLEDGMENTS

We thank Drs. Magnus Pfahl, Robert Hyman and Marianne Huet-Minkowski for cell lines, and Dr. Gunther Dennert for his generous gift of culture supernatants.

REFERENCES

1. Norman, MR and Thompson, EB (1977). Characterization of a glucocorticoid-sensitive human lymphoid cell line. Cancer Res 37:3785
2. Horibata, K and Harris, AW (1970). Mouse myelomas and lymphomas in culture. Exp Cell Res 60:61
3. Harris, AW, Bankhurst, AD, Mason, S and Warner, NL (1973) Differentiated functions expressed by cultured mouse lymphoma cells. II. Θ Antigen, surface immunoglobulin and a receptor for antibody on cells of a thymoma cell line. J Immunol 110:431.
4. Sibley, CH and Tomkins, GM (1974). Isolation of lymphoma cell variants resistant to killing by glucocorticoids. Cell 2:213.
5. Bourgeois, S and Newby, R (1977). Diploid and haploid states of the glucocorticoid receptor gene of mouse lymphoid cell lines. Cell 11:423.
6. Bourgeois, S, Newby, RF and Huet, M (1978). Glucocorticoid-resistance in murine lymphoma and thymoma lines. Cancer Res 38:4279.
7. Huet-Minkowski, M, Gasson, JC and Bourgeois, S (1981). Induction of glucocorticoid resistant variants in a murine thymoma line by antitumor drugs. Cancer Res 41:4540.
8. Davidson, RL and Gerald, PS (1976). Improved techniques for the induction of mammalian cell hybridization by polyethylene glycol. Som Cell Genet 2:165.

9. Littlefield, JW (1966). The use of drug resistant markers to study the hybridization of mouse fibroblasts. Exp Cell Res 41:190.

10. Pfahl, M, Sandros, T and Bourgeois, S (1978). Interaction of glucocorticoid receptors from lymphoid cell lines with their nuclear acceptor sites. Molec Cell Endocrinol 10:175.

11. Sibley, CH and Tomkins, GM (1974). Mechanisms of steroid resistance. Cell 2:221.

12. Pfahl, M, Kelleher, RJ and Bourgeois, S (1978). General features of steroid resistance in lymphoid cell lines. Molec Cell Endocrinol 10:193.

13. Bourgeois, S and Newby, RF (1979). Correlation between glucocorticoid receptor and cytolytic response of murine lymphoid cell lines. Cancer Res 39:4749.

14. Francke, U and Gehring, U (1980). Chromosome assignment of a murine glucocorticoid receptor gene (Grl-1) using intraspecies somatic cell hybrids. Cell 22:657.

15. Huet-Minkowski, M, Gasson, JC and Bourgeois, S (1982) Glucocorticoid resistance in lymphoid cell lines. In Bruchovsky, N, Goldie, JH (eds): "Drug and Hormone Resistance in Neoplasia," Boca Raton, Florida: CRC Press, Inc., in press.

16. Yamamoto, KR, Gehring, U, Stampfer, MR and Sibley, CH (1976). Genetic approaches to steroid hormone action. In Greep, RO (ed): "Recent Progress in Hormone Research," Volume 32, New York: Academic Press, p. 3.

17. Gasson, JC and Bourgeois, S (1981). Glucocorticoid-induced increase in viral gp70 immunoreactive protein in a lymphoid cell line. Fed Proc 40:1851.

18. Gasson, JC and Bourgeois, S (1982). Induction of murine leukemia virus proteins and mRNA by glucocorticoid hormones via lymphoid cell lines. Manuscript submitted.

19. Gasson, JC and Bourgeois, S (1981). Genetic evidence for a function other than the receptor involved in the cytolytic response to dexamethasone. J Cell Biol 91:210a.

20. Gasson, JC and Bourgeois, S (1982). A new determinant of glucocorticoid sensitivity in lymphoid cell lines. Manuscript submitted.

21. Ehrlich, M and Wang, RYH (1981). 5-methylcytosine in eukaryotic DNA. Science 212:1350.

22. Taylor, SM and Jones, PA (1979). Multiple new phenotypes induces in 10T1/2 and 3T3 cells treated with 5-azacytidine. Cell 17:771.

23. Gillis, S, Crabtree, GR and Smith, KA (1979). Gluco-
    corticoid-induced inhibition of T cell growth factor
    prediction. I. The effect on mitogen-induced lymphocyte
    proliferation. J Immunol 123:1624.
24. Farrar, WL, Mizel, JG and Farrar, JJ (1980). Partici-
    pation of lymphocyte activating factor (interleukin 1)
    in the induction of cytotoxic T cell responses. J
    Immunol 124:1371.
25. Dennert, G, Yoguswaran, G and Yamagata, S (1981).
    Cloned cell lines with natural killer activity:
    Specificity, function and cell surface markers.
    J Exp Med 153:545.
26. Smith, KA, Gilbride, KJ and Favata, MF (1980). Lympho-
    cyte activating factor promotes T-cell growth factor
    production by cloned murine lymphoma cells. Nature
    287:853.
27. Harmon, JM and Thompson, EB (1981) Isolation and
    characterization of dexamethasone-resistant mutants
    from human lymphoid cell line CEM-C7. Molec Cell
    Endocrinol 1:512.

Rational Basis for Chemotherapy, pages 177–193
© 1983 Alan R. Liss, Inc., 150 Fifth Avenue, New York, NY 10011

EFFECTS OF TAMOXIFEN ON THE CELL CYCLE KINETICS OF MCF 7 HUMAN MAMMARY CARCINOMA CELLS IN CULTURE

Robert L. Sutherland, Roger R. Reddel, Rosemary E. Hall,
Pamela J. Hodson and Ian W. Taylor
Ludwig Institute for Cancer Research (Sydney Branch),
University of Sydney,
N.S.W. 2006,
Australia

ABSTRACT   Experiments were undertaken to define the effects of tamoxifen within the cell cycle. When asynchronous MCF 7 cells, in exponential growth phase, were treated with tamoxifen, a dose-dependent inhibition of cell growth was observed and this was accompanied by a dose-dependent increase in the percentage of G_0/G_1 cells at the expense of S phase cells. At doses of tamoxifen below 5 um, simultaneous administration of estradiol completely reversed the effects of tamoxifen on cell growth and the cell cycle kinetic parameters. The effects of higher doses of tamoxifen were not completely reversed by estradiol. Cells that accumulated in G_0/G_1 following tamoxifen treatment could be stimulated to enter S phase in a semi-synchronous manner when "rescued" with estradiol. Studies with synchronized cells indicated that tamoxifen decreased the proportion of G_1 cells that were able to enter S phase. These data are compatible with tamoxifen being a cell cycle phase-specific growth inhibitory agent, causing cells to accumulate in G_1.

INTRODUCTION

There are no detailed studies on the effects of the synthetic nonsteroidal antiestrogen, tamoxifen, on cell cycle kinetic parameters of human breast cancer cells, although some preliminary data have been presented (1-3). Documentation of these effects is not only essential to an understanding of the molecular mode of action of this drug as an antitumor agent, but may be of benefit in planning combination chemotherapeutic regimens containing tamoxifen and cell cycle phase-specific cytotoxic agents.

Studies, employing human mammary carcinoma cells in culture and the technique of flow cytometry, have been undertaken in this laboratory to further define the effects of tamoxifen within the cell cycle. In this chapter some of the experiments contributing to our present understanding of the subject are presented briefly.

METHODS

All experiments described herein were performed on the estrogen receptor positive human mammary carcinoma cell line, MCF 7 (4,5), utilizing cells in the exponential growth phase. MCF 7 cells in their 299th passage were supplied by Dr. Charles M. McGrath, Meyer L. Prentis Cancer Center, Detroit, Mi. The cells used in the current experiments were from passages 305-322. Stock cells were routinely maintained in RPMI 1640 medium supplemented with 20 mM Hepes buffer, 14 mM sodium bicarbonate, 6 mM L-glutamine, 20 ug/ml gentamicin, 10 ug/ml insulin and 10% fetal calf serum (FCS). These cells were passaged at weekly intervals when 3×10^5 cells were plated into 150 cm² flasks in 50 ml of the above medium. Seven days later cell numbers had reached $1-2 \times 10^7$ cells/flask. Such a subculturing procedure ensured the production of truly exponentially growing cells.

Experimental cells were harvested from day 5 or 6 flasks when cell numbers were $0.5-1.0 \times 10^7$ cells/flask. These cells were plated into 25 cm² flasks at densities ranging from 5×10^4 to 2×10^5 cells/flask in 5 ml of the above medium except that the FCS concentration was reduced to 5%. No attempt was made to remove endogenous steroids from the FCS. The design of individual experiments is discussed in the text or in the legends to figures.

Estradiol-17 β was obtained from Sigma, St. Louis, Mo. and tamoxifen base was supplied by ICI Pharmaceuticals Division, Macclesfield, Cheshire, U.K. Both compounds were stored as stock solutions in ethanol and were added directly to the culture medium. The final ethanol concentration in all experimental flasks was 0.1%. ICRF 159 (Razoxane) was supplied by ICI Pharmaceuticals Division. A stock solution of 10 mg/ml was prepared in 0.4 M HCl, and the drug was diluted 100 fold in culture medium to give a final concentration of 100 ug/ml.

Cells were harvested from the monolayer with 0.05% trypsin, 0.02% EDTA in phosphate buffered saline, viable cell counts were made under phase-contrast on a hemocytometer and a sample of cells was stained for flow cytometry (FCM) using an ethidium bromide/mithramycin staining technique (6). Flow cytometry was performed with an ICP 22 pulse cytometer (Ortho Instruments, Westwood, Ma.) with excitation at 360-460 nm and fluorescence detection at greater than 550 nm. Estimates of the proportion of cells in the G_0/G_1, S and G_2 + M phases of the cell cycle were calculated from the DNA histograms using a planimetric method of analysis (7).

RESULTS

Factors Affecting the Response to Tamoxifen <u>In Vitro</u>

Studies in this and other laboratories have shown that the response of human breast cancer cell lines to tamoxifen <u>in vitro</u> is stongly influenced by the culture conditions employed (8). In addition to the obvious parameters such as the concentration of drug used, the time of exposure and the particular cell line under study, we have observed that a number of other factors influence the magnitude of the response to a particular dose of tamoxifen e.g. the concentration of FCS employed and whether or not it has been charcoal-treated to remove endogenous steroids, whether or not the medium and/or drug is replenished during the course of the experiment, the phase of growth when the drug is added and the presence or absence of other hormones and growth factors e.g. insulin. These variables make it difficult to compare various studies in the literature on tamoxifen sensitivity and the situation may be further complicated in the case of MCF 7 cells where it appears that different clones may have arisen with a likelihood of differing sensitivities to estrogens and antiestrogens (9).

In all experiments described below, 5% FCS was employed since it was found that this is the minimum serum concentration that can sustain exponential growth for periods up to 7 days.

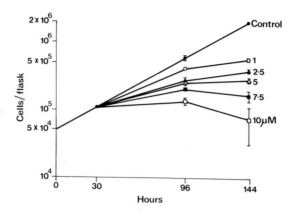

FIGURE 1. Effect of tamoxifen on the growth of MCF 7 cells. 5×10^4 MCF 7 cells in exponential growth phase were plated into 25 cm² flasks in 5 ml of medium containing 5% fetal calf serum. After 30 hr cells were treated with tamoxifen at concentrations of 1-10 uM. The experimental medium was changed daily. Data are presented as the mean ± S.E.M. of triplicate flasks from 2-3 separate experiments. From Reddel and Sutherland, submitted for publication.

Effect of Tamoxifen on Asynchronous MCF 7 Cells

MCF 7 cells in exponential growth phase were treated with varying concentrations of tamoxifen and at 96 and 144 hr cells were harvested, counted and stained for FCM analysis. Dose-response curves for cells grown in 5% FCS are shown in Fig. 1 while the cell cycle kinetic data are summarized in Fig. 2.

Tamoxifen treatment resulted in a dose-dependent decrease in cell number (Fig. 1). Since the lowest dose tested, 1 uM, reduced cell numbers to 28% of control at 144 hr, it seems likely that a significant reduction in cell number would be attained at considerably lower doses of tamoxifen under these experimental conditions. It is too early to know if the decrease in growth rate can be attributed solely to a reduction in cell proliferation rate or whether an increased cell death rate contributes to this effect.

The dose-dependent decrease in growth rate was accompanied by a dose-dependent decrease in the proportion of cells synthesizing DNA (S phase cells) with a concomitant increase in the percentage of G_0/G_1 phase cells (Fig. 2 and the CONTROL DNA histograms in Fig. 5). At the highest dose tested i.e. 10 uM tamoxifen, the percentage of S phase cells was decreased 7-fold, when compared with untreated controls.

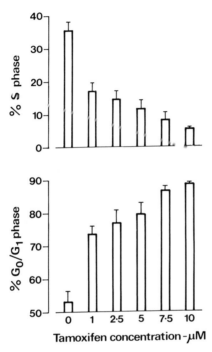

FIGURE 2. Effect of tamoxifen on the cell cycle kinetic parameters of MCF 7 cells. The cells were from the experiment described in Fig. 1. Data are presented as the mean ± S.D. of duplicate flasks from both the 96 and 144 hr time points. Redrawn from Reddel and Sutherland, submitted for publication.

Effect of Estradiol on Tamoxifen-Induced Changes in Cell Numbers and Cell Cycle Kinetic Parameters

Simultaneous treatment of cultures with tamoxifen and a 10-fold lower concentration of estradiol completely reversed the growth inhibitory effects of tamoxifen administered at doses below 5 uM. However, at higher doses of tamoxifen, the response was not reversed by estradiol (Fig. 3). A 10-fold lower dose of estradiol was chosen because the affinity of tamoxifen for the estrogen receptor has been estimated to be

between 1 and 10% that of estradiol (10-12). Increasing the
relative concentration of estradiol did not increase the
degree of reversibility of this tamoxifen effect (data not
shown).

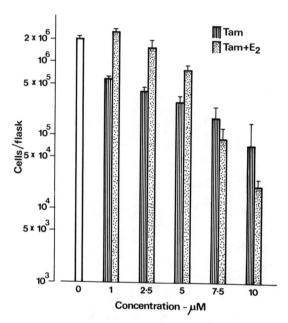

FIGURE 3. Effect of estradiol on tamoxifen-induced
changes in cell number. MCF 7 cells were grown for 114 hr in
the presence of tamoxifen, with or without a ten-fold lower
concentration of estradiol. Medium was changed every 24 hr.
Data are presented as the mean ± S.D. from triplicate flasks
from 2-3 separate experiments. Redrawn from Reddel and
Sutherland, submitted for publication.

The tamoxifen-induced decrease in the percentage of S
phase cells was completely reversed by simultaneous addition
of estradiol when the concentration of tamoxifen was 5 uM or
lower. At higher doses of tamoxifen, a 10-fold lower
concentration of estradiol had little effect on the
tamoxifen-induced decrease in the proportion of cells in S
phase (Fig. 4).

These data are interpreted as illustrating that tamoxifen,
in addition to having effects on cell proliferation which are
reversed by estrogens and are likely to be estrogen receptor

mediated, has significant effects on cell proliferation and cell cycle kinetics that are not reversed by estrogens and may involve biochemical mechanisms independent of the estrogen receptor.

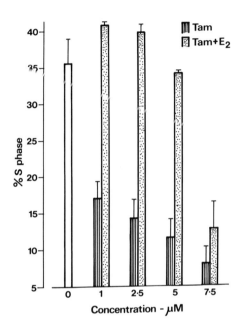

FIGURE 4.   Effect of estradiol on tamoxifen-induced changes in the percentage of S phase cells. MCF 7 cells were grown for 114 hr under the conditions described in Fig. 3. The percentage of S phase cells was calculated from DNA histograms obtained by flow cytometry. The data are presented as the mean ± S.D. of duplicate flasks from 2-3 separate experiments. There were insufficient cells for analysis in flasks treated with 10 uM tamoxifen. Redrawn from Reddel and Sutherland, submitted for publication.

Effect of Tamoxifen on the Accumulation of Cells in G_1

The experiments described above illustrate that treatment of asynchronous MCF 7 cells in exponential growth phase leads to a dose-dependent accumulation of cells in the G_0/G_1 phase of the cell cycle (Figs 2 and 5). The drug ICRF 159, an inhibitor of cytokinesis (13), prevents nuclei from dividing and re-entering the G_0/G_1 peak of the DNA histogram; it can,

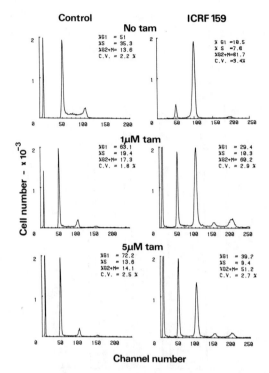

FIGURE 5. Effects of tamoxifen on the proportion of cells remaining in G_1 phase 72 hr after ICRF 159 treatment. MCF 7 cells in exponential growth phase were treated with tamoxifen for 42 hr. The medium was then replaced with medium containing 100 ug/ml ICRF 159 and 72 hr later the cells were harvested, stained and DNA histograms obtained by flow cytometry. From Sutherland et al, submitted for publication.

therefore, be used to measure the proportion of cells remaining in G_0/G_1 without the complication of cycling cells re-entering G_1.

In the experiment illustrated in Fig. 5 control cells or cells that had been exposed to 1 or 5 uM tamoxifen for 42 hr were treated with 100 ug/ml ICRF 159 and harvested 72 hr later. The proportion of cells remaining in the G_0/G_1 peak was calculated from the DNA histograms (Fig. 5). When control cells were treated with this dose of ICRF 159, i.e. 100 ug/ml, cell numbers remained static over a 154 hr period indicating that the drug completely inhibited cell division without increasing cell death rate (data not shown). By 12 hr of drug treatment, only about 10% of control cells remained in the G_0/G_1 peak and this proportion did not decrease with further exposure up to 72 hr (Fig. 5). It therefore appears that even under optimal growth conditions about 10% of MCF 7 cells do not cycle and are probably in G_0 phase.

Following 72 hr of ICRF 159 treatment, the proportion of cells remaining in G_0/G_1 was increased by prior treatment with tamoxifen (Fig. 5). When account is taken of the cells with DNA contents greater than G_2 + M phase cells, 22% of cells remained in G_0/G_1 after treatment with 1 uM tamoxifen and 31% when the dose was increased to 5 uM. These data indicate that tamoxifen induces a dose dependent accumulation of cells in the G_0/G_1 phase of the cell cycle.

Estradiol "Rescue" of Tamoxifen-Induced Effects

If tamoxifen arrests cells at a specific point in G_1 and this is due to the antiestrogenic properties of this molecule, one would predict that this effect would be reversed by estrogen and that the cells might be released from the "block" in a synchronous manner. To test this hypothesis, exponentially growing MCF 7 cells were treated for 56 hr with 5 uM tamoxifen, a dose at which the kinetic effects can be completely reversed by 500 nM estradiol. This resulted in a redistribution of cells between the various phases of the cell cycle with 30% more cells situated in G_0/G_1 in the treated cultures (Fig. 6). Following 56 hr of tamoxifen treatment, the medium was removed, replenished with medium containing vehicle (0.1% ethanol) or 500 nM estradiol and the changes in the DNA histograms monitored for a further 24 hr. Vehicle containing medium failed to induce significant changes in cell cycle kinetic parameters over this period. No changes were observed during the first 6 hr of treatment with estradiol. However, by 12 hr, a significant increase in S phase cells and decrease in G_0/G_1 phase cells had occurred in the cultures "rescued" with estradiol (Fig. 6). The proportion of cells in G_0/G_1 phase continued to decrease with time. At 24 hr of estradiol treatment 62% of cells were in S + G_2 + M phases compared with 21% in the tamoxifen-treated cultures and 50% in control cultures. These data, together with the shape of the DNA histograms illustrated in Fig. 6, suggest that the cells were released from the effects of tamoxifen in a semi-synchronous manner.

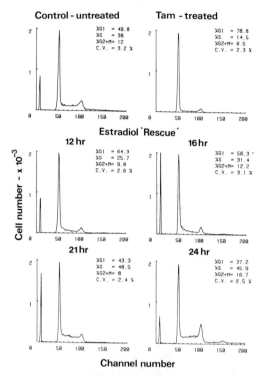

FIGURE 6. Effect of estradiol "rescue" on the progression of tamoxifen treated cells through the cell cycle. MCF 7 cells in exponential growth phase were treated with 5 uM tamoxifen for 56 hr. The medium was then replaced with medium containing no tamoxifen and 500 nM estradiol. Cells were harvested 12, 16, 21 and 24 hr later, stained and DNA histograms obtained by flow cytometry. From Sutherland et al, submitted for publication.

Effect of Tamoxifen on Synchronous MCF 7 Cells

To investigate further the effects of tamoxifen on the progression of MCF 7 cells through the cell cycle, studies were undertaken with synchronised cells. Exponentially growing MCF 7 cells were synchronised by mitotic selection (14) and plated into 25 cm² flasks in 10 ml of medium containing 5% FCS. One hour after plating 93% of cells were in the G_1 phase of the cell cycle (Fig. 7). Cells began to leave G_1 and enter S phase between 4 and 7 hrs. By 10-12 hr,

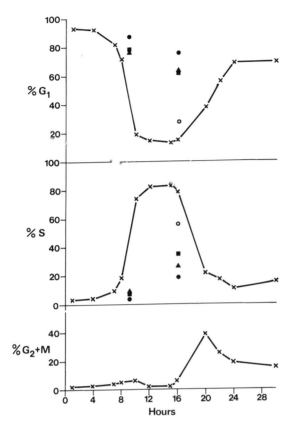

FIGURE 7. Effect of tamoxifen on the progression of synchronised MCF 7 cells through the cell cycle. MCF 7 cells in exponential growth phase were synchronised by mitotic selection and 10^5 cells were plated into 25 cm² flasks in 10 ml of medium. Control cells (x) were harvested at the times indicated and the cell cycle kinetic parameters calculated from DNA histograms obtained by flow cytometry. Treated cultures were plated in medium containing, 5 ( ), 7.5 ( ), 10 ( ) or 12.5 ( ) uM tamoxifen and harvested 9 or 16 hr later. From Taylor _et al_, submitted for publication.

the proportion of cells in G_1 phase had reached its nadir suggesting that the mean G_1 transit time was about 9 hr. The mean duration of S phase was also about 9 hr (Fig. 7). Cells began to leave S phase and enter G_2 + M after 16 hr.

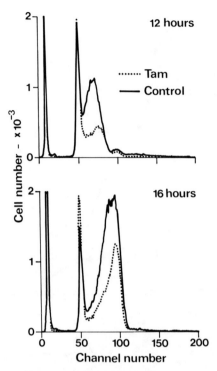

FIGURE 8.   Effect of tamoxifen on the DNA histograms of synchronous MCF 7 cells.   Synchronous MCF 7 cells were treated with 5 uM tamoxifen for 12 or 16 hr prior to harvest.   DNA histograms were prepared from treated and control cultures by flow cytometry.   From Taylor <u>et al</u>, submitted for publication.

The maximum number of cells in G_2 + M was reached at 20 hr (Fig. 7).

When these synchronous G_1 cells were cultured in the presence of tamoxifen, the proportion of cells remaining in the G_1 phase was increased and the percentage of cells entering S phase was decreased when compared with untreated cultures 9 and 16 hr after plating (Fig. 7).   The magnitude of this response was related to the dose of tamoxifen administered.   5 uM tamoxifen reduced the percentage of S phase cells from 77% to 56% at 16 hr while the highest dose. tested i.e. 12.5 uM almost completely inhibited the entry of cells into S phase with less than 20% of cells entering this phase of the cell cycle by 16 hr.

When the DNA histograms from control cells were compared with those from tamoxifen-treated cells it became apparent that those cells that entered S phase in tamoxifen treated cultures were able to traverse S phase at a similar rate to untreated cells. This is illustrated in Fig. 8 where the leading edges of the DNA histograms from control and treated cells are superimposable at both 12 and 16 hr. The major difference between the DNA histograms of control and treated cells therefore appears to be the proportion of cells that enter S phase. Such a result is compatible with tamoxifen inducing an accumulation of cells in G_0/G_1, the magnitude of which is related to the dose of tamoxifen administered.

DISCUSSION

The experiments described above were designed to further define the effects of tamoxifen within the cell cycle. Since tamoxifen may have differential effects on cycling and noncycling tumor cells, culture conditions were chosen to ensure that the cells were in exponential growth phase with the maximum proportion of cells in cycle. Studies on the effects of tamoxifen on quiescent plateau phase cells will be presented elsewhere.

The effects of tamoxifen on the growth and cell cycle kinetics of MCF 7 cells under these conditions are in general agreement with our preliminary findings (1-3). Tamoxifen causes a dose-dependent decrease in cell growth rate but as yet it has not been possible to establish whether this is due to a decrease in the rate of cell proliferation , an increase in cell death rate or both. Preliminary data indicate that cloning efficiency is significantly reduced after exposure to 10 uM tamoxifen for 24 hr while exposure to lower doses for a similar period is without effect. This implies that doses of 10 uM or higher are needed before cell death rate is increased and that growth inhibition seen at lower doses probably results from a decrease in cell proliferation rate. However, we have no data on the cloning efficiency of MCF 7 cells following exposure to doses lower than 10 uM for periods exceeding 24 hr.

Growth inhibition is associated with marked changes in the distribution of cells between the various phases of the cell cycle with cells accumulating in G_0/G_1 at the expense of S phase (Fig. 2). Reddel and Sutherland (manuscript submitted for publication) have demonstrated that at doses of 5 uM tamoxifen and below, the rate of cell growth, calculated from the mean doubling time, is highly correlated with the percentage of S phase cells while at higher doses, this correlation is less obvious. These data could be interpreted as evidence for decreased cell proliferation rate in the presence of a constant death rate at doses of 5 uM and below, while at higher doses both decreased proliferation rate and increased death rate are implicated in the observed changes in cell number. Further experimentation is clearly required to clarify this situation.

The observation that not all effects of tamoxifen on cell growth and cell cycle kinetics are reversed by the simultaneous administration of tamoxifen and estrogen also substantiates our previous findings with MCF 7 cells grown under less favorable conditions (3). These data, in conjunction with the observation that micromolar concentrations of tamoxifen can inhibit the growth of some estrogen receptor negative breast cancer cells lines in vitro with similar changes in cell cycle kinetic parameters, add support to the notion that tamoxifen can exert growth inhibitory effects through mechanisms that do not involve the estrogen receptor. Other published data which illustrate that estrogen deprivation is less effective than tamoxifen administration in inhibiting the growth of human breast cancer cells both in vitro (15) and in vivo (16) can also be interpreted as evidence for effects of tamoxifen on tumor cell proliferation that are unrelated to the estrogen receptor system. There are, of course, alternative explanations for these experimental findings.

The accumulation of cells in the G_0/G_1 peak of DNA histograms following tamoxifen treatment of asynchronous cells could be explained by preferential killing of cells as they entered S phase or it could be due to a true accumulation of cells in the G_1 phase of the cell cycle. Studies with synchronous cells which show tamoxifen-induced inhibition of cell cycle progression in the presence of static cell numbers (data not shown) argue against specific S phase killing while the experiments with ICRF 159, illustrated in Fig. 5, clearly demonstrate that tamoxifen causes a dose-dependent accumulation of cells in G_0/G_1 phase. This "block" of cells in G_1 is not irreversible since it was demonstrated that subsequent addition of estradiol allowed tamoxifen "arrested" cells to proceed through the cell cycle in an apparently semi-synchronous manner (Fig. 6).

If the reversal of antiestrogenic effects by estrogen is rapid, and there are data to suggest that this is the case (17), it appears that tamoxifen causes cells to accumulate in early G_1 phase. This conclusion is based on the observation that G_1 is about 9 hr long in exponentially growing MCF 7 cells and that no increase in S phase cells was seen during the first 6 hr (data not shown) after tamoxifen treated cells are "rescued" with estradiol (Fig. 6).

Our studies on the cell cycle effects of tamoxifen are far from complete. From the data presented here we can conclude that tamoxifen inhibition on MCF 7 cell proliferation in vitro is accompanied by an accumulation of cells in the G_1 phase of the cell cycle. Both estrogen-reversible and estrogen-irreversible effects were documented suggesting the presence of at least two biochemical pathways contributing to the changes in cell proliferation and cell cycle kinetics. The recent demonstration of differential structural requirements for estrogen-reversible and estrogen-irreversible antitumor activity of nonsteroidal antiestrogens in vitro (18) further supports the existence of two separate mechanisms of antiestrogen action as an antitumor agent.

More detailed studies are required to fully understand the biochemical and cellular mechanisms leading to the accumulation of cells in early G_1 phase. It would be interesting to know whether the cells that accumulate in G_1 are actually arrested there or whether they merely accumulate because the rate at which they can traverse a critical point in G_1 is significantly decreased by drug treatment. It is also important to examine the mechanisms by which tamoxifen causes an increase in cell death rate since this probably contributes to its growth inhibitory effect at high concentrations ($>$ 5 uM) in vitro.

The techniques required to answer these questions are currently available in this laboratory and further studies in this area are being actively pursued.

ACKNOWLEDGEMENTS

The authors thank ICI Pharmaceutical Division for supply of tamoxifen and Razoxane. The technical assistance of Narelle Hobbis and the helpful comments of Dr Leigh Murphy and Colin Watts are gratefully acknowledged.

REFERENCES

1. Sutherland RL, Taylor IW (1981). Effect of tamoxifen on the cell cycle kinetics of cultured human mammary carcinoma cells. In "Reviews on Endocrine-Related Cancer" Suppl. 8, ICI Pharmaceuticals Division, p 8

2. Green MD, Whybourne AM, Taylor IW, Sutherland RL (1981). Effects of antioestrogens on the growth and cell cycle kinetics of cultured human mammary carcinoma cells. In Sutherland RL, Jordan VC (eds): "Non-Steroidal Antioestrogens" Academic Press, Sydney, p 143.

3. Sutherland RL, Whybourne AM, Taylor IW (1981). Cell cycle effects of tamoxifen on MCF 7 human mammary carcinoma cells in culture. In "Reviews on Endocrine-Related Cancer" Suppl. 9, ICI Pharmaceuticals Division, p 169.

4. Soule HD, Vasquez J, Long A, Albert S, Brennan M (1973). A human cell line from a pleural effusion derived from a breast carcinoma. J Natl Cancer Inst 51:1409.

5. Brooks SC, Locke ER, Soule HD (1973). Estrogen receptor in a human cell line (MCF 7) from breast carcinoma. J Biol Chem 248:6251.

6. Taylor IW (1980). A rapid single step staining technique for DNA analysis by flow microfluorimetry. J Histochem Cytochem 28:1021.

7. Milthorpe BK (1980). FMFPAKI: A program package for routine analysis of single parameter flow microfluorimetric data on a low cost mini-computer. Comput Biomed Res 13:417.

8. Butler WB, Kelsey WH, Goran N (1981). Effects of serum and insulin on the sensitivity of the human breast cancer cell line MCF-7 to estrogens and antiestrogens. Cancer Res 41:82.

9. Horwitz KB, Zava DT, Thilagar AK, Jensen EM, McGuire WL (1978). Steroid receptor analyses of nine human breast cancer cell lines. Cancer Res 38:2434.

10. Lippman M, Bolan G, Huff K (1976). Interactions of antiestrogens with human breast cancer in long-term tissue culture. Cancer Treat Rep 60:1421.

11. Wakeling AE, Slater SR (1980). Estrogen-receptor binding and biologic activity of tamoxifen and its metabolites. Cancer Treat Rep 64:741.

12. Sutherland RL, Whybourne AM (1981). Binding of tamoxifen and its metabolites 4-hydroxytamoxifen and N-desmethyltamoxifen to oestrogen receptors from normal and neoplastic tissues. In Sutherland RL and Jordan VC (eds):"Non-Steroidal Antioestrogens" Academic Press, Sydney, p 75.

13. Hallowes RC, West DG, Hellmann K (1974). Cumulative cytostatic effect of ICRF 159. Nature 247:487.

14. Terasima T, Tolmach LJ (1963). Growth and nucleic acid synthesis in synchronously dividing populations of HeLa cells. Exp Cell Res 30:344.

15. Allegra JC, Lippman ME (1978). Growth of a human breast cancer cell line in serum-free hormone-supplemented medium. Cancer Res 38:3073.

16. Shafie SM, Grantham FH (1981). Role of hormones in the growth and regression of human breast cancer cells (MCF-7) transplanted into athymic nude mice. J Natl Cancer Inst 67:51.

17. Palmiter RD, Mulvihill ER, McKnight GS, Senear AW (1978). Regulation of gene expression in the chick oviduct by steroid hormones. Cold Spring Harbor Symp Quant Biol 42:639.

18. Murphy LC, Watts CKW, Sutherland RL (1982). Structural requirements for binding of antiestrogen to a specific high affinity site in MCF 7 human mammary carcinoma cells: correlation with antitumor activity in vitro. This volume p

Rational Basis for Chemotherapy, pages 195–210
© 1983 Alan R. Liss, Inc., 150 Fifth Avenue, New York, NY 10011

STRUCTURAL REQUIREMENTS FOR BINDING OF ANTIESTROGENS TO A
SPECIFIC HIGH AFFINITY SITE IN MCF 7 HUMAN MAMMARY CARCINOMA
CELLS: CORRELATION WITH ANTITUMOR ACTIVITY <u>IN VITRO</u>

Leigh C. Murphy, Colin K.W. Watts and Robert L. Sutherland

Ludwig Institute for Cancer Research (Sydney Branch),
University of Sydney,
N.S.W. 2006,
Australia

ABSTRACT   The structural features of nonsteroidal antiestrogens which determine affinity for a specific microsomal 'antiestrogen binding site' have been studied and
compared to those which determine affinity for the estrogen receptor. The structure of the aminoether side chain
of these compounds was shown to be a major determinant of
binding to the antiestrogen binding site but had markedly
less effect on binding affinity for the estrogen receptor. Antitumor activity of a series of structurally related triphenylethylene derivatives was estimated by their
ability to inhibit proliferation of MCF 7 human breast
cancer cells in culture. At low doses of drug, when the
growth inhibitory effects were reversible by estrgoen,
the antitumor activity was best correlated with affinity
for the estrogen receptor, but at higher estrogen irreversible doses, antitumor activity was correlated with
affinity for the antiestrogen binding site. It is
suggested that those structural features of triphenylethylene derivatives which determine binding affinity for
the estrogen receptor also determine the magnitude of
estrogen reversible antitumor activity <u>in vitro</u> while
those features which determine binding affinity for the
antiestrogen binding site also determine their estrogen
irreversible antitumor activity <u>in vitro</u>.

INTRODUCTION

Synthetic nonsteroidal antiestrogens, such as tamoxifen,
bind to the estrogen receptor (ER) (1,2), an interaction which

is considered to be intimately involved with the mechanism by which these compounds exert their antiestrogenic and/or anti-tumor effects at the cellular level. There is, however, evidence to suggest that some of the effects of these compounds, particularly the antitumor action, may not be mediated entirely via the ER (3,4,5,6,7,8).

A previous study from this laboratory (9), which has been confirmed in other laboratories (10,11), has documented the presence of a high affinity binding site for tamoxifen in estrogen target tissues, which does not bind estrogen and is distinct from the ER. This binding site displays a high degree of specificity for synthetic nonsteroidal compounds structurally related to tamoxifen (9,12). These data, together with the observation that the structural requirements for the binding of these synthetic compounds to the 'antiestrogen binding site' (AEBS) appear to be different from those for binding to the ER (12,13), have led us to investigate in more detail those characteristics of the ligand which determine binding to the AEBS and to study the antitumor activity of analogs with markedly different affinities for this site.

                              METHODS

    Materials and methods were as previously described (12), with the following additions:

Subcellular Fractions.

    Cytosol was prepared as previously described (12). The microsomal fraction was obtained by centrifugation of the crude MCF 7 cell homogenate at 13,000 x g for 15 mins. The resulting post-mitochondrial supernatant was diluted 1 in 8 with homogenisation buffer before use in the competitive binding assays or for ^{3}H-tamoxifen saturation analysis.

Estimation of Antitumor Activity in vitro.

    MCF 7 human breast cancer cells were maintained as described in the accompanying paper (14). 5 x 10^4 cells in exponential growth phase were plated into 75 cm² flasks in 15 ml medium (RPMI 1640 supplemented with 20 mM Hepes buffer, 14 mM sodium bicarbonate, 6 mM L-glutamine, 20 ug/ml gentamicin, 10 ug/ml insulin and 5% fetal calf serum). When cell numbers were approximately 10^5 per flask, the medium was changed and the drugs were added from ethanolic stock solutions such that the final ethanol concentration was 0.1% in all flasks, a concentration without effect on cell growth. After six population doublings of control cultures, the cells were harvested with 0.05% trypsin, 0.02% EDTA in phosphate buffered saline, viable cell counts were made under phase-contrast on a hemocytometer and the cells stained for flow cytometry (15). The percentage of cells in S phase of the cell cycle was calculated from the resultant DNA histograms (16).

RESULTS

Interaction of ³H-Tamoxifen with a Saturable High Affinity Binding Site in the Microsomal Fraction of MCF 7 Human Breast Cancer Cells.

The high affinity AEBS has been studied previously in the cytosol fraction of estrogen target tissues. It has now been

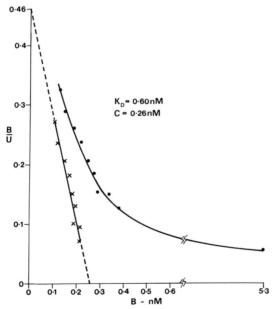

$K_D = 0.60 nM$
$C = 0.26 nM$

$\frac{B}{U}$

B - nM

FIGURE 1.   A Scatchard plot of ³H-tamoxifen binding to the microsomal fraction of MCF 7 breast cancer cells. The saturation analysis was performed and the binding parameters estimated before (●) and after (x) correction for nonspecific binding as previously described (12).   From Watts <u>et al.</u> submitted for publication.

found, at approximately 10-fold greater concentrations, on a
per mg protein basis, in the microsomal fraction of MCF 7
human breast cancer cells.

Saturation analysis of ^{3}H-tamoxifen binding to the
microsomal fraction prepared from MCF 7 cells is presented as
a Scatchard plot in Figure 1. The data are consistent with
tamoxifen being bound to a single population of binding sites
with a mean apparent equilibrium dissociation constant (K_a) of
1.0 nM (range 0.6 - 1.4 nM), which is in good agreement with
the K_d of 0.6 nM calculated from the association rate constant
(1.4×10^5 M^{-1} sec^{-1}) and the dissociation rate constant (8.5
$\times 10^{-5}$ sec^{-1}, $t_{1/2}$ = 136 mins). The binding site for
tamoxifen in the microsomal fraction displays similar
specificity to that previously reported for the binding site
in the cytosol fraction (Fig. 2).

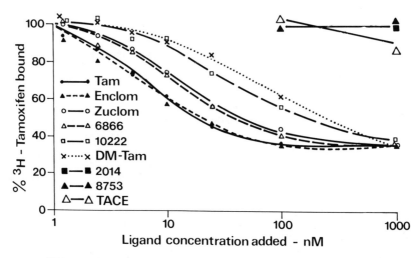

FIGURE 2. Specificity of the saturable antiestrogen
binding site in the microsomal fraction from MCF 7 breast
cancer cells. The estradiol presaturated microsomal fraction
was diluted 1 in 8 and the assay performed as previously
described (12). Data are presented as the amount of
^{3}H-tamoxifen bound as a percentage of ^{3}H-tamoxifen bound in
the absence of added ligand against the concentration of added
ligand. From Watts et al. submitted for publication.

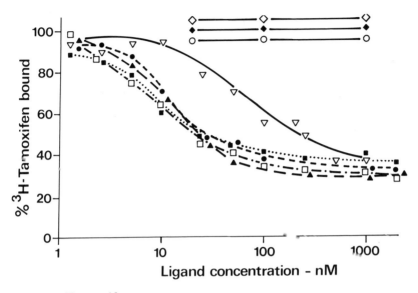

FIGURE 3. Specificity of the saturable antiestrogen binding site in the cytosol fraction from MCF 7 human breast cancer cells. The assay was performed as previously described (12). From Sutherland et al. (9).

Ligand Specificity of the 'Antiestrogen Binding Site'.

The AEBS displays a high degree of specificity for a series of structurally related synthetic non-steroidal antiestrogens, and has no affinity for several steroid hormones (Fig. 3, Tables 1 and 2).

Cis isomers of compounds binding to the AEBS show similar (ICI 47699 vs tamoxifen, Table 1) or slightly reduced (zuclomiphene vs enclomiphene, Table 2) affinities when compared to the corresponding trans isomers. In marked contrast to this the affinities of the cis isomers for the ER are considerably less than those of the trans isomers (Tables 1 and 2).

Demethylation of the alkylaminoether side chain of tamoxifen, to form N-desmethyltamoxifen, results in a marked

TABLE 1

THE RELATIVE BINDING AFFINITIES OF TAMOXIFEN METABOLITES AND
ANALOGS WITH NONBASIC SIDE CHAINS FOR THE 'ANTIESTROGEN
BINDING SITE' AND ESTROGEN RECEPTOR OF MCF 7 CELLS[a].

Code	Structure	R_1	R_2	R_3	Relative binding affinity	
					AEBS Tam=100%	ER E_2=100%
Tamoxifen (trans)		H	H	$OCH_2CH_2N(CH_3)_2$	100	2
ICI 47699 (cis)		H	H	$OCH_2CH_2N(CH_3)_2$	98	0·05
Monohydroxytamoxifen		OH	H	$OCH_2CH_2N(CH_3)_2$	63	41
Desmethyltamoxifen		H	H	$OCH_2CH_2NHCH_3$	15	1
ICI 90069		H	H	OCH_3	0	0·2
ICI 140447		H	H	$OCH_2CH=CH_2$	0	0·1
ICI 145458		H	H	$OCHCH=CH_2$ CH_3	0	0·1
ICI 145663		H	H	$OCHCHCH_2OH$ CH_3OH	0	0·3
ICI 145680		H	H	$OCH_2CHCHOH$ OH CH_3	0	1·2

[a] From Watts et al. submitted for publication.

reduction in affinity for the AEBS (Fig. 2, Table 1) with no
effect on affinity for the ER. Aromatic hydroxylation, to
form 4-hydroxytamoxifen, enhances affinity for the ER with a
slightly reduced effect on the affinity for the AEBS (Tables
1, 14). Furthermore, TACE, a nonsteroidal estrogen similar in
structure to clomiphene but without the aminoether side chain
(Fig. 4) has no affinity for the AEBS. These data suggested
that the aminoether side chain was of importance for binding
to the AEBS. To investigate further the importance of the

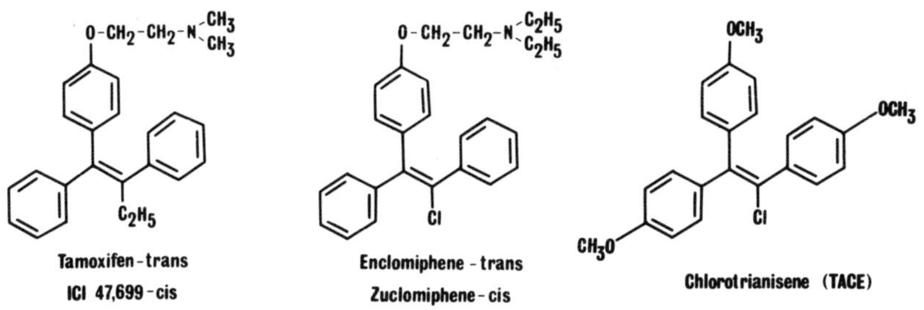

FIGURE 4. Structure of the synthetic nonsteroidal antiestrogens, tamoxifen and clomiphene, and the synthetic nonsteroidal estrogen, chlorotrianisene (TACE).

TABLE 2

THE RELATIVE BINDING AFFINITIES OF CLOMIPHENE AND CLOMIPHENE ANALOGS WITH SIDE CHAIN MODIFICATIONS FOR THE 'ANTIESTROGEN BINDING SITE' AND ESTROGEN RECEPTOR OF MCF 7 CELLS[a].

Code	Structure	R_1	R_2	R_3	Relative binding affinity	
	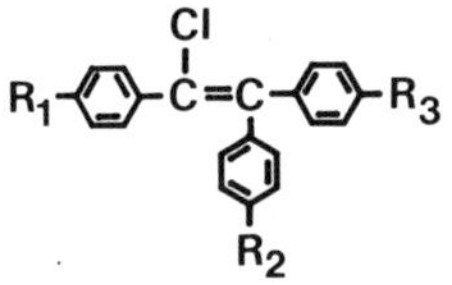				AEBS Tam=100%	ER E_2=100%
2014		H	H	H	0	0·2
8753		H	H	OCH_3	0	0·3
TACE		OCH_3	OCH_3	OCH_3	0	0·5
Enclomiphene (trans)		H	H	$OCH_2CH_2N(C_2H_5)_2$	109	2
Zuclomiphene (cis)		H	H	$OCH_2CH_2N(C_2H_5)_2$	49	0·05
9599		H	H	$OCH_2CH_2NH C_2H_5$	37	0·6
6866		H	H	$OCH_2CH_2CH_2N(C_2H_5)_2$	43	4
8650		H	H	$OCH_2CH_2N(C_3H_7)_2$	10	0·3
10222		H	H	$N HCH_2CH_2N(C_2H_5)_2$	16	4

[a] From Murphy and Sutherland (12).

aminoether side chain in determining binding affinity for the AEBS, a series of clomiphene derivatives, in which the triphenylchloroethylene moiety remained unaltered but the side chain had undergone a series of modifications, was studied. A summary of the results is presented in Table 2.

The parent compound enclomiphene was as potent as tamoxifen in inhibiting the binding of ^{3}H-tamoxifen to its saturable binding site in MCF 7 cells. This result is probably a reflection of their similar structures (Fig. 4). The presence of an aminoether side chain was an absolute requirement for binding; its removal (2014) or substitution with a methoxy group (8753, TACE, ICI 90069) resulted in complete loss of affinity for the AEBS (Tables 1 and 2). Changes in length of the side chain (6866) and changes in the number (9599) and size (8650) of the substitutions on the terminal amino group modified binding affinity (Table 2). Conversion of the ether linkage to an amine (10222) also markedly reduced affinity. Substitution of the basic aminoether side chain with non-basic side chains (ICI 140447, 145458, 145663, 145680, Table 1) resulted in complete loss of affinity for the AEBS. Together, these data demonstrate that the basic ether side chain is a major structural determinant for binding of nonsteroidal antiestrogens of the triphenyl-ethylene series to the AEBS.

The structure of the lipophilic portion of the molecule also influences binding affinity. The <u>cis</u> isomer of clomi-phene (zuclomiphene) showed slightly reduced affinity and some bibenzyl and stilbene derivatives with diethylaminoether side chains identical to that of clomiphene generally displayed weak affinity for the AEBS (data not shown)

Antitumor Activity of Some Triphenylethylene Derivatives.

In order to investigate which structural characteristics of these synthetic compounds are related to their antitumor activity <u>in vitro</u>, and with the above observations on structural requirements for binding to ER and AEBS in mind, a group of compounds with comparable affinities for the ER but widely varying affinities for the AEBS were selected and tested for their ability to inhibit the growth of exponentially growing MCF 7 cells in culture. Enclomiphene, 6866 and 10222 have relative binding affinities(RBA) of 2, 4 and 4% respectively for the ER (Table 2) and RBA of 109, 43 and 16% respectively for the AEBS (Table 2). The effects of varying doses of these compounds on viable cell number and their reversibility by estrogen are illustrated in Figure 5A.

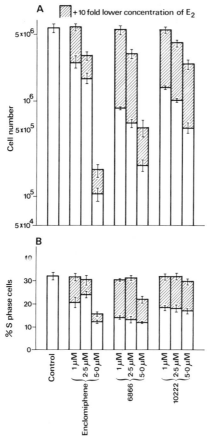

FIGURE 5. A) The effect of enclomiphene, 6866 and 10222, in the presence or absence of estradiol, on MCF 7 cell growth. Cells were grown for 6 population doublings of control cultures in the presence of varying concentrations of drug with or without a 10-fold lower dose of estradiol. Data are presented as the mean ± SEM of duplicate flasks from 3 separate experiments. B) The effect of enclomiphene, 6866 and 10222 in the presence or absence of a 10-fold lower dose of estradiol on the percentage of MCF 7 cells in S phase of the cell cycle. Cells were from the experiments described in Fig. 5A and the percentage of S phase cells was calculated from the DNA histograms obtained by flow cytometry. Data are presented as the mean ± SEM of single observations from 3 separate experiments. From Murphy et al. submitted for publication.

Under the conditions of these experiments, estradiol alone had no effect on viable cell numbers (data not shown). All compounds induced a dose-dependent growth inhibitory effect (Fig. 5) but the potencies of the compounds were not equal. At doses of 2.5 uM or below, the order of growth inhibition was 6866 > 10222 > enclomiphene, while at 5 uM, the order became enclomiphene > 6866 > 10222.

The ability of estradiol to reverse the growth inhibition induced by these drugs was assessed by the simultaneous addition of a 10-fold lower concentration of estradiol with each drug. The effects on cell number induced by 1 uM of these drugs were completely reversed by estradiol and the effects on cell number induced by 2.5 uM of all drugs and 5 uM 10222 were almost completely reversed. However, growth inhibition by 5 uM 6866 and enclomiphene was only partially reversed by estradiol (Fig 5A).

Changes in cell cycle kinetic parameters are summarized in Figure 5B and were generally consistent with the effects observed when cell number was monitored. Again, effects seen at 1 and 2.5 uM 6866 or enclomiphene and all doses of 10222 were completely reversed by estrogen, while the decrease in % S phase cells produced by 5 uM enclomiphene and 6866 was only partially reversible. Figure 6 illustrates dose/response curves, with and without estradiol, for the three compounds tested. A dramatic change in potency of enclomiphene was seen at the high, estrogen irreversible concentration. At 5 uM, in the presence or absence of estradiol, the potencies of the drugs fell into the same order as their RBA for the AEBS, while at lower estrogen reversible concentrations, the order of potencies was more closely correlated with their RBA for ER. However, at these lower concentrations, 10222 was less potent than 6866 despite the fact that their RBA for the ER were identical.

DISCUSSION

The data summarized above illustrate that the microsomal AEBS has similar characteristics (K_d, ligand specificity) to those previously described for the AEBS, present in the cytosol fraction of MCF 7 cells (9,12). It appears likely that the presence of AEBS in cytosol can be accounted for by microsomal contamination due to the homogenisation and centrifugation techniques employed. The subcellular distribution of the AEBS is in marked contrast to that of the

ER where the molecule is predominantly cytosolic or nuclear

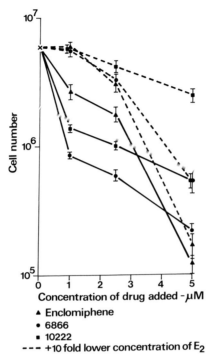

▲ Enclomiphene
● 6866
■ 10222
--- +10 fold lower concentration of E_2

FIGURE 6. Dose response curves of the effect of enclomiphene, 6866 and 10222, in the presence or absence of a 10-fold lower dose of estradiol, on the growth of MCF 7 cells in culture. Data are presented as the mean ± SEM of duplicate flasks from 3 separate experiments. From Murphy et al. submitted for publication.

depending on the degree of estrogen stimulation. Further localisation of the AEBS within the microsomal fraction is currently being pursued.

The studies presented here and elsewhere (12), show that the structural features of the triphenylethylene derivatives necessary for binding to the AEBS are different from those for binding to the ER. The basic ether side chain is a major structural determinant for binding to the AEBS, while the nature of the substitutions on the aromatic ring corresponding to the A ring of estradiol is a major structural determinant for binding to the ER (13). X-ray crystallographic studies on the 3-dimensional structure of estrogens and antiestrogens

(13) show that the aminoether side chain extends beyond the
dimensions of natural steroidal estrogens and is some distance
from the major points of interactions between the estrogen or
antiestrogen molecule and the estradiol binding site of the
ER. These studies provide an explanation as to why
modifications in the aminoether side chain usually only result
in minor alterations in binding affinity for the ER (e.g.
6866, 10222, enclomiphene) but marked changes in affinity for
the AEBS, while changes in the substituents on the aromatic
ring analogous to the A ring of estradiol can substantially
alter affinity for the ER (e.g. 4-hydroxytamoxifen) without
significant effects on affinity for AEBS.

   The significance of our observations in vitro with
respect to the antiestrogenic and antitumor activity in vivo
is unknown. That the side chain is a requirement for the
antiestrogenic activity of the triphenylethylene compounds
(18,19) raises the possibility of a functional role for the
AEBS. The removal of the side chain e.g. TACE or U 11584 (20)
is accompanied by expression of estrogenic but not antiestrogenic activity (19). In addition, restriction of the
number of positions that the aminoether side chain can adopt
in space reduces antiestrogenic activity (21,22). Both of the
modifications of the triphenylethylene derivatives described
above also result in loss of or reduced affinity for the AEBS
(10). However,other observations suggest that affinity for
the AEBS is not always correlated with antiestrogenicity e.g.:
1) the cis isomers of some of these compounds are often
estrogenic (19,23) while displaying similar (ICI 47699 vs
tamoxifen) or slightly reduced affinity (zuclomiphene vs
enclomiphene) for the AEBS, 2) 4-hydroxytamoxifen while
having a similar (17) or slightly reduced affinity compared
with tamoxifen for the AEBS has been reported to be a more
potent antiestrogen (24) and 3) some compounds with non-basic
side chains, which one would predict from our data (Table 1)
to have no affinity for the AEBS, have antiestrogenic activity
(25,26).

   Although it has long been inferred that the antitumor
activity of the triphenylethylene derivatives is due to their
antiestrogenicity, this has not been proved and the poor
correlation between the antifertility and the antiestrogenic
activities of these compounds (27) should warn against such an
assumption. We have initiated structure-activity studies with
respect to antitumor activity of these compounds, using MCF 7
human breast cancer cells in culture, a system reported not to
metabolise these compounds (28). Initially, we have taken a
group of compounds which are structurally related, have a

basic aminoether side chain, have comparable affinity for the ER but markedly different affinities for the AEBS (6866, 10222 and enclomiphene) and tested their ability to inhibit the growth of MCF 7 cells in culture. Initial studies (unpublished observation) had shown that enclomiphene displayed similar potency to tamoxifen. As was the case with tamoxifen (14) two different effects on cell growth were seen. At concentrations of 2.5 uM or below of all three compounds and at 5 uM 10222, the growth inhibitory effects were completely or almost completely estrogen reversible with an accumulation of cells in G_0/G_1, at the expense of S phase cells. At 5 uM, 6866 and enclomiphene caused an estrogen-irreversible growth inhibition with similar kinetic changes to those observed for the estrogen-reversible effect. Interestingly, the potency of the drugs with respect to the estrogen-reversible growth inhibition is similar to their order of affinity for the ER, while their potency in relation to the estrogen-irreversible growth inhibition is correlated with affinity for the AEBS. With the exception of enclomiphene we have no data on the estrogenic and/or antiestrogenic activities of these compounds.

These data indicate that further structure-activity studies of the antitumor effects of the nonsteroidal antiestrogens and their derivatives are warranted. They also support the existence of effects of tamoxifen that are not reversed by estrogen and may not be ER mediated (3,4,5,6,7,8,14). This cautions against interpreting all the effects of these nonsteroidal compounds as estrogen agonist and/or antagonist effects. It is proposed to investigate further the possibility that the characteristics which determine binding to the AEBS are related to the antitumor activity of these compounds.

ACKNOWLEDGEMENTS

The authors thank ICI Ltd, Pharmaceuticals Division for supply of tamoxifen and its analogs, and Merrell-Dow Pharmaceuticals for supply of clomiphene and its analogs. The technical assistance of Rosemary Hall and Narelle Hobbis is gratefully acknowledged, as is the helpful comment and criticism of our colleague Dr Roger Reddel.

REFERENCES

1. Skidmore J, Walpole AL, Woodburn J (1972). Effect of some triphenylethylenes on oestradiol binding in vitro to macromolecules from uterus and anterior pituitary. J Endocr 52:289.

2. Jordan VC, Koerner S (1975). Tamoxifen (ICI 46474) and the human carcinoma 8S oestrogen receptor. Europ J Cancer 11:205.

3. Ragaz J (1981). Combination of hormones for metastatic carcinoma of the breast - aminoglutethimide + Tamoxifen in combination vs aminoglutethimide alone vs Tamoxifen alone. In "Reviews on Endocrine-Related Cancer, Supplement 9, Antihormones and Breast Cancer", ICI Pharmaceuticals Division, p 547.

4. Patterson JS, Battersby LA, Edwards DG (1981). Review of the clinical pharmacology and international experience with tamoxifen in advanced breast cancer. In "Reviews on Endocrine-Related Cancer, Supplement 9, Antihormones and Breast Cancer", ICI Pharmaceuticals Division, p 563.

5. Green MD, Whybourne AM, Taylor IW, Sutherland RL (1981). Effects of antioestrogens on the growth and cell cycle kinetics of cultured human mammary carcinoma cells. In Sutherland RL, Jordan VC (eds): "Nonsteroidal Antioestrogens" Academic Press, Sydney, p 397.

6. Martin L (1981). Effects of antioestrogens on cell proliferation in the rodent reproductive tract. In Sutherland RL, Jordan VC (eds): "Nonsteroidal Antioestrogens" Academic Press, Sydney, p 143.

7. Allegra JC, Lippman ME (1978). Growth of a human breast cancer cell line in serum-free hormone-supplemented medium. Cancer Res 38:3823.

8. Shafie SM, Grantham FH (1981). Role of hormones in the growth and regression of human breast cancer cells (MCF-7) transplanted into athymic nude mice. J Natl Cancer Inst 67: 51.

9. Sutherland RL, Murphy LC, Foo MS, Green MD, Whybourne AM, Krozowski ZS (1980). High-affinity anti-oestrogen binding site distinct from the oestrogen receptor. Nature 288:273.

10. Faye JC, Lasserre B, Bayard F (1980). Antiestrogen specific, high affinity saturable binding sites in rat uterine cytosol. Biochem Biophys Res Comm 93:1225.

11. Gulino A, Pasqualini JP (1980). Specific binding and biological response of antiestrogens in the fetal uterus of the guinea pig. Cancer Res 40:3821.

12. Murphy LC, Sutherland RL (1981). Modifications in the aminoether side chain of clomiphene influence affinity for a specific antiestrogen binding site in MCF 7 cell cytosol. Biochem Biophys Res Comm 100:1353.

13. Duax WL, Weeks CM (1980). Molecular basis of estrogenicity: X-ray crystallographic studies. In McLachlan JA (ed): "Estrogens in the Environment" Elsevier/North Holland, New York p 11.

14. Sutherland RL, Reddel RR, Hall RE, Hodson PJ, Taylor IW (1982). Effects of tamoxifen on the cell cycle kinetics of MCF 7 human mammary carcinoma cells in culture. This volume p

15. Taylor IW (1980). A rapid single-step staining technique for DNA analysis by flow microfluorimetry. J Histochem Cytochem 28:1021.

16. Milthorpe BK (1980). FMFPAKI: A program for routine analysis of single parameter flow microfluorimeter data on a low cost minicomputer. Comput Biomed Res 13:417.

17. Sutherland RL, Whybourne AM (1981). Binding of tamoxifen and its metabolites 4-hydroxytamoxifen and N-desmethyltamoxifen to oestrogen receptors from normal and neoplastic tissues. In Sutherland RL, Jordan VC (eds): "Nonsteroidal Antioestrogens" Academic Press, Sydney, p 75.

18. Lednicer D, Lyster SC, Duncan GW (1967). Mammalian antifertility agents. IV. Basic 3,4-dihydronaphthalenes and 1,2,3,4-tetrahydro-1-naphthols. J Med Chem 10: 78.

19. Jordan VC, Clark ER, Allen KE (1981). Structure-activity relationships amongst non-steroidal antioestrogens. In Sutherland RL, Jordan VC (eds): "Nonsteroidal Antioestrogens" Academic Press, Sydney, p 31.

20. Lednicer D, Lyster SC, Aspergren BD, Duncan GW (1966). Mammalian antifertility agents. III. 1-Aryl-2-phenyl-1,2,3,4-tetrahydro-1-naphthols, 1-aryl-2-phenyl-3,4-dihydronaphthalenes and their derivatives. J Med Chem 9: 172.

21. Abbott AC, Clark ER, Jordan VC (1976). Inhibition of oestradiol binding to oestrogen receptor proteins by a methyl-substituted analogue to tamoxifen. J Endocr 69: 445.

22. Clark ER, Jordan VC (1976). Oestrogenic, anti-oestrogenic and fertility effects of some triphenylethanes and triphenylethylenes related to ethamoxytriphetol (MER25). Br J Pharmacol 57:487.

23. Harper MJK, Walpole AL (1967). A new derivative of triphenylethylene: effect on implantation and mode of action in rats. J Reprod Fert 13:101.

24. Jordan VC, Collins MM, Rowsby L, Prestwich G (1977). A monohydroxylated metabolite of tamoxifen with potent antioestrogenic activity. J Endocr 75:305.

25. Ferguson ER, Katzenellenbogen BS (1977). A comparative study of antiestrogen action: temporal patterns of antagonism of estrogen stimulated uterine growth and effects on estrogen receptor levels. Endocrinol 100: 1242.

26. Robertson DW, Katzenellenbogen JA, Hayes JR, Katzenellenbogen BS (1982). Antiestrogen basicity-activity relationships: a comparison of the estrogen receptor binding and antiuterotrophic potencies of several analogues of (Z)-1,2-diphenyl-1-[4-[2-(di-methylamino)ethoxy]phenyl]-1-butene (Tamoxifen, Nolvadex) having altered basicity. J Med Chem 25:167.

27. Emmens CW (1970). Antifertility agents. Ann Rev Pharmacol 10:237.

28. Horwitz KB, Koseki Y, McGuire WL (1978). Estrogen control of progesterone receptor in human breast cancer: role of estradiol and antiestrogen. Endocrinol 103:1742.

Rational Basis for Chemotherapy, pages 211–238

HETEROGENEITY OF HUMAN T AND B CELL NEOPLASMS

Kenneth C. Anderson, Michael P. Bates, Edward K. Park, Robert C.F. Leonard, Stuart F. Schlossman and Lee M. Nadler

Division of Tumor Immunology, Sidney Farber Cancer Institute, Boston, Massachusetts 02115

INTRODUCTION

Human leukemias and lymphomas have been recognized as heterogeneous diseases by morphologic appearance, clinical presentation, and response to therapy (1-3). Their classification has been traditionally based on the histologic appearance and cytochemical properties of the tumor cell (4-9). Specifically, lymphomas have been classified on the basis of lymph node histologic architecture as either nodular (N) or diffuse (D) and according to the cytologic appearance of the individual tumor cell as well differentiated lymphocytic (WD), poorly differentiated lymphocytic (PDL), mixed lymphocytic histiocytic (M) or histiocytic (H) (5). Within each subgroup, there is considerable clinical heterogeneity based on primary site of tumor involvement, extent of disease and response to therapy. Additional heterogeneity has recently been identified using immunologic markers which relate the malignant cell to its T, B or null cell lineage (10-19). To date, current classification schemes have failed to clearly correlate histopathology and immunologic cellular origin with the clinical course of these diseases.

The nodular lymphomas are B cell derived tumors which are frequently widely disseminated at presentation. Although most nodular poorly differentiated lymphocytic lymphomas (N-PDL) are Stage IV at presentation, they tend to have long survivals (20). In contrast to the other non-Hodgkin's lymphomas, the survival for nodular lymphomas has not significantly changed with the institution of single or multi-agent chemotherapy, or the combination of chemothera-

py and radiation therapy (20-26). Most patients with nodular mixed (NM) or nodular histiocytic (NH) lymphomas, in
contrast, require early aggressive therapy which may result
in long disease free intervals and even cures (27-29). Although delineation of the heterogeneity of the histopathologic groups of nodular lymphomas has significant clinical
importance, an immunologically based classification scheme
may further identify groups of nodular lymphoma patients
who would respond to particular therapeutic regimens.

Even greater heterogeneity has been observed within
diffuse lymphomas. Diffuse well differentiated lymphomas
(DWDL) have a natural history similar to patients with chronic lymphocytic leukemia (CLL) with average survival in excess of 6 years regardless of therapeutic approach (21,30,
31). In contrast, diffuse poorly differentiated lymphocytic (DPDL), mixed (DM), and histiocytic (DHL) lymphomas all
require aggressive combination chemotherapy for long survival (22,23,27,31-48). Within the DPDL subgroup, some patients with tumor cells of B cell origin may have a survival
equivalent to that of NPDL (16,49), in contrast to the T
cell subset of DPDL which is usually a highly aggressive disease with a short survival(37,43).

Diffuse histiocytic lymphomas (DHL) demonstrate the
greatest clinical heterogeneity in disease presentation and
response to therapy. They have generally been regarded as
aggressive neoplasms with short survivals prior to the advent of chemotherapy. However, with aggressive combination
chemotherapy approximately 50% of the patients with advanced
stage DHL have experienced long disease free intervals or
even cures (31-48). To identify the subgroups of DHL which
respond to therapy, several investigators have undertaken
histopathological and immunologic studies (12,16,50-59).
Strauchen and his colleagues (51) attempted to identify morphologic features which correlate with prognosis. Five morphologically distinct subgroups of DHL were proposed which
appeared to have different prognoses. Immunologic marker
studies of DHL have also demonstrated heterogeneity: 75% are
of B cell, 10% of T cell, 10% of "null" cell and <5% are of
a true histiocytic origin (14,50,52-54). Although no large
definitive study of the immunologic heterogeneity of DHL has
been published, several groups have reported that B cell DHL
has a better prognosis than T cell or null cell DHL (50).
In recent studies, Warnke and his colleagues (60) found significant immunologic heterogeneity within DHL using surface
immunoglobulin, Ia antigens and T cell antigens. Eight immunologic phenotypes of DHL were identified and retrospective

clinical analysis suggested shorter survival and more advanced disease in patients with surface Ig+ tumor cells. As is generally true for other studies of immunologic markers, treatment was not standardized and therefore no definitive conclusions could be drawn. More recent reports include those of Gajl-Pezalska (61), Barcos (62) and Ford (63) in which marked heterogeneity of immunologic phenotype was demonstrated using monoclonal reagents. To date, however, the immunologic heterogeneity of the leukemias and lymphomas as defined by cell surface markers has not been studied in a large enough patient sample to provide a meaningful correlation with either histology, clinical course or response to therapy.

In the present report, we will attempt to summarize the immunologic heterogeneity of leukemias and lymphomas. The enumeration of cell surface determinants, which are both lineage restricted and identify discrete stages of differentiation, should now permit us to relate the malignant cell to its normal cellular counterpart. By relating the malignant cell to normal differentiative steps, it may be possible to more precisely understand the heterogeneity of leukemias and lymphomas as well as to more precisely define the cell populations, ontogeny and function of normal hematopoietic cells. We will review the ontogeny of T and B cell development and attempt to relate the stages of differentiation with the histopathologically defined malignancies. Although this work is preliminary, it is hoped that the heterogeneity defined by lineage restricted differentiation antigens will allows us to more precisely understand both the biologic and clinical aspects of leukemias and non-Hodgkin's lymphomas.

TUMORS OF T CELL LINEAGE

Normal T Lymphocyte Differentiation

Functionally distinct subpopulations of normal human T cells have been defined by heteroantisera (64,65) and more recently, monoclonal antisera against T cell antigens. Reinherz et al. have developed a series of monoclonal antibodies which identify antigens expressed on human T cells at distinct stages of differentiation (Table 1, Fig. 1)(66). Anti-T1, anti-T3 and anti-T12 defined molecularly distinct antigens which are expressed on all peripheral T cells (67-72). Anti-T4 defines the phenotype of the helper/inducer cell and

TABLE 1
MONOCLONAL ANTIBODIES TO HUMAN T CELL SURFACE ANTIGEN

Monoclonal antibodies	Cell surface expression (% reactivity with antibodies)			Reference
	Thymocytes	T cells	Non-T cells	
Anti-T1	10[a]	100	0	67-69
Anti-T3	10	100	0	69,70
Anti-T12	10	100	0	71
Anti-T4	75	60	0	73,75
Anti-T5	80	25	0	74,75
Anti-T8	80	30	0	74,75
Anti-T6	70	0	0	76,77
Anti-T9	10	0	0	76,77
Anti-T10	95	5	10	76,77
Anti-T11	100	100	<5	78

[a]% reactivity with monoclonal antibodies was assessed by flow cytometry. T cells are E rosette positive and non-T cells are E rosette negative.

anti-T5/8 that of the cytotoxic/suppressor cell (73-75); T6 is a unique antigen since it is only found on thymocytes within the lymphoid system (76,77) and is not expressed on more mature T cells. T9 and T10, while non-lineage specific, are expressed within the T cell series on early thymocytes (76,77). The E rosette receptor, defined by anti-T11, is expressed on all thymocytes as well as on mature T lymphocytes (78).

A hypothetical model of normal T cell differentiation is seen in Fig. 1 (66). The early thymocyte is thought to originate in the normal bone marrow and migrate to the thymus. Many more prothymocytes enter the thymus than the number of mature T cells. The sequence of maturation within the thymus is as follows: early thymocyte (T10, T9/T10), common thymocyte (T4, T5/8, T6 and T10), and mature thymocytes (T1, T3, T4, T10 and T1, T3, T5/8, T10)(76). Early, common and mature thymocytes constitute 10, 70 and 10% of thymocytes, respectively. Early and common thymocytes are cortical and mature thymocytes are medullary in location. Circulating peripheral T lymphocytes are either of the

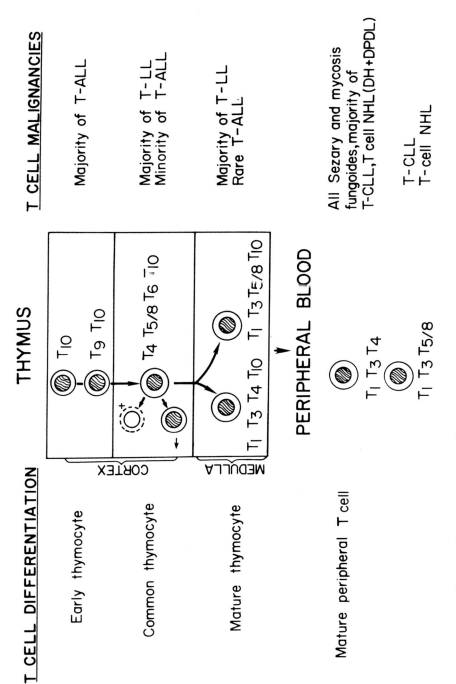

Figure 1. Stages of Normal and Malignant T Cell Differentiation

helper/inducer (T1,T3,T4) or cytotoxic/suppressor (T1,T3, T5/8) phenotype (73-75).

Stage I and Stage II T Cell Malignancies

The cell surface phenotype of T cell leukemias and lymphomas permits one to relate them to the above mentioned stages of normal thymic maturation (Fig. 1)(79,80). For example, the majority of patients with T cell acute lymphoblastic leukemia (T-ALL) have the phenotype of an early thymocyte and only rarely have the phenotype of either a common or mature thymocyte (81,82). This observation is consistent with the clinical presentation of T-ALL with primarily bone marrow infiltration. In contrast, patients with T cell lymphoblastic lymphoma (T-LL) have the phenotype of the common or mature thymocyte (82) and clinically present with mediastinal masses (37,43,83). This is consistent with the notion that this tumor has an intrathymic origin. Moreover, T-ALL and T-LL differ clinically in that those patients with T-LL have significantly prolonged survival compared to T-ALL patients treated with similar strategies. The phenotypic diversity between T-LL and T-ALL therefore seems to correlate with clinical presentation, survival, and response to therapy.

Stage III T Cell Malignancies

In contrast to T-ALL and T-LL, the malignancies which correspond to the mature T cell phenotype appear to be the adult leukemias and lymphomas (Fig. 1). The majority of tumor cells isolated from patients with Sezary syndrome, mycosis fungoides, T cell chronic lymphocytic leukemia (T-CLL) and T cell non-Hodgkin's lymphomas share the phenotype of mature peripheral T cells (84,85). As was true for malignancies of Stage I and Stage II thymocytes, each of these diseases has a characteristic clinical presentation and response to therapy which is distinct from T-ALL and T-LL. Sezary patients have a classical cutaneous presentation only later extending to viscera and CNS. T-CLL patients present initially with bone marrow involvement, and in contrast to B cell CLL (B-CLL), demonstrate early skin and CNS involvement. Finally, the NHL's of T cell lineage (DPDL or DH) frequently present in non-lymphoid tissue (e.g. skin, GI tract, CNS, lung, etc.) with rapid dissemination to other viscera. All patients so far reported with Sezary syndrome and most other T cell leukemias and lymphomas have the helper/inducer (T1,T3,T4) phenotype (Fig. 1)(73,75). Further heterogeneity will certainly be identified as subpopulations of helper/inducer cells are immunologically defined.

TUMORS OF B CELL LINEAGE

B Cell Associated Surface Determinants

The human B lymphocyte expresses a large number of cell surface and cytoplasmic determinants. The sine qua non of a B cell is either integral cell surface (86,89) or cytoplasmic immunoglobulin (88). Pre-B cells express cytoplasmic Ig heavy chains without detectable surface Ig. True B cells express the complete Ig molecule on the cell surface. Following exportation of Ig to the cell surface, heavy chain isotype diversity occurs. Finally, immunoglobulin molecules are lost from the cell surface at the time when the cells become secretory and differentiate toward the plasma cell (89). Excluding integral surface Ig, most cell surface determinants expressed on B lymphocytes are not B lineage restricted (Fig. 2). For example, the HLA-D/DR related Ia-like antigens (Ia)(90,91) are strongly expressed on B lymphocytes but are also found on monocytes, activated T cells, and myeloid precursors (CFU-C). Receptors for the Fc portion of IgG and the complement receptor C3 (92-95) are expressed at discrete stages of B cell differentiation, but are also expressed on monocytes, granulocytes and subpopulations of T lymphocytes. At the terminal stages of B cell differentiation, these determinants are lost and a new antigen termed T10 (70,89,96), initially defined on Stage I thymocytes, is then expressed (Fig. 2). T10 expression, although not B lineage restricted, is clearly limited to the terminal stages of differentiation.

Other than integral cell surface immunoglobulin and its isotypes, there are no other B cell specific surface determinants. In the past several years, several laboratories have reported monoclonal antibodies reactive with human B cell antigens distinct from conventional human immunoglobulins, Ia-like antigens, and Fc and C3 receptors (97-101). These monoclonal antibodies were derived from immunizations with normal B lymphocytes, B cell lines and B cells derived from patients with leukemias and lymphomas. In our laboratory, we have recently characterized two B cell asso-

HYPOTHETICAL MODEL FOR B-CELL ANTIGEN EXPRESSION

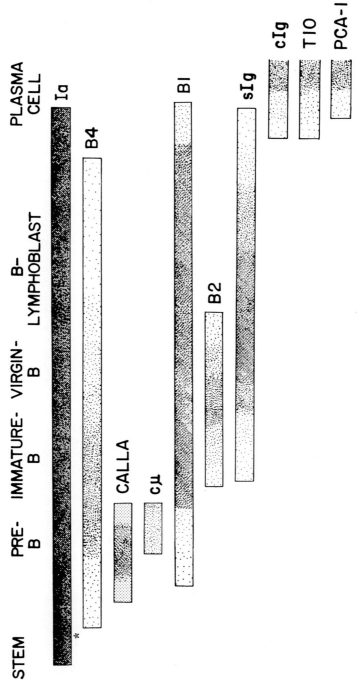

Figure 2. Stages of Normal B Cell Differentiation.

*Stippling reflects intensity of antigen expression as measured by flow cytometry.

ciated monoclonal antibodies. The first of these, B1 (98), is a nonglycosylated phosphorylated protein with the molecular weight of 35,000 daltons expressed on >95% of B cells and peripheral blood and lymphoid organs, but is absent from resting or activated T cells, monocytes, null cells, granulocytes, erythrocytes or platelets. B1 is primarily restricted to the B cell regions (follicles) of lymphoid organs. Functional experiments have demonstrated that all B lymphocytes capable of being induced to secrete immunoglobulin by pokeweed mitogen are contained within the B1 reactive population (89). In vitro stimulation experiments demonstrate that B1 is a unique differentiation antigen. When surface Ig bearing B cells are stimulated with PWM to secrete immunoglobulin, the B1 antigen is lost. The loss of B1 is accompanied by the development of presecretory cytoplasmic IgG and surface T10 staining (89). This suggests that the B1 antigen spans B cell differentiation and is lost at the plasma cell stage (Fig. 2).

A second B cell associated antigen termed B2 (99) is a glycosylated nonphosphorylated protein of a molecular weight of 140,000 daltons. In contrast to the B1 antigen, the B2 antigen is very weakly expressed on peripheral blood B cells but is more strongly expressed on B cells isolated from lymph node, tonsil or spleen. Like B1, B2 is restricted in its expression to B cells and is not expressed on other fractionated lymphoid cells. In a pokeweed mitogen driven model of B cell differentiation (Fig. 2)(89), B2 was lost from the cell surface at a time when surface IgD was lost, lymphoblast transformation occurred and the cells developed presecretory cytoplasmic IgM. These experiments suggest that B2 is a more restricted differentiation antigen than is B1 (Fig. 2).

Confirmatory evidence that the B1 and B2 antigens are B cell restricted is derived from examining leukemias and lymphomas of several lineage derivations (15,98,99,102). The B1 and B2 antigens are not found on leukemias or lymphomas of T cell origin. In addition, acute myeloblastic leukemia and chronic myelocytic leukemia cells did not express B1 or B2. These observations further confirmed the observations that B1 and B2 are not expressed on cells of T cell or myeloid origin. The B1 antigen was expressed on tumor cells isolated from all patients with B cell lymphomas and the B2 antigen was found on approximately 1/3 of patients with B cell lymphoma (Table 2). The B1 antigen was found on all patients with B cell derived chronic lymphocytic leukemia and the B2 antigen was found on a great majority of these

TABLE 2

EXPRESSION OF B CELL ASSOCIATED ANTIGENS ON B CELL TUMORS

	Non-T ALL (35)*	B-CLL (50)	N-PDL (30)	D-PDL△ (15)	NH (5)	DH△ (20)	Myeloma (20)
Ia	100[+]	100	100	100	100	100	>50
B4	100	95	100	100	ND[§]	ND	0
CALLA	80	0	90	0	>75	0	0
B1	50	100	100	100	100	100	0
cIg	30	ND	ND	ND	ND	ND	100
B2	<10	75	75	75	<5	<20	0
sIg	0	75[+]	90	>95	>90	100	0
T10	ND	ND	ND	ND	ND	ND	100
PCA-1	0	0	0	0	0	0	100
PCA-2	0	0	0	0	0	0	100

*Number in parentheses = number of patients tested.

[+]Approximate % of patients reactive with monoclonal antisera as summarized from multiple studies, assessed by flow cytometry

[§]ND = not done

△All D-PDL or DH included were B cell tumors

patients. Within the B cell series, the only tumor which
did not express B1 was plasma cell myeloma, thus confirming
the observation that B1 is not expressed on the terminal
stage of B cell differentiation.

Sequence of Normal B Cell Differentiation

     In contrast to the large body of evidence so far accu-
mulated for T cell differentiation and ontogeny, the development of B cells is not well understood in either murine or
human systems. The earliest defined B cell is the pre-B
cell which contains cytoplasmic μ heavy chain without light
chains (Figs. 2 and 3)(88,103). This cell has been identified in small numbers within the fetal liver and normal
adult bone marrow (88,104-106). The pre-B cell appears to
express the Ia antigen but is not known to express receptors
for Fc or C3 or a receptor for monkey red blood cells (105,
107). The next stage of B cell differentiation is termed
the immature B cell which now is defined by the presence of
cell surface IgM (sIgM)(104). These cells expressed weak
surface immunoglobulin (sIg), Ia, Fc and C3 receptors, and
have a receptor for monkey red blood cells (Fig. 3)(108,109).
The next several stages of B cell differentiation include the
development of immunoglobulin isotype diversity (88). It is
believed that cells first express sIgM (110-112), then sIgD
(112,113) and finally undergo a commitment to the individual
isotype which they will ultimately secrete (114-117). The
intensity of sIg, C3 and Fc receptor on the cell surface
increases over the next several stages of differentiation
(Fig. 4). The differentiation from the pre-B cell to the
virgin B cell (Fig. 4) is considered to be antigen independent. The B1 antigen is expressed on most cells of the pre-B
cell stage and is only lost at the plasma cell stage whereas
B2 antigen appeared at the stage of the immature B cell and
is lost at the lymphoblast (98,99). The B lymphoblast is
transformed, and thereafter committed to differentiate into
a secretory plasma cell. As seen in Fig. 2, sIg and B1 are
lost prior to the plasma cell stage (90). The T10 antigen
appears shortly before the plasma cell and is the only known
B cell associated surface determinant expressed on the plasma cell (90,97).
     Confirmation of this differentiation scheme can be seen
from the distribution of B1 and B2 in normal lymphoid tissues (89,98,99,118). The B1 and B2 antigens are expressed
on the majority of cells in the primary follicle and the

mantle zone of the secondary follicle expressing cell surface antigens similar to those of circulating B cells (IgM,
IgD, Ia, Bl and B2). In contrast, the germinal center cells
of the secondary follicles (IgM, IgG, Bl stronger B2, Ia but
not IgD) indicated that the generation of the germinal center in a lymphoid follicle involves phenotypic changes analogous to those observed after antigenic or mitogenic activation of B cells.

     The expression of the B2 antigen on leukemias and lym-
phomas further confirmed the hypothesis that the expression
of B2 was limited to the discrete stages of B cell differentiation (99). The Bl antigen is expressed on all B cell tumors and half of null cell diffuse histiocytic lymphomas,
but is unreactive with myelomas (Table 2)(98,102). In contrast, the B2 antigen is found on B cell tumors from the
immature B cells (CLL) to the virgin B cell (nodular or diffuse PDL)(Table 2, Fig. 4)(99). The B2 antigen was not
found on tumors isolated from patients with either nodular
or diffuse histiocytic lymphomas which correspond to the
transformed or lymphoblastic B cells, or to those which correspond to the secretory phase of B cell differentiation,
including Waldenstroms macroglobulinemia and myeloma (Table
2, Fig. 4). These observations of the heterogeneous expression of B2 on non-Hodgkin's lymphomas confirm the in vitro
evidence that the B2 antigen is lost at approximately the
time of transformation of the virgin B cell and to the B
lymphoblast.

"Pre-B" Cell Tumors

     Leukemic cells from approximately 80% of patients with
acute lymphoblastic leukemia (ALL) lack both cell sIg and T
cell antigens. Although these cells are devoid of conventional B or T cell antigens, they express a variety of cell
surface markers including the common acute lymphoblastic
leukemia antigen (CALLA)(119-124) and the Ia-like antigens
(Ia)(91). The cellular origin of these non-T ALL's has been
the subject of numerous studies which, for the most part,
suggest that they are of B cell origin. Several laboratories
have demonstrated that tumor cells from approximately 20-30%
of patients with non-T ALL have a pre-B cell phenotype since
they express intracytoplasmic μ chain but lack cell sIg (107,
125,126). We have previously shown that approximately 50%
of non-T cell ALL's and CML in blast crisis were reactive
with anti-Bl (98,102). Moreover, the non-T cell ALL's and

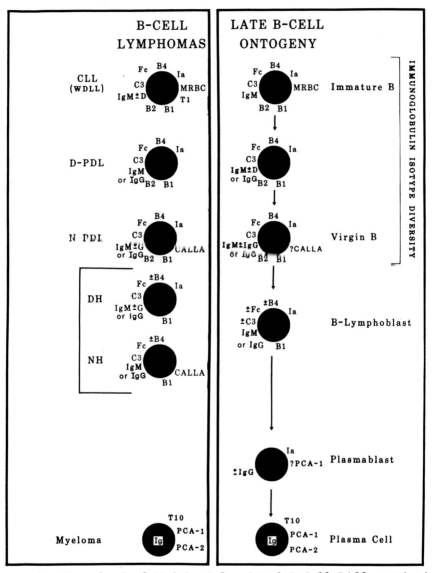

Figure 3.   Hypothetical Model of Committed B Cell Differentiation

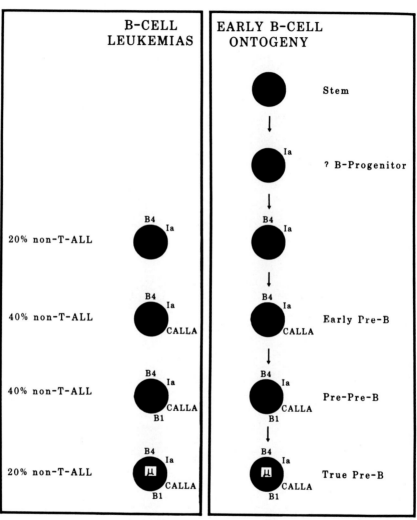

Figure 4. Hypothetical Model of Early B Cell Differentiation

CML in blast crisis can be divided into the following sub-
groups: 1) Ia+CALLA+B1+; 2) Ia+CALLA+B1-; and 3) Ia+CALLA-
B1-. A small number of non-T cell ALL's also co-express the
B2 antigen suggesting that they are more differentiated (99).
These studies provide evidence for the B cell lineage and
heterogeneity of non-T cell ALL.

The cellular origin of the Ia+CALLA+B1- non-T cell ALL's
has also been further investigated (127). Non-T cell ALL
lines and tumor cells isolated from patients with non-T cell
ALL (Ia+CALLA+B1- cytoplasmic μ negative) were studied in
vitro with a variety of agents known to promote cellular
differentiation. Phorbol diester (TPA) or phytohemagglutinin conditioned lymphocyte culture media (PHA-LCM) were capable of inducing the expression of B1 on four non-T cell
ALL lines and the expression of both B1 and cytoplasmic
on 9 patients with non-T cell ALL. In contrast, 5 patients
with Ia+CALLA+B1- cytoplasmic μ negative non-T cell ALL
could not be induced with TPA to express CALLA, B1, or cytoplasmic μ. These studies suggest that non-T cell ALL's are
heterogeneous and represent a spectrum of early B cell differentiation including the pre-pre-B cell (Ia+CALLA+B1-cμ-),
the intermediate pre-B cell (Ia+CALLA+B1+cμ-), and the "true"
pre-B cell (Ia+CALLA+B1+cμ+). Recent studies by Hokland et
al. (128) strongly suggest that CALLA+ fetal hematopoietic
cells are the normal counterparts of non-T ALL.

The cellular origin of the remaining Ia+CALLA-B1- form
of non-T ALL (20%) is still unknown. However, in recent
studies, we have identified another B cell specific antigen,
termed B4, which appears to identify the cell of origin in
most of these patients (Table 2, Figs. 2-4)(129). By indirect immunofluorescence and quantitative absorption, the B4
antigen is also expressed exclusively on Ig+ B cells isolated from peripheral blood and lymphoid tissues. B4 is
weakly expressed on peripheral blood B cells and like B2, is
strongly expressed on lymph node, tonsil and splenic B cells.
By examination of cellular populations in normal bone marrow
and fetal tissue, it appears that B4 is expressed earlier
than B1. Of 35 patients with non-T ALL, 10 co-expressed
both B1 and B4. The 25 patients who did not express B1 did
express B4 and therefore were also of B cell lineage. Thus,
35 of 35 patients (100%) with non-T ALL were of B cell lineage, accounting for the majority of non-T cell ALL, both
CALLA+ and CALLA- (Table 2).

"Early" B Cell Leukemias and Lymphomas

The concomitant expression of sIg, Ia, B1 and B2 on
most B cell chronic lymphocytic leukemia suggests that these
cells may correspond to the immature B cell (Table 2, Fig.4)
(98,99). The T1 antigen, usually expressed on thymocytes
and peripheral blood T lymphocytes, is also found on almost
all CLL cells, but not on peripheral blood B lymphocytes
(130-134). The precise meaning of the expression of T1 on
CLL cells is unknown, but the absence of T1 on most normal
peripheral blood B cells provides one line of evidence that
B cell CLL is not the neoplastic counterpart of these cells.

"Virgin" B and "Transformed" B Cell Tumors

The cellular origin of poorly differentiated lymphocytic lymphoma (PDL) has also been recently studied and is
apparently the "virgin" B cell (Fig. 2). Patients with
nodular lymphoma express moderate amounts of monoclonal sIg,
B1 and Ia, and weaker expression of B2 (Table 2). Of great
interest is the observation that nodular PDL's (NPDL) also
express CALLA, in contrast to the diffuse PDL's (DPDL) which
have an identical phenotype but do not express CALLA (15).
These observations suggest that the nodular and diffuse PDL's
may be derived from distinct populations of B cells. Moreover, preliminary data suggests that the CALLA antigen is
expressed very weakly on germinal center B cells, further
evidence that these tumors are derived from germinal center
B cells. Extracellular cytoplasmic staining for the B2 antigen within nodular lymphoma which exactly reproduces the
pattern observed in normal lymph node germinal centers also
suggests that nodular lymphomas are of germinal center origin (99). Moreover, within nodular lymphomas, those of
phenotype sIg+B2+ were primarily NPDL, while those of Ig+B2-
phenotype were primarily NH, suggesting a correlation between histopathologic subtype and immunologic phenotype (135).
Cases of nodular mixed lymphoma, which are intermediary by
histopathologic characteristics between NPDL and NH, expressed both sIg+B2+ and sIg+B2- phenotypes. Within NPDL,
B2 cell surface staining was most constant on the small cell
types (NPD and NM) whereas extracellular staining was predominant where larger transformed cells were present. This
distribution of staining is consistent with the speculation
that B2 is shed from the surface of larger transformed B
cells and therefore may accumulate extracellularly. It fur-

ther suggests that PDL does correspond to "virgin" B cell
by virtue of its B2 cell surface staining.

In contrast to the poorly differentiated lymphomas,
the diffuse histiocytic lymphomas almost never express B2
and strongly express sIg, B1 and Ia (Table 2)(98,99). They
correspond to the "transformed" B cells or B cell lymphoblast (Figs. 2 and 3). As was true in PDL, nodular histiocytic lymphomas do express CALLA but diffuse histiocytic
lymphomas do not.

Plasma Cell Tumors

Finally, B1, B2 and B4 are B cell specific antigens
which are not expressed at the terminal stage of B cell differentiation, the plasma cell (Figs. 2 and 3). Plasma cells
lack all B cell surface determinants but do express cytoplasmic immunoglobulin (cIg) and a 45,000 molecular weight
surface protein (T10)(89,96). We have recently described
two plasma cell associated antigens (PCA-1 and PCA-2)(136)
that are distinct from previously described B and plasma
cell determinants. Moreover, within the spectrum of B cell
differentiation, PCA-1 and PCA-2 are uniquely expressed on
plasma cells. In a pokeweed mitogen driven model of B cell
differentiation, PCA-1 expression correlates with the appearance of plasma cells whereas PCA-2 was not induced suggesting
that PCA-2 may come later in B cell differentiation. All
plasma cell leukemias, myelomas, and plasmacytomas thus far
tested express both PCA-1 and PCA-2 antigens and do not express other B lineage determinants including B1, B2 and B4
(Table 2). PCA-1 and PCA-2 may therefore prove to be useful for the study of normal and abnormal plasma cells as well
as the definition of heterogeneity within plasma cell dys-
crasias, analogous to the utility of B1 and B2 in the study
of B lymphocytes and their corresponding malignancies.

OVERVIEW

In conclusion, cell surface markers have identified
considerably greater heterogeneity within the human T and B
cell lymphoid neoplasms than was evident by standard morphologic and histochemical techniques. Utilizing markers specific for lineage and state of differentiation, it is now
possible to correlate the malignant lymphocyte with its normal cellular counterpart. Considering the complexity of the

immune system in regard to ontogeny, differentiation, function and migration, it is not surprising that the lymphoid malignancies reflect this degree of diversity. Moreover, the biologic and clinical heterogeneity of these diseases is clearly greater than has been identified by presently employed histopathologic and immunologic classification schemes. The challenge of the next several years is to integrate our understanding of the diversity of the immune system with the clinical and histopathologic heterogeneity of the leukemias and lymphomas in an attempt to devise a more rational classification scheme. Hopefully, this scheme will not only be biologically accurate but more importantly, will identify clinically relevant subgroups of patients.

REFERENCES

1. Hayhoe FGJ, Flemans RJ. (1970). "An Atlas of Haematological Cytology." New York, Wiley-Interscience, p 710.
2. Galton DAG, Catovsky D, Wiltshaw E (1978). Clinical spectrum of lymphoproliferative diseases. Cancer 42:901.
3. Frei E III, Sallan SE (1978). Acute lymphoblastic leukemia: treatment. Cancer 42:828.
4. Hayhoe FGJ, Quagliano M, Doll R (1964). The cytology and cytochemistry of acute leukemias: a study of 140 cases. London: Her Majesty's Stationery Office.
5. Rappaport, H (1966). Tumors of the hematopoietic system. In: "Atlas of Tumor Pathology, Section 3, Fascicle 8" Washington, D.C., Armed Forces Institute of Pathology, p 13.
6. Braylan RC, Jaffe ES, Berard CW (1975). Malignant lymphomas: current classification and new observations. Pathol Annu 10:213.
7. Bennett JM, Catovsky D, Daniel MT, et al (1976). Proposals for the classification of the acute leukemias. Br J Haematol 33:451.
8. Gralnick HR, Galton DAG, Catovsky D, Sulton C, Bennett JM (1977). Classification of acute leukemia. Ann Intern Med 87:740
9. Dorfman RF (1977). Pathology of the non-Hodgkin's lymphomas: new classification. Cancer Treat. Rep 61:945.
10. Aisenberg AC, Bloch KJ (1972). Immunoglobulins on the

surface of neoplastic lymphocytes. N Engl J Med 287:272.

11. Borella L, Sen L (1973). T cell surface markers on lymphoblasts from acute lymphocytic leukemia. J Immunol 111:1257.

12. Brouet JC, Seligmann M (1978). The immunological classification of acute lymphoblastic leukemia. Cancer 42:817.

13. Siegal FP (1978). Cytoidentity of the lymphoreticular neoplasms. In: Twomey JJ, Good RA (eds): "The Immunopathology of Lymphoreticular Neoplasms." New York, Plenum Press, p 281.

14. Mann RB, Jaffe ES, Berard CW (1979). Malignant lymphomas: a conceptual understanding of morphologic diversity. Review Am J Pathol 94:104.

15. Nadler LM, Ritz J, Griffin JD, Todd RF, Reinherz EL, Schlossman SF (1981). Diagnosis and treatment of human leukemias and lymphomas utilizing monoclonal antibodies. Prog Hematol XII:187.

16. Bloomfield CA, Kersey JH, Brunning RD, Gajl-Peczalska KJ (1976). Prognostic significance of lymphocyte surface markers in adult non-Hodgkin's malignant lymphoma. Lancet 2:1330.

17. Chessells JM, Hardisty RM, Rapson NT, Greaves MF (1977). Acute lymphoblastic leukemia in children: classification and prognosis. Lancet 2:1307.

18. Bloomfield CD, Gajl-Peczalska KJ, Frizzera G, Kersey JH, Goldman AI (1979). Clinical utility of lymphocyte surface markers combined with the Lukes-Collins histologic classification in adult lymphoma. N Engl J Med 301:512.

19. Chess L, Schlossman SF (1977). Human lymphocyte subpopulations. In: Dixon FJ, Kunkel HG (eds): "Advanced Immunology, Vol. 25" New York, Academic Press, p 213

20. Portlock CS, Rosenberg SA (1979). No initial therapy for stage III and IV non-Hodgkin's lymphomas of favorable histologic types. Ann Intern Med 90:10.

21. Jones SE, Rosenberg SA, Kaplan HS et al. (1972). Non-Hodgkin's lymphomas. II. Single agent chemotherapy. Cancer 30:31.

22. Bagley CM, DeVita VT, Berard CW, Canellos GP (1972). Advanced lymphosarcoma: intensive cyclical combination chemotherapy with cyclophosphamide, vincristine and prednisone. Ann Intern Med 76:227.

23. Stein RS, Moran EM, Desser RK et al (1974). Combination chemotherapy of lymphomas other than Hodgkin's disease. Ann Intern Med 81:601.

24. Portlock CS, Rosenberg SA, Glatstein E, Kaplan HS (1976).

Treatment of advanced non-Hodgkin's lymphomas with favorable histologies: Preliminary results of a prospective trial. Blood 47:747.

25. Bender RA, DeVita VT (1978). Non-Hodgkin's lymphoma.
In: Staquet MJ (ed): "Randomized Clinical Trials in
Cancer: A Critical Review by Sites." New York, Raven
Press, p 77.

26. Chabner BA (1979). Nodular non-Hodgkin's lymphomas:
the case for watchful waiting. Ann Intern Med 90:115.

27. Anderson T, Bender RA, Fisher RI et al (1977). Combination chemotherapy in non-Hodgkin's lymphoma: Results
of long term follow up. Cancer Treat Rep 61:1057.

28. Osborne CK, Norton L., Young RC et al (1980). Nodular
histiocytic lymphoma: An aggressive nodular lymphoma
with potential for prolonged disease free survival.
Blood 56:98.

29. Portlock CS (1980). Management of indolent non-Hodgkin's
lymphomas. Sem Oncol 7:292.

30. Pangalis GA, Nathwani BN, Rappaport H (1977). Malignant
lymphoma, well differentiated lymphocytic. Its relationship with chronic lymphocytic leukemia and macroglobulinemia of Waldenstrom. Cancer 39:999.

31. Schein PS, Chabner BA, Canellos GP et al (1974). Potential for prolonged disease free survival following combination chemotherapy of non-Hodgkin's lymphoma. Blood
43:181.

32. Luce JK, Delaney FC, Gehan EA (1973). Remission induction chemotherapy of malignant lymphoma with combination bleomycin, cyclophosphamide, vincristine and prednisone. Proc Am Assoc Cancer Res 14:66.

33. Bonadonna G, Berretta G, Tancini G et al. (1974). Adriamycin in combination and in combined treatment modalities. Tumori 60:393.

34. DeVita VT, Chabner B, Hubbard SP et al. (1975). Advanced
diffuse histiocytic lymphoma, a potentially curable
disease. Lancet 1:248.

35. Durant JR, Loeb VJ, Dorfman R, Chan YK (1975). 1,3-bis
(2-chloroethyl)-1-nitrosourea (BCNU), cyclophosphamide
vincristine and prednisone (BCOP). A new therapeutic
regimen for diffuse histiocytic lymphoma. Cancer 36:1936.

36. Berd D, Cornog J., DeConti RC et al (1975). Long term
remission in diffuse histiocytic lymphoma treated with
combination sequential chemotherapy. Cancer 35:1050.

37. Nathwani BN, Kim H, Rappaport H (1976). Malignant lymphoma, lymphoblastic. Cancer 38:964.

38. Schein PS, DeVita VT, Hubbard S et al (1976). Bleomycin,

adriamycin, cyclophosphamide, vincristine, and prednisone (BACOP) combination chemotherapy in the treatment
of advanced diffuse histiocytic lymphoma. Ann Intern
Med 85:417.

39. McKelvey EM, Gottlieb JA, Wilson HE (1976). Hydroxyl-
daunomycin (Adriamycin) combination chemotherapy in
malignant lymphoma. Cancer 38:1484.

40. Rodriguez V, Cabanillas F, Burgess MA et al (1977).
Combination chemotherapy ("CHOP-Bleo") in advanced
(non-Hodgkin's) malignant lymphoma. Blood 49:325.

41. Skarin AT, Rosenthal DS, Maloney WC, Frei E III (1977).
Combination chemotherapy of advanced non-Hodgkin's lymphoma with bleomycin,adriamycin, cyclophosphamide,vin-
cristine, and prednisone (BACOP). Blood 49:759.

42. Elias L, Portlock CS, Rosenberg SA (1978). Combination
chemotherapy of diffuse histiocytic lymphoma with cyclophosphamide, adriamycin, vincristine and prednisone
(CHOP). Cancer 42:1705.

43. Rosen PJ, Feinstein DI, Pattengale PK et al(1978).
Convoluted lymphocytic lymphoma in adults. A clinico
pathologic entity. Ann Intern Med 89:319.

44. Harrison DT, Neiman PE, Sullivan K et al (1978). Combined modality therapy for advanced diffuse lymphocytic
and histiocytic lymphomas. Cancer 42:1697.

45. Sweet DL, Golomb HM, Mann JE et al (1980). Cyclophosphamide, vincristine, methotrexate with leukovorin rescue, and cytosine arbinoside (COMLA) combination sequential chemotherapy in the treatment of advanced diffuse
histiocytic lymphoma. Ann Intern Med 92:785.

46. Fisher RI, DeVita VT, Hubbard SM et al (1980). Pro-
MACE-MOPP combination chemotherapy: Treatment of diffuse
lymphomas. Proc. ASCO 16:468.

47. Sweet DL, Golomb HM (1980). The treatment of histiocytic lymphoma. Sem Oncol 7:302.

48. Canellos GP, Leonard RCF (1982). Management of non-
Hodgkin's lymphomas of unfavorable prognosis. Cancer
Topics 3(12):137.

49. Stein RS, Cousar J, Flexner JM et al (1979). Malignant
lymphomas of follicular center origin in man. III.
Prognostic features. Cancer 44:2236.

50. Stein RS, Cousar J, Flexner JM, Collins RD (1980). Correlations between immunologic markers and histopathologic classifications: clinical implications. Sem Oncol
7:244.

51. Strauchen JA, Young RC, DeVita VT et al (1978). Clinical relevance of the histopathological subclassifica-

tion of diffuse "histiocytic" lymphoma. N Engl J Med 299:1382.

52. Gajl-Peczalska KJ, Bloomfield CD, Coucia PF et al. (1975). B and T cell lymphomas. Analysis of blood and lymph nodes in 87 patients. Am J Med 59:674.

53. Brouet JC, Labaume S, Seligmann M (1975). Evaluation of T and B lymphocyte membrane markers in human non-Hodgkin's malignant lymphomas. Br J Cancer 31:121.

54. Davey FR, Goldberg J, Stockman J, Gottlieb AJ (1976). Immunologic and cytochemical cell markers in non-Hodgkin's lymphomas. Lab Invest 35:430.

55. Berard CW, Jaffe ES, Braylon RC et al (1978). Immunologic aspects and pathology of malignant lymphomas. Cancer 42:911.

56. Filippa DA, Lieberman PH, Erlandson RA et al (1978). A study of malignant lymphomas using light and ultra-microscopic, cytochemical and immunologic techniques. Am J Med 64:259.

57. Li C, Harrison EG (1978). Histochemical and immunohis-tochemical study of diffuse large cell lymphomas. Am J Clin Pathol 70:721.

58. Epstein AL, Levy R, Kim H et al (1978). Biology of the human malignant lymphomas. IV. Functional characteri-zation of ten diffuse histiocytic lymphoma cell lines. Cancer 42:2379.

59. Said JW, Hargreaves HK, Pinkus GS (1979). Non-Hodgkin's lymphomas: An ultrastructural study correlating mor-phology with immunologic cell type. Cancer 44:504.

60. Warnke R, Miller R, Grogan T, Pederson M, Dilley J, Levy R (1980). Immunologic phenotype in 30 patients with diffuse large cell lymphoma. N Engl J Med 303:293.

61. Gajl-Peczalska JK, Bloomfield CD, Frizzera G et al. (1982). Diversity of phenotypes of malignant lymphomas (ML) defined by a panel of 14 monoclonal antibodies and other lymphocyte markers. Proc AACR 23:115.

62. Barcos M, Minato K, Minowada J et al (1982). Monoclonal and heterologous reagents in the phenotyping of lympho-mas. Proc AACR 23:255.

63. Ford RJ, Davis F, Kusy KC et al (1982). Cell surface phenotype and functional characterization of non-Hodg-kin's lymphomas. Proc AACR 23:251.

64. Evans RL, Lazarus H, Penta AC et al (1978). Two func-tionally distinct subpopulations of human T cells that collaborate in the generation of cytotoxic cells respon-sible for cell-mediated lympholysis. J. Immunol. 120:1423.

65. Reinherz EL, Schlossman SF (1979). Con A inducible suppression of MLC: evidence for mediation by the TH2+ T cell subset in man. J Immunol 122:1335.

66. Reinherz EL, Schlossman SF (1980). The differentiation and function of human T lymphocytes: A review. Cell 19:821.

67. Reinherz EL, Kung PC, Goldstein G, Schlossman SF (1979). A monoclonal antibody with selective reactivity with functionally mature thymocytes and all peripheral human T cells. J Immunol 123:1312.

68. Reinherz EL, Kung PC, Pesando JM et al (1979). Ia determinants on human T cell subsets defined by monoclonal antibody: activation stimuli required for expression. J.Exp Med 150:1472.

69. van Agthoven A, Terhorst C, Reinherz EL et al (1981). Characterization of T cell surface glycoproteins T1 and T3 present on all human peripheral T lymphocytes and functionally mature thymocytes. Eur J Immunol 11:18.

70. Reinherz EL, Hussey RE, Schlossman SF (1980). A monoclonal antibody blocking human T cell function. Eur J Immunol 10:758.

71. Meuer S, Schlossman SF, Reinherz EL (1982). Clonal analysis of human cytotoxic T lymphocytes: T4+ and T8+ effector T cells recognize products of different major histocomatibility complex regions. Proc Natl Acad Sci USA 79:4395.

72. Reinherz EL, Kung PC, Goldstein G et al (1979). Separation of functional subsets of human T cells by a monoclonal antibody. Proc Natl Acad Sci USA 76:4061.

73. Reinherz EL, Kung PC, Goldstein G, Schlossman SF (1979). Further characterization of the human inducer T cell subset defined by monoclonal antibody. J Immunol 123: 2894.

74. Reinherz EL, Kung PC, Goldstein G, Schlossman SF (1980). A monoclonal antibody reactive with the human cytotoxic/ suppressor T cell subset previously defined by a heteroantiserum termed TH2. J Immunol 124:1301.

75. Terhorst C, van Agthoven A, Reinherz EL, Schlossman SF (1980). Biochemical analysis of human T lymphocyte differentiation antigens T4 and T5. Science 209:520.

76. Reinherz EL, Kung PC, Goldstein G et al (1980). Discrete stages of human intrathymic differentiation: analysis of normal thymocytes and leukemic lymphoblasts of T lineage. Proc Natl Acad Sci USA 77:1588.

77. Terhorst C, van Agthoven A, LeClair K et al (1981). Biochemical studies of human thymocyte cell surface

antigens T6, T9 and T10. Cell 23:771.

78. von Wauwe J, Goossens J, DeCock W et al (1981). Suppression of human T cell mitogenesis and E rosette formation by the monoclonal antibody OKT11A. Immunol 44:865.

79. Nadler LM, Reinherz EL, Weinstein HJ, D'Orsi CJ, Schlossman SF (1980). Heterogeneity of T cell lymphoblastic malignancies. Blood 55:806.

80. Nadler LM, Reinherz EL, Schlossman SF (1980). The T lymphoblastic malignancies: a review. Cancer Chemother Pharmacol 4:11.

81. Reinherz EL, Nadler LM, Sallan SE, Schlossman SF (1979). Subset derivation of T cell acute lymphoblastic leukemia in man. J Clin Invest 64:392.

82. Bernard A, Boumsell L, Reinherz EL et al (1981). Malignant T cells from acute lymphoblastic leukemia and from malignant lymphomas exhibit different patterns of surface antigens. Blood 57:1105.

83. Jaffe ES, Berard CW (1978). Lymphoblastic lymphoma, a term rekindled with new precision. Ann Int Med 89:415.

84. Reinherz EL, Nadler LM, Rosenthal DS et al (1979). T cell subset characterization of human T-CLL. Blood 53:1066.

85. Boumsell L, Bernard A, Reinherz EL et al (1981). Surface antigens on malignant Sezary and T-CLL cells correspond to those of mature T cells. Blood 57:526.

86. Froland SS, Natvig JB (1970). Effect of polyspecific rabbit anti-immunoglobulin antisera on human lymphocytes in vitro. Int Arch Allerg Appl Immunol 39:121.

87. Froland SS, Natvig JB, Berdal P (1971). Surface bound immunoglobulin as a marker of B lymphocytes in man. Nature New Biol (Lond) 234:251.

88. Gathings WE, Lawton AR, Cooper MD (1977). Immunofluorescent studies of the development of pre-B cells, B lymphocytes and immunoglobulin isotype diversity in humans. Eur J Immunol 7:804.

89. Stashenko P, Nadler LM, Hardy R, Schlossman SF (1981). Expression of cell surface markers after human B lymphocyte activation. Proc Natl Acad Sci USA 78:3848.

90. Winchester RJ, Fu SM, Wernet P et al (1975). Recognition by pregnancy serum of non-HLA alloantigen selectivity expressed on B lymphocytes. J Exp Med 141:924.

91. Schlossman SF, Chess L, Humphreys RE, Strominger JL (1976). Distribution of Ia-like molecules on the surface of normal and leukemic human cells. Proc Natl Acad Sci USA 73:1288.

92. Huber H, Douglas SD, Fudenberg HH (1969). The IgG re-

ceptor: an immunological marker for the characterization of mononuclear cells. Immunology 17:7.

93. Bianco C, Patrick R, Nussenzweig V (1970). A population of lymphocytes bearing a membrane receptor for antigen-antibody complement complexes. J Exp Med 132:702.

94. Dickler HB, Kunkel HG (1972). Interaction of the aggregated γ globulin with B lymphocytes. J Exp Med 136:191.

95. Ross GD, Rabellino EM, Polley MJ, Grey HM (1973). Combined studies of complement receptor and surface immunoglobulin bearing cells in normal and leukemic human lymphocytes. J Clin Invest 52:377.

96. Reinherz EL, Schlossman SF (1981). Regulatory T cell subsets in man. Immunol Today 2:69.

97. Brooks DA, Beckman I, Bradley J et al (1980). Human lymphocyte markers defined by antibodies derived from somatic cell hybrids. I. A hybridoma secreting antibody against a marker specific for human B lymphocytes. Clin Exp Immunol 39:477.

98. Stashenko P, Nadler LM, Hardy R, Schlossman SF (1980). Characterization of a human B lymphocyte specific antigen. J. Immunol 125:1678.

99. Nadler LM, Stashenko P, Hardy R et al (1981). Characterization of a human B cell specific antigen (B2) distinct from B1. J Immunol 126:1941.

100. Greaves MF, Verbi W, Kemshead J, Kennet R (1980). A monoclonal antibody identifying a cell surface antigen shared by common acute lymphoblastic leukemias and B lineage cells. Blood 56:1141.

101. Abramson C, Kersey J, Lebien T (1981). A monoclonal antibody (BA-1) reactive with cells of human B lymphocyte lineage. J Immunol 126:83.

102. Nadler LM, Stashenko P, Ritz J et al (1981). A unique cell surface antigen identifying lymphoid malignancies of B cell origin. J Clin Invest 67:134.

103. Raff MC, Wegson J, Owen JJT, Cooper MD (1976). Early production of intracellular IgM by B lymphocyte precursors in mouse. Nature 259:224.

104. Cooper MD (1981). Pre-B cells: normal and abnormal development. J Clin Immunol 1:81.

105. Okos AT, Gathings WE (1977). Characterization of precursor B cells in human bone marrow. Fed Proc 36:1294A.

106. Osmond DG (1980). Production and differentiation of B lymphocytes in the bone marrow. In: Battisto JR, Knight KL (eds): "Immunoglobulin Genes and B Cell Differentiation." Elsevier/North Holland, New York, p 135.

107. Vogler LB, Crist WM, Blockman DE et al (1978). Pre-B

cell leukemia: a new phenotype of childhood lymphoblastic leukemia. N Engl J Med 298:872.

108. Pellegrino MA, Ferrone S, Theofilopoulous AW (1975). Rosette formation on human lymphoid cells with monkey red blood cells.

109. Gupta S, Grieco MH (1976). Rosette formation with mouse erythrocytes: Probable marker for human B lymphocytes. Int Arch Allergy Appl Immunol 49:734.

110. Gupta S, Pahwa R et al (1976). Ontogeny of lymphocyte subpopulations in human fetal liver. Proc Natl Acad Sci USA 73:919.

111. Vossen JM, Hijmans W (1975). Membrane associated immunoglobulin determinants on bone marrow and blood lymphocytes in the pediatric age group and on fetal tissues. Ann NY Acad Sci 254:262.

112. Abney E, Parkhouse RME (1974). Candidate for immunoglobulin D present on murine lymphocytes. Nature (Lond) 252:600.

113. Vitetta ES, Melcher V, McWilliams M et al (1975). Cell surface immunoglobulin. XI. The appearance of an IgD-like molecule on murine lymphoid cells during ontogeny. J Exp Med 141:206.

114. Coffman RL, Cohn M (1977). The class of surface immunoglobulin on virgin and memory B lymphocytes. J Immunol 118:1806.

115. Parkhouse RME, Cooper MD (1977). A model for the differentiation of lymphocytes with implications for the biological role of IgD. Immunol Rev 37:105.

116. Bourgois A, Kitajima K, Hunger IR, Askonas BA (1977). Surface immunoglobulins of lipopolysaccharide stimulated spleen cells. The behavior of IgM, IgD and IgG. Eur J Immunol 7:151.

117. Parkhouse RME, Dresser DW (1978). In: "Advances in Experimental Medicine and Biology: Secretory Immunity." Plenum Press, New York, p 43.

118. Bhan AK, Nadler LM, Stashenko P, Schlossman SF (1981). Stages of B cell differentiation in human lymphoid tissues. J Exp Med 154:737.

119. Greaves MF, Brown G, Rapson NT, Lister TA (1975). Antisera to acute lymphoblastic leukemia cells. Clin Immunol Immunopathol 4:67.

120. Pesando JM, Ritz J, Lazarus H et al (1979). Leukemia-associated antigens in ALL. Blood 54:1240.

121. Billing R, Minowada J, Cline M et al (1978). Acute lymphocytic leukemia associated cell membrane antigen. J Natl Cancer Inst 61:423.

122. Ritz J, Pesando JM, Notis-McConarty J et al (1980). A monoclonal antibody to human acute lymphoblastic antigen. Nature 283:583.

123. Greaves MF (1981). Monoclonal antibodies as probes for leukemic heterogeneity and hemapoietic differentiation. In: Knapp W (ed): "Leukemia Markers" Academic Press, New York, p 19.

124. Nadler LM, Ritz J, Reinherz EL, Schlossman SF (1981). Cellular origins of human leukemias and lymphomas. In: Knapp W (ed): "Leukemia Markers" Academic Press, New York, p 10.

125. Brouet JC, Preud'homme JL, Peut C et al (1979). Acute lymphoblastic leukemia with pre-B cell characteristics. Blood 54:269.

126. Greaves MF, Verbi FW, Vogler LR et al (1979). Antigenic and enzymatic phenotypes of the pre-B subclass of acute lymphoblastic leukemias. Leuk Res 3:353.

127. Nadler LM, Ritz J, Bates MP et al (1982). Induction of human B cell antigens in non-T cell acute lymphoblastic leukemia. J Clin Invest (In press).

128. Hokland P, Rosenthal P, Griffin JD et al (1982). Purification and characterization of fetal hematopoietic cells which express the common acute lymphoblastic leukemia antigen (CALLA). J Exp Med (Submitted).

129. Nadler LM, Bates MP, Park EK et al (1982). Unique stages of early B cell differentiation defined by a B cell specific monoclonal antibody (B4). In preparation.

130. Boumsell L, Coppin H, Pham D et al (1980). An antigen shared by a human T cell subset and B cell chronic lymphocytic leukemic cells. J Exp Med 152:229.

131. Kamoun M, Kadis M, Martin P et al (1981). A novel human T cell antigen preferentially expressed on mature T cells and shared by both well and poorly differentiated B cell leukemias and lymphomas. J Immunol 127:987.

132. Royston I, Jagda JA, Baird SM et al (1980). Human T cell antigens defined by monoclonal antibodies: the 65,000 dalton antigen of T cells (T 65) is also found on chronic lymphocytic leukemia cells bearing surface immunoglobulin. J Immunol 125:725.

133. Foon KA, Billing RJ, Terasaki PI (1980). Dual B and T markers in acute and chronic lymphocytic leukemia. Blood 55:16.

134. Martin PJ, Hansen JA, Siadale AW, Nowinski RC (1981). Monoclonal antibodies recognizing normal and human T lymphocytes and malignant human B lymphocytes: a comparative study. J Immunol 127:1920.

135. Nadler LM, Bhan AK, Harris NL et al (1982). Nodular lymphomas correspond to discrete phases of B cell differentiation. J Clin Invest (Submitted).
136. Anderson KC, Park EK, Bates MP et al (1982). Antigens on human plasma cells identified by monoclonal antibodies. J Immunol (Submitted).

ACKNOWLEDGEMENTS

We would like to thank John F. Daley and Lori Palley for their excellent technical assistance.

Rational Basis for Chemotherapy, pages 239–247
© 1983 Alan R. Liss, Inc., 150 Fifth Avenue, New York, NY 10011

MECHANISM OF ACTION OF DEOXYADENOSINE/ADENOSINE DEAMINASE
INHIBITOR COMBINATIONS: LYMPHOTOXICITY
IN G_1 AND G_0 PHASES OF THE CELL CYCLE

Richard M. Fox and Richard F. Kefford

Ludwig Institute for Cancer Research (Sydney Branch)
Blackburn Building, University of Sydney
Sydney. N.S.W. 2006. Australia

ABSTRACT   DNA flow cytometry has been used to
investigate the mechanism of deoxyadenosine (dAdo)
toxicity in cultured lymphoid cells. dAdo was shown to
cause a G_1 block in T lymphoblasts, and cells in S-
phase exposed to dAdo were able to complete that S-
phase, pass through G_2 +M and return to the G_1 phase.
By contrast, dAdo resistant B lymphoblasts were blocked
in S-phase. Human peripheral blood lymphocytes (PBL)
showed elevation of their dATP pools on incubation with
dAdo, to a similar extent as T lymphoblasts. Furthermore, these G_0 PBL were killed by μM concentrations of
dAdo. T cell and PBL dATP pool rises were prevented
by coincubation with deoxycytidine which also prevented cytotoxicity. The exact biochemical mechanism
of G_1/G_0 lymphoid toxicity, which appears to be dATP
mediated, is not known.

INTRODUCTION

Drugs which inhibit the enzyme Adenosine Deaminase
(ADA), in particular deoxycoformycin used in the treatment of
T cell and other leukemias, have stimulated interest in dAdo
mediated cytotoxicity (1). The recognition that human combined immune deficiency is associated with inborn ADA deficiency has also focused attention on the importance of
purine nucleoside metabolism and toxicity in the lymphoid
system (2). Cultured human T leukemic lymphoblasts (in the
presence of ADA inhibitors) are highly sensitive to dAdo
induced cytotoxicity; while Epstein-Barr Virus (EBV) trans-

formed B cell lines are resistant. These cell lines have
proven valuable models to study dAdo metabolism and toxicity
(3).

Several mechanisms have been postulated to explain the
selective toxicity of dAdo to T cells. The first of these
reflects excessive intracellular accumulation of dATP
following dAdo phosphorylation. This high dATP pool has been
considered to allosterically inhibit ribonucleotide reductase with consequent cessation of DNA replication (2). An
alternative nucleotide independent mechanism of toxicity has
been proposed based on dAdo inactivation of S-adenosylhomocysteine hydrolase resulting in inhibition of methylation(4).

We have investigated dAdo mediated toxicity in cultured
T leukemic and EBV-transformed B-lymphocyte lines as well as
human PBL. We demonstrate that dAdo induces a specific G_1
arrest in T lymphocytes, and kills G_0 PBL, associated with
rises in their respective dATP pools. The G_1 arrest, PBL
toxicity and elevations in dATP pools were prevented by
deoxycytidine (dCyd) indicating a nucleotide dependent
toxicity. These findings imply dATP mediated toxicity independent of DNA replication and ribonucleotide reductase
inhibition.

METHODS

Human lymphocyte lines and PBL were cultured as previously described (5,6). DNA flow cytometry and fluorescent
staining for DNA was performed using established techniques
(7,8). Deoxyribonucleoside triphosphate pools were measured
using the DNA polymerase assay (5), and centrifugal
elutriation fractionation as previously described by us (9).
S-adenosylhomocysteine hydrolase was assayed by the method
of Hershfield (4).

RESULTS

DNA Flow Cytometry Studies of dAdo Growth Inhibition of Cultured T cells

Human leukemic CCRF-CEM cells (T type) were incubated with 3μM dAdo (with 5μM erythro-9-(3-(2-hydroxynonyl) adenine, (EHNA), an ADA inhibitor). At this dAdo concentration, the number of viable cells remain constant over 48 hours. DNA flow cytometry, using 33342 Hoechst dye, was performed at selected time intervals after addition of dAdo. This fluorescent benzimidazole compound binds specifically to thymine bases in DNA. Four hours after addition of dAdo, disappearance of cells with an early S-phase content of DNA was apparent. At 8 hours after addition of dAdo the majority of cells were in G_1, with residual late S-phase and G_2 -M cells. By 16 hours, predominantly G_1 phase cells remained (Fig. 1).

When cells are grown in media containing bromodeoxy-uridine (BrdUrd), this is incorporated into newly synthe-sised DNA strands. Bromouracil bases are larger than thymine and will not bind 33342 Hoechst. Cells completing a replication cycle in the presence of BrdUrd will thus have their DNA tagged Hoechst fluorescence reduced to 50% of original intensity. Thus, studies identical to those above were carried out with the addition of BrdUrd (5μM) to the medium. By 16 - 24 hours, there was the progressive appearance of cells with fluorescence in channel 30 - 40 (i.e. less than "G_1" DNA fluorescence (Fig. 2).

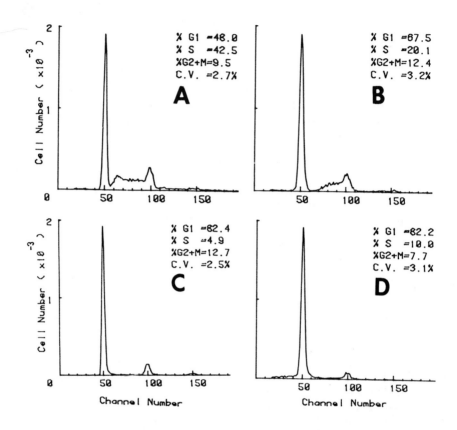

FIGURE 1.   DNA distribution of CCRF-CEM cells following
exposure to dAdo (3μM), in the presence of 5μM EHNA.
Cells were stained with 33342 Hoechst dye prior to
flow cytometry.   Channel number corresponds to relative
fluorescence intensity (DNA content).   Number of cells
is shown on the ordinate.   A - 4 hrs, B - 8 hrs,
C - 16 hrs and D - 24 hrs.

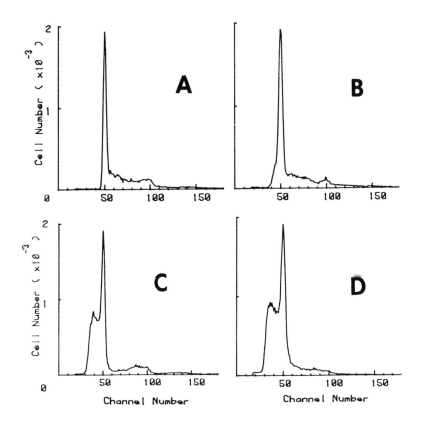

FIGURE 2. DNA distribution of CCRF-CEM cells following exposure to dAdo (3µM), in the presence of 5µM EHNA, using BrdUrd (5µM) to quench 33342 Hoechst dye fluorescence. Channel number corresponds to relative fluorescence intensity (DNA content). Number of cells is shown on the ordinate. A - 4 hrs, B - 8 hrs, C - 16 hrs and D - 24 hrs.

These studies indicate that dAdo, at a cytostatic concentration, has induced a G_1 block and those cells in S were capable of continuing that round of DNA replication, pass through G_2 -M and reaccumulate in G_1. These findings were confirmed in 2 other human T cell lines and 3 murine T cell lines.

By contrast, EBV-B cell lines exposed to cytostatic concentrations of dAdo (400μM in the presence of 5μM EHNA) and stained with Hoechst stain demonstrated accumulation of cells in the S-phase (data not shown).

dAdo Toxicity to Human Peripheral Blood Lymphocytes

Unstimulated PBL were killed by incubation with dAdo (with 5μM EHNA). This toxicity was both dAdo concentration and time dependent. For instance, 1μM dAdo killed 50% of cells after 72 hours of incubation and 90% by 96 hours. Increasing the concentration of dAdo killed a greater percentage of cells, but did not kill cells within the first 24 hours of incubation. DNA flow cytometry studies indicate these cells are not replicating their DNA, i.e. are in G_0.

The toxicity of 1μM dAdo was entirely prevented by coincubation with dCyd (50μM), while cells treated with 30μM and coincubated with 50μM dCyd, protection was only partial with 30% of cells alive at 96 hours, compared to 8% of cells treated with dAdo alone.

Deoxynucleoside Triphosphate Pool Changes Following Incubation with dAdo

When CCRF-CEM cells were exposed to 3μM dAdo (in the presence of 5μM EHNA), there was a time dependent rise in the dATP pool to almost 10-fold by 24 hours. This was not associated with a fall in the dCTP pool. In cells exposed simultaneously to dAdo (3μM) and dCyd (100μM), the rise in the dATP pool was prevented. Similarly, unstimulated PBL incubated with dAdo in the presence of 5μM EHNA elevated their dATP pools. After 4 hours incubation with 1μM dAdo, the dATP pool was elevated 2 x, and with 100μM dAdo, there was a 40 x elevation.

CCRF-CEM cells were enriched for various phases of the cell cycle by centrifugal elutration. In cells exposed to dAdo (4 hours) prior to elutration, the dATP pools were elevated approximately 4-fold, independent of their position in the cell cycle (Table 1).

TABLE 1

EFFECT OF dAdo ON CEM dATP/dCTP POOLS. CELL
CYCLE SPECIFIC ENRICHMENT BY ELUTRIATION[a]

Fraction	G_1%	$S + G_2$ -M	dATP	dCTP
			% change from control	
1	92	8	372	80
2	82	18	410	83
3	51	49	512	112
4	20	80	269	104

[a]Determinations of % of cells in various phases of
the cell cycle was made from DNA content histograms
derived by flow cytometry

Independence of dAdo Mediated Cytotoxicity and S-Adenosylhomocysteine Hydrolase Inhibition

    The pattern of inhibition of S-adenosylhomocysteine
hydrolase (AdoHcyase) (and its recovery) produced by dAdo
was studied in cultured T and B lymphoblasts and unstimulated
PBL. In the presence of 5µM EHNA, the AdoHcyase activity
was inhibited 50% after 1 hour incubation by 3µM, 10µM and
30µM dAdo for B lymphoblasts, T-lymphoblasts and PBL respectively, cytotoxicity (to 50% of controls) was effected by
600µM, 3µM and 1µM dAdo respectively. Coincubation with
50µM Cyd which protects T lymphoblasts and PBL from dAdo
cytotoxicity had no effect on the pattern of inhibition
of AdoHycase activity.

DISCUSSION

DNA flow cytometry study of dAdo induced inhibition of
leukemic cell growth demonstrate dAdo induces a G_1 block.
Of particular interest is the observation that those cells
in S-phase, during exposure to dAdo complete that S-phase,
pass through the G_2 -M phase and re-enter G_1. These
findings suggest that the dAdo is acting independently of
ribonucleotide reductase inhibition or an effect on DNA
polymerase. This is supported by the toxicity of dAdo to
unstimulated human PBL, which are in G_0.

The G_1 phase block and PBL toxicity is accompanied by a dATP pool rise, both preventable by coincubation with dCyd. It is possible that the G_1 block induced in replicating T lymphoblasts and toxicity to unstimulated PBL reflect a common biochemical mechanism. The mechanism of dCyd protection does not appear to reflect replenishment of a depleted dCTP but competition with dAdo for phosphorylation to dATP. There is strong evidence that dAdo and dCyd kinase are the same enzyme (10). Evidence that the type of dAdo toxicity described in this presentation is nucleotide dependent, i.e. presumably dATP mediated is: a) dCyd reversibility of toxicity, accompanied by a fall in dATP pool levels, b) the lack of effect of dCyd on the pattern of AdoHcyase inhibition in both cultured lymphoblasts and PBL, c) the high concentrations of dAdo required to inhibit growth of B cell lines, which correlates with a high threshold for dATP accumulation rather than AdoHcyase inhibition.

The exact biochemical mechanisms by which dAdo, presumably via dATP, induces a G_1 block of G_0 toxicity is not known. The G_1 block phenomena has some analogy with the restriction or committment points described by Pardee (11). Further analogies for dAdo lymphoid toxicity are the G_1 block induced by both dibutyryl cyclic-AMP and glucocorticoids in T lymphoblasts (12. 13). Clearly. further investigation of the mechanisms of dAdo toxicity will increase our insight into regulatory mechanisms of lymphoid cells.

REFERENCES

1.   Prentice HG, Ganeshagaru K, Bradstock KF, Goldstone AH, Smyth JF, Wonke B, Janossy G, Hoffbrand AV (1980). Remission induction with adenosine deaminase inhibitor 2'deoxycoformycin in Thy-lymphoblastic leukaemia. Lancet. 2:170.
2.   Seegmiller JE, Thompson L, Willis R, Matsumoto S, Carson D (1980). Nucleotide and nucleoside metabolism and lymphocyte function. In Gelfand EW, Dosch HM (eds): "Biochemical Basis of Immunodeficiency", New York: Raven Press, p 25.
3.   Carson DA, Kay J, Matsumoto S, Seegmiller JE, Thompson L (1979). Biochemical basis for the enhanced toxicity of deoxyribonucleosides towards malignant human T cell lines. Proc. Natl. Acad. Sci. U.S.A. 76:2430.

4.   Hershfield MS (1979). Apparent suicide inactivation of human lymphoblast S-adenosylhomocysteine hydrolase by 2'deoxyadenosine and adenine arabinoside. J. Biol. Chem. 254:22.

5.   Fox RM, Piddington SK, Tripp EH, Tattersall MHN (1981). Ecto-adenosine triphosphatase deficiency in cultured human T and Null leukemic lymphocytes. A biochemical basis for thymidine sensitivity. J. Clin. Invest. 68:544.

6.   Kefford RF, Fox RM (1982). Purine deoxynucleoside toxicity in nondividing human lymphoid cells. Cancer Research. 42:324.

7.   Taylor IW, Milthorpe BK (1980). An evaluation of DNA fluorochromes, staining techniques and analysis for flow cytometry: I. Unperturbed cell populations. J. Histochem. Cytochem. 28:1224.

8.   Bulmor RM (1979). Flow cytometric cell cycle analysis using the quenching of 33258 Hoechst fluorescence by bromodeoxyuridine incorporation. Cell Tissue Kinet 12:101.

9.   Piper AA, Tattersall MHN, Fox RM (1980). The activities of thymidine metabolising enzymes during the cell cycle of a human lymphocyte cell line LAZ-007 synchronised by centrifugal elutriation. Biochem. Biophy. Acta. 633;400.

10. Krenitsky TA, Tuttle JV, Koszalka GW, Chen IS, Beacham LM III, Ridout JL, Elion GB (1976). Deoxy-cytidine kinase from calf thymus. Substrate and inhibitor sepcificity. J. Biol. Chem. 251:4055.

11. Pardee AB, Dubrow R, Hamlin JL, Kletzein RF (1978). Animal cell cycle. Ann. Rev. Biochem. 47:715.

12. Coffino P, Graw JW, Tomkins W (1975). Cyclic-AMP, a nonessential regulator of the cell cycle. Proc. Natl. Acad. Sci. U.S.A. 72:878.

13. Thompson EB, Harmon JB, Norman MR, Schmidt TJ (1980). Glucocorticoid actions in a human acute lymphoblastic leukemia T cell line: A model system for understanding toxicity. In Iacobelli S, King RJB, Lidner HR, Lippman ME (eds): "Hormones and Cancer", New York: Raven Press, p. 89.

Rational Basis for Chemotherapy, pages 249–259
© 1983 Alan R. Liss, Inc., 150 Fifth Avenue, New York, NY 10011

REGULATION OF DEOXYNUCLEOSIDE METABOLISM
IN T AND B HUMAN LYMPHOBLASTOID CELLS

Joanne Kurtzberg and Michael S. Hershfield

Departments of Medicine and Biochemistry,
Division of Rheumatic and Genetic Diseases,
and Department of Pediatrics,
Division of Hematology-Oncology
Duke University Medical Center
Durham, North Carolina 27710

ABSTRACT: T lymphoblasts are markedly more
sensitive than B lymphoblasts to the toxic effects
of 2' deoxyadenosine (dAdo) in the presence of an
adenosine deaminase (ADA) inhibitor. This
correlates with the more efficient accumulation of
deoxyadenosine triphosphate (dATP) from dAdo in T
cells. We fused a T lymphoblastoid cell line (CEM)
with a B lymphoblastoid cell line (WI-L2) in order
to study the dominance or recessiveness of dAdo
sensitivity, and the ability to accumulate and
catabolize dAdo nucleotides (dAXP) in the hybrid
offspring. Preliminary results indicate that
resistance to dAdo (B-ness) is dominant, probably
owing to expression of dAXP catabolizing activity
in the B cell parent and T/B hybrid offspring. We
speculate that in vivo hybrid formation could be
one mechanism for the development of drug
resistance to treatment of T cell leukemia with the
ADA inhibitor 2' deoxycoformycin (dCF).

This work was supported by NIH grant AM 20902 and
research career development award AM 00424 (M.S.
Hershfield). J. Kurtzberg was supported on NIH
training grant T32AM07015.

INTRODUCTION

Genetic ADA deficiency is associated with severe
combined immunodeficiency disease with profound
lymphopenia (1,2). Of interest is the relative sparing
of other organ systems in affected individuals. This
observation has provided a rationale for oncologists to
approach the treatment of refractory lymphoid
malignancies with inhibitors of ADA (for more detailed
discussion of this topic see paper by Dr. Hershfield
elsewhere in this volume (3)).

The sensitivity of T lymphoid cells to ADA
inhibition is primarily a function of their capacity to
accumulate dATP derived from dAdo (4-8). In contrast, B
cell lines are relatively resistant to dAdo and very
inefficient in accumulating dATP. This difference has
been postulated to be related to differences in the
activities of dAdo phosphorylating enzymes and dATP
catabolizing enzymes between these lymphocyte subsets
(9-17). The rates of dATP accumulation by T and B cell
lines cultured with dAdo in the 2-100 uM range in the
presence of ADA inhibitors, differ by about 10-100 fold,
but the activities of dAdo kinases and dAdo
nucleotidases in cytoplasmic extracts of these cells
differ by only 2-4 fold (11,17). Thus the basis for the
difference in ability of these cells to expand their
intracellular dATP pool is poorly understood. We have
attempted a series of experiments with intact cells to
directly test the hypothesis that rapid dAdo nucleotide
catabolism limits dATP accumulation in B cells.

In order to obtain more information about the
nature of the mechanisms that control dAdo nucleotide
accumulation in T and B cells, we have explored the
usefulness of the somatic cell genetic technique of cell
hybridization. We have generated T/B hybrid cell lines
by polyethylene glycol (PEG) induced fusion of CEM (T)
and WI-L2 (B) cell lines, the human cell lines that we
have previously used to examine the enzymatic basis for
dAdo phosphorylation (14,15,17). We have compared the
T/B hybrids with their parent lines with respect to
sensitivity to dAdo toxicity and ability to accumulate
and degrade intracellular dAdo nucleotides. We have
interpreted our results in terms of three simplified

hypotheses regarding the control of dATP accumulation: Hypothesis A: That dAdo kinase(s) in T cells operate more efficiently than in B cells. Hypothesis B: That B cells contain an inhibitor of dAdo phosphorylation. Hypothesis C: That B cells limit dATP accumulation by rapidly catabolizing intracellular dAdo nucleotides. Table 1 shows the phenotype that would be expected in a T/B cell hybrid for each of the postulated control mechanisms, assuming for simplicity that only one of the mechanisms was operative.

TABLE 1

Expected Hybrid Phenotype

Hypothesis	dAdo Sensitivity	dAXP Accumulation	dAXP Catabolism
A. more efficient dAdo kinase(s) in T cells.	T-like (sensitive)	T-like (efficient)	no
B. B cells possess an inhibitor of dAdo phosphorylation	B-like (resistant)	B-like	no
C. B cells catabolize dAXP	B-like	B-like or T-like	active

METHODS

The T cell parent was a hypoxanthine-guanine phosphoribosyltransferase (HGPRT)-deficient, ouabain-resistant derivative of the CEM human T cell line, which we obtained from David Howell and Peter Creswell of the Immunology Department, Duke University. The B cell parent was the WI-L2 spleen cell line. Fusion was induced with 50%PEG and hybrids were selected in 96-well culture dishes in RPMI culture medium

containing 10% horse serum and 50 nM ouabain, 100 uM
hypoxanthine, and 5 uM azaserine (OHA medium). Cells
from wells that showed growth were cloned in agarose
containing OHA medium. The use of OHA selective medium
rather than the standard HAT (Hypoxathine, Aminopterin,
Thymidine) medium was dictated by the fact that T cells
are more sensitive than B cells to growth inhibition by
thymidine as well as dAdo. We did not want to bias our
selection for thymidine-resistant cells, which might be
cross-resistant to other deoxyribonucleosides. This is
avoided by use of azaserine at a concentration that
inhibits purine synthesis alone, rather than
aminopterin, which inhibits thymidilate synthesis as
well. Sensitivity to dAdo growth inhibition and the
concentration of total intracellular dAXP (dAMP + dADP +
dATP) were measured as described (14,17).

RESULTS

The hybrid nature of the cloned fusion products was
established by nutritional, karyotypic, immunologic and
biochemical means. The fusion products (termed
"hybrids") grew in selective medium that failed to
support growth of either parent. Sensitivity of the
hybrids to thioguanine, and to azaserine in the absence
of hypoxanthine, established that they contained HGPRT
activity and were not simply azaserine-resistant mutants
of the T cell parent. The hybrids possessed a modal
chromosome number that was about the sum of that of the
parental cell lines. Cell surface antigen analysis
revealed that the HLA antigens of both parents were
expressed on the hybrids, as well as new antigens at
each HLA locus that were not expressed by either parent.
The latter phenomenon has been observed by others who
have examined regulation of HLA phenotype of hybrid
lymphocytes (18). Ecto-5'-nucleotidase, an enzyme that
WI-L2 cells express at 150 times the activity present on
CEM, was expressed on WI-L2/CEM hybrids at a level 50
times higher than on CEM. A number of other activities,
including ADA, Ado kinase, deoxycytidine kinase, and
cytoplasmic 5'-nucleotidase activity were expressed at
intermediate levels in the hybrids.

The most relevant studies that we have conducted thus far relate to a) sensitivity to dAdo-mediated growth inhibition, b) ability to accumulate dATP, and c) ability to catabolize intracellular dAdo nucleotides (Table 2, Figure 1).

Table 2

Cell line	Growth inhibition by dAdo	dAXP Catabolism
	EC-50, uM	nmol/hr/10^9 cells
CEM(T)	0.3-0.6	<30
WI-L2(B)	43	>660
T/B hybrid	25-27	740

All studies were conducted in the presence of 5 uM dCF. Growth inhibition was measured after 72 hours. To measure dAXP catabolism cell cultures were first preincubated with dAdo plus dCF to expand intracellular dAXP pools. Then the cells were chilled, washed, and resuspended in medium that contained dCF but without dAdo, and the intracellular dAXP concentration measured immediately and at several times over a 5 hour period. The preincubation conditions were chosen so as to expand the dAXP pools in CEM and WI-L2 to the same degree. To achieve this WI-L2 was incubated for 3 hours with 500 uM dAdo, and CEM for 2 hours with 20 uM dAdo. The T/B hybrid was incubated under the same conditions as WI-L2. The dAXP pool concentrations actually obtained immediately following the preincubation (nmol/10^9 cells) were 660, 820, and 2900 for WI-L2, CEM, and the hybrid, respectively. All experiments were performed in duplicate, and average values are reported.

We have examined 6 independently isolated WI-L2/CEM hybrids and 2 other T/B hybrid clones from a fusion of CEM with another human B cell line, SB (kindly provided

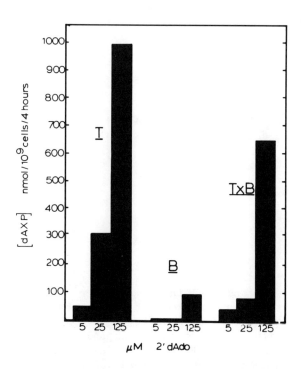

Figure 1. Accumulation of total dAdo nucleotides by CEM
(T), WI-L2 (B), and a CEM/WI-L2 hybrid clone (T x B).
Cultures were incubated with 5 uM dCF and the indicated
concentrations of dAdo for 4 hours. Total intracellular
dAdo nucleotides were measured as described (14,17).

by David Howell). In all cases the hybrids were nearly
as resistant to dAdo as their B cell parent. As
controls we have constructed hybrids by fusion of CEM x
CEM. None of these T/T fusion products were resistant
to dAdo. The T/B hybrids accumulated much less dATP
from dAdo than the T cell parent line, but more than the
B cell parent, particularly at high concentrations of dAdo
(Figure 1). The most informative results were obtained
when the capacity to degrade intracellular dAXP was

compared in the parental and hybrid cell lines. In
these studies cells were preincubated with dCF and dAdo
to expand intracellular dAXP pools, and then were washed
and incubated for 5 hours in medium that contained dCF
but no dAdo (see legend to Table 2 for details). During
this period there was almost no decrease in dAXP content
of the CEM cells, but a rapid disappearance of dAXP from
WI-L2 and the WI-L2/CEM hybrid. Similar results have
been obtained with two other hybrid clones. These
results are consistent with hypothesis C. They show
that an activity responsible for dAXP catabolism in
WI-L2, which is absent in CEM, is expressed in the
hybrid and limits its ability to maintain high levels of
dAXP.

We are currently attempting to further explore
possible differences in the regulation of dAdo
phosphorylation in T and B cells. To approach this
question we are using variants of WI-L2 and CEM that
lack deoxycytidine kinase (14-17) to construct T/B
hybrids that possess only T cell or B cell derived dAdo
phosphorylating activities, but are otherwise identical
to the T/B hybrids discussed above. Differences in
rates of dAXP accumulation between such T/B hybrids
should reflect differences due to the source of these
kinases. Studies of this sort may yield information
about intracellular function and regulation of these
enzymes that has thus far been difficult to achieve with
studies of the isolated enzymes.

Possible Role of Spontaneous Hybrid Formation in
Development of Resistance to Deoxycoformycin Therapy.

It has long been postulated that spontaneous cell
fusion might occur in vivo and contribute to the
remarkable diversity found in populations of tumor cells
(19-23). In particular, it has been speculated that
hybrid formation may be a general phenomenon in
lymphoproliferative diseases, in which several factors
may operate to promote cell fusion. For example it has
been shown that an E-B virus induced protein causes cell
fusion, and the suggestion has been made that fusion
with an EB-infected B cell may be responsible for the
expression of EB receptors on the surface of
nasopharyngeal carcinoma cells (24). Fusion of B cells

that produce antibody against tumor cell surface antigens with the tumor cell has also been proposed (20,22). Hybrid formation involving a human lymphoma propagated in hamsters has been reported (19). Thus far there is only speculation that fusion plays a role in determining important biological characteristics of tumors, and no direct evidence that the phenomenon occurs in man.

Treatment of T cell ALL with deoxycoformycin frequently produces dramatic but transitory depletion of circulating tumors cells. Whether this is due to inadequate treatment or to true acquired resistance has not been determined. As discussed earlier at this meeting (3) we have observed what we believe to be a instance of acquired resistance due to a decrease in the capacity of the patient's T lymphoblasts to accumulate dATP from dAdo in vivo (25). The explanation for the diminished accumulation of dATP in this patient has not been determined, although it did not appear to be due to any alteration in ADA activity, to inadequate exposure to dAdo, or to inability of dAdo to enter the tumor cells. Furthermore, there was no no loss or obvious alteration in tumor cell deoxycytidine kinase or Ado kinase (unpublished results). It is interesting that the T/B hybrids that we have constructed also possess normal levels of dAdo phosphorylating enzymes but diminished capacity to accumulate dATP, and are quite resistant to dAdo when ADA is inhibited. Treatment with dCF in vivo, which causes dAdo accumulation, would be expected to provide a strong selective advantage to such cells. Actual proof of in vivo hybrid formation will require careful, sequential monitoring of the karyotypes, cell surface antigenic, and biochemical properties of malignant cells of patients undergoing treatment with dCF, or with nucleoside analogs.

ACKNOWLEDGEMENTS

We had the expert technical assistance of Janet Misenheimer in conducting these studies. We appreciate the advice and assistance of Drs. David Howell, Peter Cresswell, Bart Haynes, and Emily Reisner with analyses of cell surface antigens.

REFERENCES

1. Giblett ER, Anderson JE, Cohen F, Pollara B, Meuwissen HJ (1972). Adenosine deaminase deficiency in two patients with severely impaired cellular immunity. Lancet 2:1067.

2. Kredich NM, Hershfield MS (1982). Immunodeficiency diseases associated with adenosine deaminase deficiency and purine nucleoside phosphorylase deficiency. In Stanbury JB, Wyngaarden JB, Fredrickson DS, Goldstein J, Brown M (eds): "The Metabolic Basis of Inherited Disease," New York:McGraw Hill, 5th edition, in Press.

3. Hershfield MS (1982). Biochemical consequences of inhibition of adenosine deaminase in the treatment of lymphocytic leukemias. This symposium.

4. Horibata K, Harris AW (1970). Mouse Myelomas and lymphomas in culture. Exp Cell Res 60:61.

5. Reynolds EC, Harris AW, Finch IR (1979). Deoxyribonucleoside triphosphate pools and differential thymidine sensitivities of cultured mouse lymphoma and myeloma cells. Biochim Biophys Acta 561:110.

6. Mitchell BS, Mejias E, Daddona PE, Kelly WN (1978). Purinogenic immunodeficiency diseases:selective toxicity of deoxyribonucleosides for T cells. Proc Natl Acad Sci USA 75:5011.

7. Carson DA, Kaye J, Seegmiller JE (1978). Differential sensitivity of human leukemic T cell lines and B cell lines to growth inhibition by deoxyadenosine. J Immunol 121:1726.

8. Gelfand EW, Lee JJ, Dosch HM (1979). Selective toxicity of purine deoxynucleosides for human lymphocyte growth and function. Proc Natl Acad Sci USA 76:1998.

9. Carson DA, Kaye, J, Matsumoto S, Seegmiller JE, Thompson L (1979). Biochemical basis for the enhanced toxicity of deoxyribonucleosides toward malignant human T cell lines. Proc Natl Acad Sci USA 76:2430.

10. Wortmann RL, Mitchell BS, Edwards NL, Fox IH (1979). Biochemical basis for differential deoxyadenosine toxicity to T and B lymphoblasts. Role of 5'nucleotidase. Proc Natl Acad Sci USA 76:2434.

11. Carson DA, Kaye J, Wasson WB (1981). The potential importance of soluble deoxynucleotidase activity in mediating deoxyadenosine toxicity in human lymphoblasts. J Immunol 126:348.

12. Fox RM, Tripp EH, Piddington SK, Tattersall MHN (1980). Sensitivity of leukemic human null lymhocytes to deoxynucleosides. Cancer Res 40:3383.

13. Fox RM, Piddington SK, Tripp EH, Tattersall MHN (1981). Ecto-ATPase deficiency in cultured human T and null leukemic lymphocytes. A biochemical basis for thymidine sensitivity. J Clin Invest 68:544.

14. Hershfield MS, Kredich NM (1980). Resistance of an adenosine kinase-deficient human lymphoblastoid cell line to effects of deoxyadenosine on growth, S-adenosylhomocysteine hydrolase inactivation, and dATP accumulation. Proc Natl Acad Sci USA 77:4292.

15. Ullman B, Levinson BB, Hershfield MS, Martin DW Jr (1981). A biochemical genetic study of the role of specific nucleoside kinases in deoxyadenosine phosphorylation by cultured human cells. J Biol Chem 256:848.

16. Verhoef V, Sarup J, Fridland A (1981). Identification of the mechanism of activation of 9-B-D-arabinofuranosyladenine in human lymphoid cells using mutants deficient in nucleoside kinases. Cancer Res 41:4478.

17. Hershfield MS, Fetter JE, Small WC, Bagnara AS, Williams SR, Ullman B, Martin DW Jr, Wasson DB, Carson DA (1982). Effects of mutational loss of adenosine kinase and deoxycytidine kinase on deoxyATP accumulation and deoxyadenosine toxicity in cultured CEM human T-lymphoblastoid cells. J Biol Chem 257:6380.

18. Howell DN, Berger AE, Creswell P (1982). Human T-B lymphoblast hybrids express HLA-DR specificities not expressed by either parent. Immunogenetics 15:199.

19. Goldenberg DM, Bhan RD, Pavia RA (1971). In vivo human-hamster somatic cell fusion indicated by glucose 6-phosphate dehydrogenase and lactate dehydrogenase profiles. Cancer Res 31:1148.

20. Sinkovics JG, Drewinco B, Thornell E (1970). Immunoresistant tetraploid lymphoma cells. Lancet 1:139.

21. Wiener F, Fenyo EM, Klein G, Harris H (1972).
     Fusion of tumor cells with host cells. Nature New
     Biology 238:155.
22. Sinkovics JG (1981). Early history of specific
     antibody-producing lymphocyte hybridomas. Cancer
     Res 41:1246.
23. Revoltella RP, Brahe C, Procicchiani G (1979).
     Spontaneous fusion and formation of hybrids between
     C1300 neuroblastoma cells and lymphoid cells in
     mixed cultured. Cellular Immunol 47:115.
24. Bayliss GM, Wolf H (1981). An Epstein-Barr virus
     early protein induces cell fusion. Proc Natl Acad
     Sci USA 78:7162.
25. Hershfield MS, Kredich NM, Falletta JM, Kinney TR,
     Mitchell BS, Koller CA (1981). Effects of
     deoxyadenosine and adenine arabinoside during
     deoxycoformycin therapy. Proc Am Assoc Cancer Res
     ??:157,

Rational Basis for Chemotherapy, pages 261–273
© 1983 Alan R. Liss, Inc., 150 Fifth Avenue, New York, NY 10011

DIFFERENTIAL SENSITIVITY OF HUMAN T AND B LYMPHOBLASTS TO
CYTOTOXIC NUCLEOSIDE ANALOGS[1]

Vernon L. Verhoef and Arnold Fridland

Division of Biochemical and Clinical Pharmacology
St. Jude Children's Research Hospital
Memphis, Tennessee 38101

ABSTRACT The selective cytotoxicity of purine deoxyribonucleosides for T cells is a currently proposed
mechanism for the selective dysfunction of T cells in
immunodeficiency diseases. Cytotoxic nucleoside analogs might therefore be useful agents to selectively
kill subpopulations of human lymphoid cells during
lymphoproliferative diseases. We have compared the
cytotoxic effect of ten structurally related purine
and pyrimidine nucleosides on cultured T and B lymphoblasts. On the basis of the concentration producing
50% inhibition of cell growth, deoxyadenosine (with
deoxycoformycin) and thymidine were 28–50 fold more
cytotoxic to T cells than B cells; four nucleoside
analogs – 9-β-D-arabinofuranosyladenine (with deoxycoformycin), 9-β-D-arabinofuranosyl-2-F-adenine, 1-β-D-
arabinofuranosylcytosine and 2'-O-nitro-1-β-D-arabino-
furanosylcytosine – were 2–12 fold more cytotoxic to T
cells than B cells; and the other four agents exhibited no selectivity.
     The routes of activation for the selective agents
were compared to the routes of activation for nonse-
lective agents by means of nucleoside kinase-deficient
sublines of CCRF-CEM T lymphoblasts. All agents, except adenosine, were found to require deoxycytidine
kinase, adenosine kinase or thymidine kinase for cyto-

---

[1]This work was supported by grants from NIH CA-09346, ACS
IN99H and CH52C, and by ALSAC.

toxic activity.   The T-cell selectivity of these agents did not correlate with their routes of activation.

The activated nucleosides and analogs share a common mechanism of deactivation via dephosphorylation in lymphoid cells.   The 5'-nucleotide derivatives of these agents were tested as substrates for a partially purified preparation of a soluble deoxynucleotidase of CCRF-CEM cells.   The results revealed a striking positive correlation between an agent's selectivity for T cells and the specificity of its 5'-phosphorylated derivative for the nucleotidase.   The unique specificity of this nucleotidase can be used to investigate its role in nucleoside and nucleoside-analog metabolism and the differential sensitivity of T and B cells.

INTRODUCTION

T cell growth and cell mediated immunity are more frequently and drastically perturbed than B cell growth and humoral immunity during the course of inherited immune deficiency diseases associated with loss of purine nucleoside phosphorylase or adenosine deaminase activity (1,2).   This preferential destruction of T cell function is thought to be a consequence of the increased levels of deoxynucleosides in the tissues of these individuals (3).   Studies of leukemic lymphoblasts and peripheral blood lymphocytes in culture have confirmed that T lymphoid cells are more sensitive to deoxyadenosine (dAdo) and deoxyguanosine (dGuo) than B cells, and that T cells are hypersensitive to thymidine (dThd) and 1-β-D-arabinofuranosylcytosine (araC) as well (4,5).

The molecular basis for the hypersensitivity of T lymphoid cells to nucleosides is not understood but appears to be related to a lack of deoxynucleotide catabolism in thymus lymphoid cells (6,7).   T cells in contrast to B cells, accumulate high concentrations of 5'-phosphates of dAdo, dGuo and dThd which in each case may cause cytotoxicity by disrupting the level of deoxynucleotide precursors necessary for DNA synthesis (7,8,9).   Investigations into the biochemical mechanisms of this toxicity have shown that T cells have much lower ecto-5'-nucleotidase levels, a monophosphatase present on the surface of cells, than B cells (6,7).   Similarly, T cells lack the surface enzyme, ecto-adenosine triphosphatase, an enzyme with apparent activity with dTTP, dATP, dCTP and dGTP as well as ATP (4).   Carson and coworkers, however, have found that a soluble deoxy-nucleotidase also varied inversely with deoxyadenosine toxicity in lymphoid cells (10), and suggested that this enzyme rather than the membrane-bound ecto-5'-nucleotidase may be responsible for the differential catabolism of deoxynucleotides in T and B cells.

In addition to lower levels of nucleotidase, T cells have more active nucleoside kinase activities than B cells (4,9,11,12). Moreover, we have recently shown that dAdo and 9-β-D-arabinofuranosyladenine (araA) are phosphorylated in cultured human T cells by the conserted action of two enzymes – adenosine kinase and deoxycytidine kinase (13); whereas dAdo is phosphorylated in B cells via one enzyme – adenosine kinase (14). These differences in phosphoryla-tion may contribute to the preferential T-cell toxicity of dAdo and structurally related analogs.

In this report we compare the effects of 10 struc-turally related purine and pyrimidines on cultured T and B lymphoblasts. The selective T cell toxicity of these agents appears to correlate with the specificity of their pathway of deactivation via soluble deoxynucleotidase rather than with the pathways for activation. These re-sults suggest a unique role for soluble deoxynucleotidase activity as a determinant of the T cell selectivity of nucleoside analogs.

METHODS

Materials

The sources of most of our materials have been des-cribed (13). Other agents were from the following com-panies or individuals: α,β-methyleneadenosine 5'-diphos-phate, araAMP and araCMP were from PL Biochemicals, Inc. (Milwaukee, WI); 2'-azido-araA was a gift of Dr. A.C. Sartorelli (Yale University, New Haven, CT); 2-F-araAMP was a gift of Dr. J.A. Montgomery (Southern Research Institute, Birmingham, AL); and 2'-0-nitro-araC was a gift of Dr. L. Chwang (St. Jude Children's Research Hospital, Memphis, TN).

Cells and Cell Culture

The growth and culture of CCRF-CEM T-lymphoblasts (termed CEM) has been described previously (13). Other human lines, Molt 4 (15), Raji (15) and RPMI 6410 (16) were cultured under conditions identical to CCRF-CEM cells except that RPMI 1640 medium (Gibco) was substituted for

Eagle's minimal essential medium. Doubling times for these four cell lines ranged between 15 and 20 hours.

The selection of deoxycytidine kinase-deficient and deoxycytidine kinase/adenosine kinase-deficient mutant CEM cells has been described (13). An adenosine kinase-deficient mutant was selected in a similar manner by exposing CEM cells to increasingly higher concentrations of pyrazofurin (Pyr). Cells growing in 5×10^{-5} M Pyr were cloned as described and expanded into separate populations. The clone CEM/AK⁻ used in this study has been growing more than one year in the absence of drug with a doubling time of approximately 24 hours. These cells contain less than 1% adenosine kinase of wild type levels.

Soluble Deoxynucleotidase

A single peak of deoxynucleotidase activity eluted at 0.2 M KCl when a high speed supernatant of homogenized CEM cells was applied to DEAE-cellulose (13). The enzyme was assayed by measuring the release of phosphate from enzyme-containing fractions incubated with sodium acetate pH 6.0, 5 mM $MgCl_2$ and 1 mM substrate at 37°C. The phosphate was measured by the method of Rathbun et al (17) and protein was measured by the Bio-Rad procedure (Bio-Rad Laboratories, Richmond, CA) with standard bovine gamma globulin.

RESULTS

Cytotoxic Effects of Nucleoside Analogs on Cultured T and B Lymphoblasts.

Structurally related purine and pyrimidine analogs were incubated individually or with nontoxic concentrations of deoxycoformycin with cultured T or B lymphoblasts and the concentration which caused 50% inhibition of the growth of the population was determined for each (Fig. 1). Four agents had no preferential inhibition of T or B lymphoblasts and are grouped together as Type I agents. The other six agents showed variable degrees of T cell selectivity as evidenced by the lower concentrations of these compounds required to inhibit T cell growth. The four antitumor agents - araC, 2'-O-nitro-araC, araA, and 2-F-araA - had a 2-12 fold selectivity (IC_{50} for B cells/IC_{50} for T cells) for the T cells and are classified as Type II agents. The two deoxynucleosides, dAdo and dThd had the greatest selectivity for T cells. These agents were 28-50

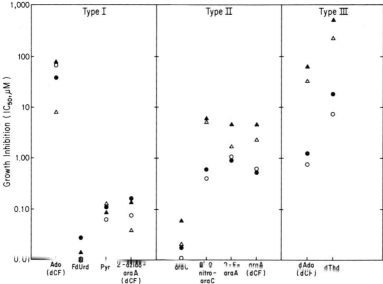

FIGURE 1. Cytotoxic effects of structurally related nucleosides on T and B lymphoblasts. The concentration producing 50% inhibition of cell growth during 48 hours (IC$_{50}$) was determined for each nucleoside and each cell line. The purine nucleosides, except 2-F-araA, were tested in combination with nontoxic concentrations of deoxycoformycin (dCF, 3.8 μM) to prevent deamination. Legend: T-lymphoblasts – CCRF-CEM ●, Molt-4 o; B-lymphoblasts – RPMI 6410 ▲, Raji Δ.

fold more effective against T than B cells and are termed Type III agents.

These results are quantitatively similar to the results of other investigators who have measured the T cell selectivity of dAdo (8,9), dThd (4), 5-fluoro-deoxyuridine (18) and 2-F-araA (19). However, in contrast to our results, araC was reported to be 45-80 fold more effective against T cell lines than B cell lines (5). The reason for this apparent discrepancy is not known.

Activation of T Cell Selective Agents.

The routes of activation of these cytotoxic nucleosides were determined by measuring the growth inhibition of

wild-type and nucleoside kinase-deficient CCRF-CEM lymphoblasts. The level of resistance of a kinase-deficient cell
to an agent is a measure of the contribution of that kinase
for activation of the agent in the intact cell. By this
criteria, Table 1 shows that all of the agents, except

TABLE 1
ROUTES OF ACTIVATION FOR T-CELL SELECTIVE AGENTS

Agent	Kinase-Deficient Lymphoblast	Resistance (IC_{50} Mutant/ IC_{50} Wild Type)
Type III		
dAdo (+dCF)	CEM/AK$^-$	0.7
	CEM/dCK$^-$	3.8
	CEM/dCK$^-$/AK$^-$	500
dThd	CEM/TK$^-$	10[a]
Type II		
araC	CEM/dCK$^-$	1800
2'-O-nitro-araC	CEM/dCK$^-$	1700
2-F-araA	CEM/dCK$^-$	300
araA (+dCF)	CEM/AK$^-$	1.2
	CEM/dCK$^-$	6.1
	CEM/dCK$^-$/AK$^-$	250
Type I		
Ado (+dCF)	CEM/AK$^-$	0.6
	CEM/dCK$^-$	2.1
	CEM/dCK$^-$/AK$^-$	1.0
F-dUrd	L1210/TK$^-$	>4000[b]
Pyrazofurin	CEM/AK$^-$	1000
2'-azido-araA (+dCF)	CEM/AK$^-$	80
	CEM/dCK$^-$	1.4
	CEM/dCK$^-$/AK$^-$	170

[a]Zielke, H.R. (1979) Cancer Res. 39:3373.
[b]Mulkins, M. and Heidelberger, C. (1980) Proc. Am.
Assoc. Cancer Res. 21:285.

adenosine (Ado), required one or more kinases for activation. Type III agents, defined as those with the greatest T cell selectivity, utilized three pathways for activation - deoxycytidine kinase, adenosine kinase and thymidine kinase; Type II agents used deoxycytidine kinase and adenosine kinase; and Type I agents were activated by adenosine kinase and thymidine kinase. Thus, selective T cell cytotoxicity was not strictly associated with any single pathway of activation by phosphorylation.

Degradation of Activated T-Cell Selective Agents.

Since these results show that the T-cell selective agents apparently require phosphorylation to cytotoxic metabolites in order to inhibit cell growth, the level and specificity of dephosphorylating enzymes in cells may determine how rapidly these agents are detoxified in a particular cell line. Carson et al. have shown that levels of soluble deoxynucleotidase activity in extracts of 19 lymphoblastoid lines varies inversely with the sensitivity of these lines to dAdo toxicity, but they did not study the substrate specificity of this enzyme in detail (10).

We partially purified the soluble deoxynucleotidase activity from CCRF-CEM T-lymphoblasts and compared it to the soluble deoxynucleotidase and ecto-5'-nucleotidase of WI-L2 B-lymphoblasts (Table 2). Acidic pH optimum, poor inhibition by α,β-methyleneadenosine 5'-diphosphate (AMPCH$_2$P), and specificity for deoxynucleotides are three properties which distinguish the soluble enzyme from the membrane-bound ecto-5'-nucleotidase. Further characterization of the substrate specificity of soluble deoxynucleotidase is shown in Table 3. The poor utilization of glycerophosphates and glucose-1-phosphate indicate that deoxynucleotidase is not simply a nonspecific acid phosphatase. Moreover, the enzyme has highest activity for deoxynucleotides, 50-75% less activity for ribonucleotides and 90-95% less activity for arabinonucleotides. Thus, it appears that the substrate specificity is determined by the sugar rather than the base portion of the molecule.

The deoxynucleotidase specificity may have important implications for the effectiveness of T-cell selective agents. The best substrates of this enzyme are the 5'-nucleotides of Type III agents (Fig. 2). Hence, Type III agents are more likely than Type II or I agents to be detoxified by this enzyme in intact cells. These results support the evidence by Carson et al. that this enzyme has

TABLE 2

DIFFERENCES OF SOLUBLE DEOXYNUCLEOTIDASES AND
ECTO-5'-NUCLEOTIDASE FROM LYMPHOID CELLS

| | SOLUBLE DEOXYNUCLEOTIDASE | | ECTO-5'-NUCLEOTIDASE |
	CCRF-CEM	WI-L2[a]	WI-L2[a]
pH Optimum	5.5	5.8-6.3	7.0-7.4
Cofactors	Mg^{++}	Mg^{++}	Mg^{++}
Inhibitors			
NaF	+	+	+
Tartrate	+	-	-
$AMP(CH_2)P$	±	±	+
K_m (dAMP)	90 µM	380 µM	210 µM
SUBSTRATE SPECIFICITY	DEOXYNUCLEOTIDES	DEOXYNUCLEOTIDES	RIBONUCLEOTIDES

[a]Carson, D.A. et al. (1981) J. Immunol. 126:348.

TABLE 3

SUBSTRATE SPECIFICITY OF SOLUBLE DEOXYNUCLEOTIDASE

Substrate (1 mM)	Specific Activity (nmoles/hr/mg)	(%)[a]
dGMP	971	100
dAMP	749	77
dIMP	726	75
dCMP	794	82
dTMP	669	69
dUMP	870	89
GMP	290	30
AMP	363	37
TMP	176	18
CMP	182	19
UMP	227	23
ara-AMP	34	3.5
ara-CMP	58	6.0
dADP	338	35
dATP	64	6.6
p-Nitro-phenylphosphate	1042	107
α-Glycerophosphate	197	20
β-Glycerophosphate	54	5.6
Glucose-1-phosphate	0	0

[a]The specific activity of dGMP is taken as 100%.

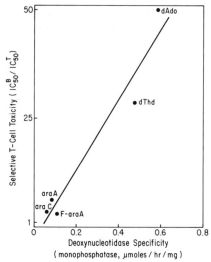

FIGURE 2.   The relationship of selective T cell toxicity and deoxynucleotidase specificity for Type II and III agents.

an important role for determining the highly selective dAdo effects on T cells (10).

DISCUSSION

The results presented here demonstrate the differences between cytotoxic nucleosides in terms of their selectivity for T cells.   The increased sensitivity of T cells to growth inhibition by nucleosides parallels the increased ability of these same cells to accumulate toxic nucleotides (7,8,9).   However, there is no close correlation between the levels of nucleoside phosphorylating activity in the T cells and their ability to sequester the nucleoside tri-phosphates (4,9).   Thus, in addition to nucleoside phos-phorylation, the increased sensitivity of T cells to cyto-toxic nucleosides may be related to low levels of dephos-phorylating ability in the same cells (7).   Early investi-gations of this possibility revealed that the cell surface enzyme ecto-5'-nucleotidase was 93-99% lower for T cells than B cells (6,7); but subsequent studies with other lym-phoblastoid cell lines showed that ecto-5'-nucleotidase de-ficiency was not always associated with high sensitivity to dAdo or dThd (20,21).   Of particular interest in this re-gard is a soluble deoxyribonucleotidase described by Carson et al. (10) which varies inversely with the toxicity of

dAdo for cell lines of different phenotype and origin, including cells with T and B characteristics.

The enzyme reported here from the CEM cells closely
resembles that studied by Carson et al. from B lymphoblasts
(10). The latter enzyme too was found in post-microsomal
supernatant, had an acidic pH optimum and reacted better
with deoxyribonucleotides than with ribonucleotides. In
addition, the present study revealed that arabinonucleotides were very poor substrates for the CEM cell enzyme.
This may be one reason why the arabinosyl nucleosides of
adenine and cytosine are not as selective for T cells as
the natural deoxyribonucleosides (Fig. 2).

A lingering question, however, is how much the soluble
nucleotidase contributes to the rate of accumulation of
toxic nucleotides in the intact cell. T cell extracts contain 30% of this enzyme activity of B cell extracts (10),
yet T cells can accumulate more than 10-fold greater concentrations of dATP than B cells (7,8,9). One possibility
is that low soluble deoxynucleotidase and high nucleoside
kinase activities contribute to the preferred accumulation
of 5'-nucleotides in T cells. Alternatively, B cells may
have additional nucleotidases, such as the ecto-adenosine
triphosphate described by Fox et al. (4) which also contributes to the catabolism of nucleotides in these cells.
In either case the unique specificity of the soluble deoxynucleotidase for deoxyribonucleotides in contrast to
arabinonucleotides can perhaps be used as a tool to determine the contribution of this enzyme to the catabolism of
toxic nucleotides in the intact cell and determine how much
the activity of this enzyme contributes to the differential
accumulation of cytotoxic nucleotides in T and B cells.

ACKNOWLEDGEMENTS

We wish to thank Michele Connelly for excellent technical asistance.

REFERENCES

1. Polmar SH (1980).   Metabolic aspects of immunode-
    ficiency disease. Sem Hematol 17:30.
2. Thompson LF, Seegmiller JE (1980).   Adenosine deami-
    nase deficiency and severe combined immunodeficiency
    disease.   In Meister A (ed): "Advances in Enzymology,"
    New York: Interscience, Vol 51:167.
3. Martin DW Jr, Gelfand EW (1981).   Biochemistry of
    diseases of immunodevelopment.   Ann Rev Biochem
    50:845.
4. Fox RM, Piddington SK, Tripp EH, Tattersall MHN
    (1981).   Ecto-adenosine triphosphatase deficiency in
    cultured human T and null leukemic lymphocytes: A bio-
    chemical basis for thymidine sensitivity.   J Clin
    Invest 68:544.
5. Ohnuma T, Arkin H, Minowada J, Holland JF (1978).
    Differential chemotherapeutic susceptibility of human
    T-lymphocytes and B-lymphocytes in culture.   J Natl
    Cancer Inst 60:749.
6. Wortmann RL, Mitchell BS, Edwards NL, Fox IH (1979).
    Biochemical basis for differential deoxyadenosine
    toxicity to T and B lymphoblasts: Role for 5'-nucleo-
    tidase.   Proc Natl Acad Sci USA 76:2434.
7. Carson DA, Kaye J, Matsumoto S, Seegmiller JE,
    Thompson L (1979).   Biochemical basis for the enhanced
    toxicity of deoxyribonucleosides toward malignant
    human T cell lines.   Proc Natl Acad Sci USA 76:2430.
8. Mitchell BS, Mejias E, Daddona PE, Kelley WN (1978).
    Purinogenic immunodeficiency diseases: Selective
    toxicity of deoxyribonucleosides for T cells.   Proc
    Natl Acad Sci USA 75:5011.
9. Carson DA, Kaye J, Seegmiller JE (1978).   Differential
    sensitivity of human leukemic T cell lines and B cell
    lines to growth inhibition by deoxyadenosine.   J
    Immunol 121:1726.
10. Carson DA, Kaye J, Wasson DB (1981).   The potential
    importance of soluble deoxynucleotidase activity in
    mediating deoxyadenosine toxicity in human lympho-
    blasts. J Immunol 126:348.
11. Carson DA, Kaye J, Seegmiller JE (1977).   Lymphospe-
    cific toxicity in adenosine deaminase deficiency and
    purine nucleoside phosphorylase deficiency: Possible
    role of nucleoside kinase(s).   Proc Natl Acad Sci USA
    74:5677.
12. Cohen A, Lee JWW, Dosch H-M, Gelfand EW (1980).   The
    expression of deoxyguanosine toxicity in T lymphocytes

at different stages of maturation. J Immunol 125:1578.

13. Verhoef V, Sarup J, Fridland A (1981). Identification of the mechanism of activation of 9-β-D-arabinofurano-syladenine in human lymphoid cells using mutants deficient in nucleoside kinases. Cancer Res 41:4478.

14. Hershfield MS, Kredich NM (1980). Resistance of an adenosine kinase-deficient human lymphoblastoid cell line to effects of deoxyadenosine on growth, 5-adenosylhomocysteine hydrolase inactivation, and dATP accumulation. Proc Natl Acad Sci USA 77:4292.

15. Minowada J, Janossy G, Greaves MF, Tsubota T, Srivastava BIS, Morikawa S, Tatsumi E (1978). Expression of an antigen associated with acute lymphoblastic leukemia in human leukemia-lymphoma cell lines. J Natl Cancer Inst 60:1269.

16. Minowada J, Nonoyama M, Moore GE, Rauch AM, Pagano JS (1974). The presence of the Epstein-Barr viral genome in human lymphoblastoid B-cell lines and its absence in a myeloma cell line. Cancer Res 34:1898.

17. Rathbun WB, Betlach MV (1969). Estimation of enzymically produced orthophosphate in the presence of cysteine and adenosine triphosphate. Anal Biochem 28:436.

18. Piper AA, Fox RM (1981). Differential metabolism of fluorouracil (FU) in cultured human T and B lymphocyte cell lines: Modulation of sensitivity by purine nucleosides and bases. In Tattersall MHN, Fox RM (eds): "Nucleosides and Cancer Treatment: Rational Approaches to Antimetabolite Selectivity and Modulation," Sydney: Academic Press, p. 251.

19. Carson DA, Wasson DB, Kaye J, Ullman B, Martin DW Jr, Robins RK, Montgomery JA (1980). Deoxycytidine kinase-mediated toxicity of deoxyadenosine analogs toward malignant human lymphoblasts in vitro and toward murine L1210 leukemia in vivo. Proc Natl Acad Sci USA 77:6865.

20. Fox RM, Tripp EH, Piddington SK, Tattersall MHN (1980). Sensitivity of leukemic human null lymphocytes to deoxynucleosides. Cancer Res 40:3383.

21. Boss GR, Thompson LF, O'Connor RD, Ziering RW, Seegmiller JE (1981). Ecto-5'-nucleotidase deficiency: Association with adenosine deaminase deficiency and nonassociation with deoxyadenosine toxicity. Clin Immunol Immunopathol 19:1.

Rational Basis for Chemotherapy, pages 275–290
© 1983 Alan R. Liss, Inc., 150 Fifth Avenue, New York, NY 10011

BIOCHEMICAL CONSEQUENCES OF INHIBITION OF ADENOSINE
DEAMINASE IN THE TREATMENT OF LYMPHOCYTIC LEUKEMIAS

Michael S. Hershfield

Departments of Medicine and Biochemistry,
Division of Rheumatic and Genetic Diseases,
Duke University Medical Center
Durham, North Carolina 27710

ABSTRACT The rationale for the use of
2'-deoxycoformycin, a potent inhibitor of adenosine
deaminase, in the treatment of lymphoid
malignancies is discussed in terms of the
biochemical actions of the substrates for adenosine
deaminase, adenosine and 2'-deoxyadenosine, and of
their analogs. Factors that may influence the
sensitivity of specific classes of lymphoblasts to
treatment with 2'-deoxycoformycin are considered,
along with factors that may predispose to
nonlymphoid toxicity.

INTRODUCTION

About 20% of acute lymphoblastic leukemia involves
T cells. However, this cell type is over-represented
among patients in the category termed 'high risk' (1).
This group has a poor prognosis, with an estimated 80%
probability of disease recurrence within a year of
induction of first remission. According to a recent
review, acquired drug resistance and the lack of drugs
effective in treating relapse of disease remain as major
challenges to these patients and their physicians (1).
Because of this situation it is important to consider a
new, rational approach to the treatment of lymphoid

This work was supported by NIH grant AM 20902 and
research career development award AM 00424.

malignancies that involves the use of inhibitors of adenosine deaminase (ADA), alone or in combination with analogs of adenosine (Ado) and 2'-deoxyadenosine (dAdo), the substrates for this enzyme.

Genetic deficiency of ADA is associated with profound and selective depletion of lymphoid cells, causing severe combined immunodeficiency disease (2). (For a recent review of genetic ADA deficiency see reference 3). The selectivity of the lymphopenia suggests a uniquely important role for ADA in lymphocytes, which is further indicated by the fact that lymphocytes and particularly T cells, possess the highest tissue levels of ADA activity (4).

Tight binding inhibitors of ADA, including coformycin, 2'-deoxycoformycin (dCF), and EHNA (erythro-9-(2-hydroxy-3-nonyl)adenine (5) have enabled study of the effects of ADA deficiency in cultured cells and animals. The potential for use of these drugs as rational chemotherapeutic and immunosuppressive agents has led in the last few years to initial clinical trials of dCF alone, or recently in combination with adenine arabinoside (Ara-A), in the treatment of lymphocytic leukemias (6-12). ADA inhibitors can also be used to potentiate the effects of other drugs such as xylosyladenine, cordycepin (3'-dAdo), and other Ado analogs that are rapidly converted by ADA to their inactive inosine derivates.

BASIS FOR TOXICITY OF ADO AND dADO

It appears that ADA serves a detoxifying function, protecting lymphoid cells from exposure to Ado and dAdo. This conclusion arises from the finding that ADA inhibition is not per se toxic to cultured lymphoid cell lines or mitogen-stimulated peripheral blood lymphocytes, but it greatly potentiates the cytotoxic effects of Ado and dAdo in the micromolar range. In contrast, the ADA products inosine and deoxyinosine are not toxic, even at millimolar concentration. Several effects of Ado, dAdo, and their metabolites have been identified that may contribute in varying degree to their toxicity to cultured lymphoid cell lines (3). The occurrence of some of these effects has been observed in the erythrocytes and circulating lymphoblasts of patients undergoing treatment with dCF. These include the accumulation of dATP, depletion of ATP, and decrease in the activity of the enzyme S-adenosylhomocysteine (AdoHcy hydrolase).

There have been several recently published reviews of the pharmacology of dCF (13-15). I would like to review our own recent studies that deal with 1) the enzymatic basis for, and regulation of dATP accumulation from dAdo in lymphoid cells, 2) the mechanism responsible for ATP depletion during dCF treatment, and 3) the effects of dCF treatment on AdoHcy hydrolysis in lymphoid cells in vivo.

Control of dATP Accumulation from dAdo.

It appears that there are inherent differences in the sensitivity to ADA inhibition among lymphoid neoplasms derived from the various lymphocyte subclasses. Cultured T lymphoblastoid cells of both murine and human origin are much more sensitive to the toxic effects of dAdo than are B cell lines, and this correlates with the much greater efficiency with which T cell lines are able to trap dAdo as intracellular dATP (16-21). We have examined the basis for this difference using a somatic cell genetic approach.

In extracts of both T and B cell lines there are two enzymatic activities capable of phosphorylating dAdo (22-25). The major activity, which has the higher affinity for dAdo and Ara-A, is associated with deoxycytidine kinase; the minor activity is associated with Ado kinase (Figure 1). To determine the relative contributions of these enzymes to dAdo accumulation we have isolated mutants that lack these kinases from the CEM human leukemic T cell line (25) and from the WI-L2 human B cell line (22,23). In the case of the T cell line, we found that deoxycytidine kinase is primarily responsible for phosphorylation of dAdo at the lowest concentration of the nucleoside required to inhibit growth when ADA is inhibited (0.5-3 uM). Ado kinase becomes increasingly involved in phosphorylation of dAdo above a concentration of about 20 uM. Sensitivity to dAdo growth inhibition was diminished by about 3 fold by loss of deoxycytidine kinase, and by less than 2 fold by loss of Ado kinase; loss of both enzymes decreased sensitivity to dAdo about 100 fold (Figure 2). These results agree with similar studies of the CEM cell line by Verhoef et al. (24), and they indicate that the toxicity of dAdo below about 100 uM arises from its conversion to nucleotides. Ara-A is also

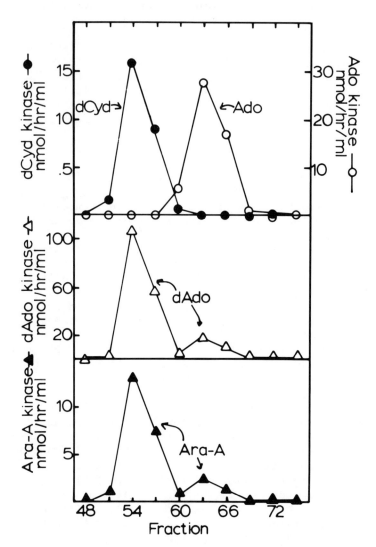

Figure 1.   Ultrogel AcA 34 gel filtration chromatography of an extract of CEM T lymphoblasts showing the pattern of nucleoside kinase activities.   The phosphorylation of radioactively labeled deoxycytidine (dCyd), adenosine (Ado), deoxyadenosine (dAdo), and arabinosyladenine (Ara-A) were measured as described (25).   A similar pattern of kinases is found in extracts of WI-L2 B cells (22).

phosphorylated by both deoxycytidine kinase and Ado kinase
(Fig. 1, reference 24)

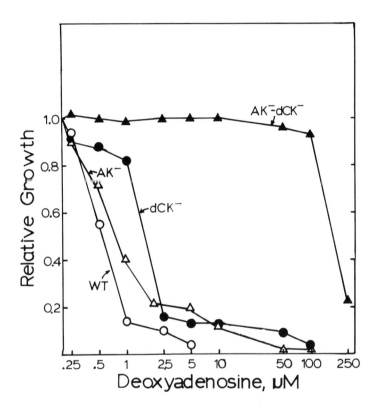

Figure 2.   Effect of dAdo on growth of mutants of the CEM
T cell line that are deficient in nucleoside kinase activities.   All cultures were incubated with 5 uM dCF in addition
to dAdo.   WT = wild type (with respect to nucleoside
kinases) AK⁻ = Ado kinase deficient; dCK⁻ = dCyd kinase
deficient; AK⁻ - dCK⁻ = deficient in both Ado and dCyd
kinases (from reference 25).

The results obtained with the WI-L2 B cell line differ
from the above in that loss of Ado kinase had a much greater
effect than loss of deoxycytidine kinase on dATP accumulation
and dAdo sensitivity (22,23). WI-L2 in fact behaves as if
deoxycytidine kinase plays very little role in trapping dAdo
as nucleotide: the higher concentrations of dAdo required to
produce dATP accumulation and growth inhibition in WI-L2
reflect the higher Km for dAdo of Ado kinase compared with
deoxycytidine kinase. In addition, exogenous deoxycytidine
has less ability to block dAdo toxicity in WI-L2 (22) than in
CEM (25). These differences between WI-L2 and CEM are not
explained simply by differences in their levels of Ado and
deoxycytidine kinases, which differ by no more than 3 fold in
extracts of the two cell lines (19,25). The findings with
CEM and WI-L2 are similar to those obtained with a number of
other human T and B cell lines, in which capacity to
accumulate dATP did not correlate with the level of dAdo
phosphorylating activities present in cell extracts (19).

It has been proposed that greater rates of catabolism of
deoxyadenosine nucleotides in B than T cells could account
for the limited ability of B cells to accumulate dATP
(21,26,27). B cell lines possess much higher levels of
ecto-5'-nucleotidase (21,26) and ecto-ATPase (28) activities
than T cells. However, there is little evidence that these
ecto enzymes can act on intracellular nucleotides. Human
null lymphoblastoid cell lines, which like B cells have high
ecto-5'-nucleotidase activity, are as sensitive as T cell
lines to dAdo and are efficient at accumulating dATP (29). A
cytoplasmic deoxyribonucleotidase has been proposed as the
catabolic activity that might prevent dATP accumulation by B
cell lines (27). However, the levels of this activity were
on the average only about 2-3 fold higher in T than in B cell
lines. The characteristics of a cytoplasmic nucleotidase
that may be involved in dATP degradation are discussed
elsewhere in this symposium (30).

We have recently attempted to test the hypothesis that
enhanced ability of B cells to catabolize intracellular dATP
accounts for their inefficient accumulation of this toxic
nucleotide. Dr. Joanne Kurtzberg will discuss these
preliminary studies in which we asked whether the capacity to
accumulate and degrade intracellular dATP, and the level of
sensitivity to dAdo, are expressed in a B-like or T-like
manner in hybrid cell lines formed by fusing WI-L2 and CEM

cell lines. Our results show that such hybrids are B-like, and that their ability to accumulate dATP is indeed limited by a rapid rate of dATP catabolism (31). Demonstration of rapid breakdown of intracellular dATP by lymphoblasts isolated directly from leukemic patients would be useful in establishing that this is an important mechanism that determines sensitivity to dCF treatment in vivo.

We have had the opportunity to closely monitor the serial clinical and biochemical responses to 9 courses of dCF given at 3 weekly intervals to a young man with refractory T cell ALL (32). He initially, responded to dCF, and after the third course of the drug a remission was obtained that persisted until disease recurred 9 weeks later. During the first two courses of dCF peripheral lymphoblasts from this patient accumulated 360-530 nmol dATP per 10^9 cells in vivo, in the presence of 1-2 uM dAdo in plasma. However, following relapse, during the last 3 courses of dCF, his lymphoblasts accumulated dATP to only 20-30 nmol per 10^9 cells, despite plasma dAdo concentrations up to 12 uM. The coincidence of relapse with emergence of a population of lymphoblasts that had greatly diminished capacity to accumulate dATP in vivo supports the conclusion of in vitro studies that dATP pool expansion is the primary determinant of response to ADA inhibition.

Our studies of the basis for the loss of capacity to accumulate dATP in this patient are still in progress, although we have excluded as possibilities the loss of ability to transport dCF or dAdo, alteration in lymphoblast ADA activity, or loss of the enzymes that phosphorylate dAdo. We are considering as one possibility, to be discussed further by Dr. Kurtzberg (31), that resistance resulted from formation in vivo of a hybrid cell line with "B-like" properties, similar to the T cell-B cell hybrids discussed above. Treatment with dCF would provide strong selective advantage to such a hybrid owing to its acquisition of the ability to degrade dATP. Spontaneous in vivo hybrid formation has been proposed over the years as an explanation for the generation of tumor cell diversity in lymphoproliferative diseases (33-35), although to date there is no definitive evidence of the occurrence of this phenomenon in human cancer. Other possible mechanisms of resistance to dCF therapy might include alteration of elements of the nucleoside transport system; overproduction

of ADA (possibly through gene amplification); or loss of
deoxycytidine kinase or Ado kinase. Resistance of various
cellular targets of dAdo, Ara-A or their nucleotide
derivatives could also confer resistance. The latter might
include ribonucleotide reductase or DNA polymerase activities
in the case of the nucleotides, or AdoHcy hydrolase in the
case of dAdo and Ara-A (see below). As will be discussed by
Dr. Richard Fox (36), there are likely to be additional
targets that mediate the toxic effects of dATP and probably
Ara-ATP, but these remain to be identified.

In addition to the inherent capacities of individual
populations of lymphoblasts to trap dAdo as dATP, differences
among patients in the ability to elevate plasma dAdo will
also be a determinant of dATP accumulation, since dAdo
probably arises from the degradation of DNA in senescent
cells, rather than from any metabolic route within living
cells (3). Some studies of response to dCF have focused upon
ability to achieve a high degree of inhibition of lymphoblast
ADA as an index of adequacy of dCF dosage, but have not
considered the primary importance of inhibiting total body
ADA activity in elevating plasma dAdo to a toxic level. As
pointed out above, dCF is not toxic to lymphoblasts cultured
in the absence of exogenous Ado or dAdo.

The major route of dAdo elimination is renal; and far
more dAdo is excreted in urine than is trapped as
intracellular nucleotide during treatment with dCF.
Significant impairment in renal function therefore can lead
to marked elevation in plasma dAdo. Levels of dAdo in the
20-100 uM range have been observed in some patients
undergoing treatment with dCF (6-11,32), far higher than have
been reported in genetic ADA deficiency (1-2 uM) (3). As
discussed above, at low concentrations of dAdo found in
genetic ADA deficiency its phoshorylation is primarily
catalyzed by deoxycytidine kinase, an enzyme found in highest
levels in lymphoid tissues (37,38). At higher concentrations
phosphorylation of dAdo by Ado kinase which has a more
uniform tissue distribution, may lead to enhanced dATP
accumulation in nonlymphoid tissues, possibly contributing to
the renal, hepatic, and central nervous toxicity seen in some
patients.

A third factor to be considered is the effect of cell lysis on dAdo generation from the DNA of dying cells. In the patient referred to above (32) we observed the effect of administering the same total dose of dCF (1 mg/kg infused over 48 hours) when the patient had a large burden of tumor cells, and then when he was in remission. During treatment in remission plasma dAdo rose to about 1-1.5 uM but during treatment of active disease cell lysis caused plasma dAdo to rise to 8-12 uM, with a proportionately large increase in appearance of dAdo in the urine, and of dATP in the patient's erythrocytes (a cell that possesses Ado kinase, but which lacks deoxycytidine kinase). Accumulation of dATP in other nonlymphoid organs has been observed during dCF treatment (9). If nonlymphoid toxicity is to be avoided, it may be wisest to lower the tumor burden by other means before using dCF, and to closely monitor plasma levels of dAdo when treating patients with active disease.

Mechanism of ATP Depletion.

A striking consequence of dCF treatment, which has not been observed to the same degree in genetic ADA deficiency, is the depletion of intracellular ATP in erythrocytes (39) and lymphoblasts (40) that accompanies accumulation of dATP. We have examined the basis for this phenomemon in cultured CEM cells (41). We found that inhibition of ADA alone did not cause ATP depletion, nor did the combination of dCF and dAdo in a mutant of CEM that was incapable of phosphorylating dAdo. In CEM cells that could accumulate dATP, dCF plus dAdo caused a time and dAdo dose dependent fall in total adenine ribonucleotides. Catabolism proceded via a route that involved deamination of AMP to IMP, followed by dephosphorylation of IMP to inosine, and phosphorolysis of inosine to hypoxanthine, with diffusion of inosine and hypoxanthine from the cells. Little if any degradation of AMP ocurred by direct dephosphorylation to Ado. dATP and ATP were both found to be potent activators of lymphoblast AMP deaminase and of a cytoplasmic nucleotidase that dephosphorylates IMP. dAMP was a poor substrate for lymphoblast AMP deaminase. dATP accumulation also inhibited de novo purine synthesis and the conversion of IMP to AMP. Taken together, these findings suggested the following explanation for dAdo mediated ATP catabolism: dATP formation from dAdo, which results in the generation of AMP from ATP, activates AMP catabolism to inosine by maintaining the active

state of AMP deaminase and of the cytoplasmic nucleotidase
that dephosphorylates IMP to inosine. Presumably, under
normal metabolic conditions, conversion of ATP to AMP would
lead to diminished activity of these enzymes, which would
favor the reconversion of AMP to ATP. A similar mechanism
could account for the ATP depletion observed in erythrocytes
(39). In the latter case AMP catabolism would further be
enhanced since these cells lack the ability to reconvert IMP
to AMP, and cannot synthesize purines de novo.

Although dATP toxicity has been attributed by some
solely to allosteric inhibition of ribonucleotide reductase,
dCF treatment causes rapid depletion of peripheral blood
lymphocytes in individuals with nonlymphoid malignancies
(13). These cells are largely nondividing and lack
ribonucleotide reductase activity (42). Furthermore, dATP
accumulation in T cells causes a block in the G 1 phase of
the cell cycle rather than the S phase (43) and is toxic to
nondividing lymphocytes (44). It is possible that ATP
depletion could contribute to this toxity to nonreplicating
cells. It is unclear whether significant depletion of ATP in
lymphoblasts is a common or uncommon consequence of dCF
treatment, nor whether it occurs in nonlymphoid cells other
than erythrocytes. Nevertheless, depletion of ATP to any
degree should potentiate any toxic effects that are due to
the ability of dATP to act as a competitive analog of ATP.

Effect of dCF Treatment on Catabolism of
S-Adenosylhomocysteine (AdoHcy).

For several years Dr. Nicholas Kredich and I have been
interested in actions of Ado, dAdo and Ara-A that can lead to
accumulation of AdoHcy, which is both a product and potent
inhibitor of S-adenosylmethionine (AdoMet)-dependent
transmethylation reactions. In mammalian cells the enzyme
AdoHcy hydrolase catalyzes the hydrolytic degradation of
AdoHcy to Ado and homocysteine (45). However, this reaction
is freely reversible with an equilibrium that greatly favors
AdoHcy formation. Kredich first proposed that when
deamination of Ado is prevented Ado will cause the
accumulation of AdoHcy, resulting in inhibition of sensitive
and possibly essential transmethylation reactions (46). This
mechanism is largely responsible for the toxicity of Ado at
micromolar concentrations to ADA-inhibited cultured lymphoid
cells (47). In addition we have shown that AdoHcy hydrolase

is a high affinity Ado binding protein (48), and that binding
of dAdo causes the "suicide-like" inactivation of purified
(49) and intracellular AdoHcy hydrolase (22). This effect of
dAdo is responsible for the finding that erythrocytes of
children with ADA deficiency possess <2% of normal
erythrocyte AdoHcyase activity (50). AdoHcy hydrolase is
also rapidly inactivated when dAdo accumulates in dCF treated
patients (7,8,32).

We have attempted to determine whether these effects of
Ado and dAdo actually cause accumulation of AdoHcy in the
lymphoblasts of patients undergoing treatment with dCF. In
the case of the T cell ALL patient mentioned above, we made
serial measurements of the concentrations in his lymphoblasts
of AdoMet and AdoHcy, and of the activity of AdoHcy hydrolase
(32). We observed a rapid increase in intracellular AdoHcy
within hours of administering dCF, probably resulting
primarily from the effect of Ado since it occurred before
there was inactivation of more than 50% of lymphoblast AdoHcy
hydrolase activity. The accumulation of AdoHcy persisted
during the period of extensive (85-98%) hydrolase
inactivation, which occurred as dAdo levels in plasma rose to
concentrations above 1 uM. The greatest degree of
inactivation occurred during treatment with dCF and Ara-A,
which is a more potent inactivator of AdoHcy hydrolase than
dAdo. Combined treatment with dCF and Ara-A caused a
decrease in the ratio of intracellular concentration of
AdoMet to that of AdoHcy, sometimes called the 'methylation
index', from pretreatment values of >20:1 to as low as 3:1.
In cultured lymphoid cell lines a decrease of this magnitude
in this ratio is associated with inhibition of some RNA
methylation reactions, and inhibition of cell growth (47,51).
We observed partial inhibition of the methylation of
pyrimidine residue in newly synthesized RNA when lymphoblasts
freshly isolated from this patient during treament were
incubated in vitro. During the period of relapse when
lymphoblast dATP pool expansion was greatly diminished, dCF
infusion alone still caused lymphoblast lysis, though not
sufficient to control disease. This occurred when plasma
dAdo in this patient rose to 8-12 uM, which caused a
sustained inactivation of lymphoblast AdoHcy hydrolase by
93-95% and a decrease in the AdoMet:AdoHcy ratio to <5:1.
These results suggest that AdoHcy accumulation itself may
have a lymphopenic effect, though less than that caused by
dATP accumulation. Such an effect could result from

inhibition of any of several types of transmethylation reactions, possibly those that modify bases in ribosomal, messenger, or small nuclear RNA. Further studies of the consequences of dCF treatment may provide valuable information about the effects of Ado and dAdo on specific transmethylation reactions, and on the importance of these reactions to lymphocyte viability. In addition it is possible that inhibition of AdoHcy catabolism may contribute to the hepatic and central nervous system toxicity that has been oserved in some ptients receiving dCF.

REFERENCES

1. Mauer AM (1980). Therapy of acute lymphoblastic leukemia in chilhood. Blood 56:1.
2. Giblett ER, Anderson JE, Cohen F, Pollara B, Meuwissen HJ (1972). Adenosine deaminase deficiency in two patients with severely impaired cellular immunity. Lancet 2:1067.
3. Kredich NM, Hershfield MS (1982). Immunodeficiency diseases associated with adenosine deaminase deficiency and purine nucleoside phosphorylase deficiency. In Stanbury JB, Wyngaarden JB, Fredrickson DS, Goldstein J, Brown M (eds): "The Metabolic Basis of Inherited Disease," New York:McGraw Hill, 5th edition, in Press.
4. Adams A, Harkness RA (1976). Adenosine deaminase activity in thymus and other human tissues. Clin Exp Immunol 26:647.
5. Agarwal RP, Spector T, Parks RE Jr (1977). Tight binding inhibitors IV. Inhibition of adenosine deaminases by various inhibitors. Biochem Pharmacol 26:359.
6. Koller CA, Mitchell BS, Grever MR, Mejias E, Malspeis L, Metz EN (1979). Treatment of acute lymphoblastic leukemia with 2'-deoxycoformycin: Clinical and biochemical consequences of adenosine deaminase inhibition. Cancer Treatment Reports 63:1949.
7. Mitchell BS, Koller CA, Heyn R (1980). Inhibition of adenosine deaminase activity results in cytotoxicity to T lymphoblasts in vivo. Blood 56:556.
8. Russell NH, Prentice HG, Lee N, Piga A, Ganeshaguru K, Smyth JF (1981). Studies on the biochemical sequelae of therapy in thy-acute lymphoblastic leukemia with the adenosine deaminase inhibitor 2'-deoxycoformycin. Brit J Haematol 49:1.

9. Grever MR, Siaw MFE, Jacob WF, Neidhart JA, Miser JS, Coleman MS, Hutton JJ, Balcerzak SP (1981). The biochemical and clinical consequences of 2'-deoxycoformycin in refractory lymphoproliferative malignancy. Blood 57:406.

10. Prentice HG, Lee N, Blacklock H, Smyth JF, Russell NH, Ganeshaguru K, Piga A, Hofbrand AV (1981). Therapeuutic selectivity of and prediction of response to 2'-deoxycoformycin in acute leukemia. Lancet 2:1250.

11. Poplack DG, Sallan SE, Rivera G, Holcenberg J, Murphy SB, Blatt J, Lipton JM, Venner P, Glaubiger DL, Ungerleider R, Johns D (1981). Phase I study of 2'-deoxycoformycin in acute lymphoblastic leukemia. Cancer Res 41:3343.

12. Gray DP, Grever MR, Siaw MFE, Coleman MS, Balcerzak SP (1982). 2'-deoxycoformycin and 9-B-D-arabinofuranosyladenine (Ara-A) in the treatment of acute myelocytic leukemia. Cancer Treatment Reports 66:253.

13. Smyth JF, Paine RM, Jackman AL, Harrap KR, Chassin MM, Adamson RH, Johns DG (1980). The clinical pharmacology of the adenosine deaminase inhibitor 2'-deoxycoformycin. Cancer Chemother Pharmacol 5:93.

14. Poster DS, Penta JS, Bruno S, Macdonald JS (1981). 2'-Deoxycoformycin. A new anticancer agent. Cancer Clin Trials 4:209.

15. Major PP, Agarwal RP, Kufe DW (1981). Clinical pharmacology of deoxycoformycin. Blood 58:91.

16. Horibata K, Harris AW (1970). Mouse Myelomas and lymphomas in culture. Exp Cell Res 60:61.

17. Reynolds EC, Harris AW, Finch LR (1979). Deoxyribonucleoside triphosphate pools and differential thymidine sensitivities of cultured mouse lymphoma and myeloma cells. Biochim Biophys Acta 561:110.

18. Mitchell BS, Mejias E, Daddona PE, Kelly WN (1978). Purinogenic immunodeficiency diseases: selective toxicity of deoxyribonucleosides for T cells. Proc Natl Acad Sci USA 75:5011.

19. Carson DA, Kaye J, Seegmiller JE (1978). Differential sensitivity of human leukemic T cell lines and B cell lines to growth inhibition by deoxyadenosine. J Immunol 121:1726.

20. Gelfand EW, Lee JJ, Dosch HM (1979). Selective toxicity of purine deoxynucleosides for human lymphocyte growth and function. Proc Natl Acad Sci USA 76:1998.

21. Carson DA, Kaye J, Matsumoto S, Seegmiller JE, Thompson L
     (1979). Biochemical basis for the enhanced toxicity of
     deoxyribonucleosides toward malignant human T cell lines.
     Proc Natl Acad Sci USA 76:2430.
22. Hershfield MS, Kredich NM (1980). Resistance of an
     adenosine kinase-deficient human lymphoblastoid cell line
     to effects of deoxyadenosine on growth,
     S-adenosylhomocysteine hydrolase inactivitation, and dATP
     accumulation. Proc Natl Acad Sci USA 77:4292.
23. Ullman B, Levinson BB, Hershfield MS, Martin DW Jr
     (1981). A biochemical genetic study of the role of
     specific nucleoside kinases in deoxyadenosine
     phosphorylation by cultured human cells. J Biol Chem
     256:848.
24. Verhoef V, Sarup J, Fridland A (1981). Identification of
     the mechanism of activation of
     9-B-D-arabinofuranosyladenine in human lymphoid cells
     using mutants deficient in nucleoside kinases. Cancer
     Res 41:4478.
25. Hershfield MS, Fetter JE, Small WC, Bagnara AS, Williams
     SR, Ullman B, Martin DW Jr, Wasson DB, Carson DA (1982).
     Effects of mutational loss of adenosine kinase and
     deoxycytidine kinase on deoxyATP accumulation and
     deoxyadenosine toxicity in cultured CEM human
     T-lymphoblastoid cells. J Biol Chem 257:6380.
26. Wortmann RL, Mitchell BS, Edwads NL, Fox IH (1979).
     Biochemical basis for differential deoxyadenosine
     toxicity to T and B lymphoblasts. Role for 5'
     nucleotidase. Proc Natl Acad Sci USA 76:2434.
27. Carson DA, Kaye J, Wasson DB (1981). The potential
     importance of soluble deoxynucleotidase activity in
     mediating deoxyadenosine toxicity in human lymphoblasts.
     J Immunol 126:348.
28. Fox RM, Piddington SK, Tripp EH, Tattersall MHN (1981).
     Ecto-ATPase deficiency in cultured human T and null
     leukemic lymphocytes. A biochemical basis for thymidine
     sensitivity. J Clin Invest 68:544.
29. Fox RM, Tripp EH, Piddington SK, Tattersall MHN (1980).
     Sensitivity of leukemic human null lymphocytes to
     deoxynucleosides. Cancer Res 40:3383.
30. Verhoef VL, Fridland A (1982). Differential sensitivity
     of human T and B lymphoblasts to cytotoxic nucleoside
     analogs. J Cellular Biochem Suppl 6, p. 381.

31. Kurtzberg J, Hershfield MS (1982). Deoxynucleoside metabolism in T/B hybrid lymphoblasts. J Cellular Biochem Suppl 6, p. 380.

32. Hershfield MS, Kredich NM, Falletta JM, Kinney TR, Mitchell BS, Koller CA (1981). Effects of deoxyadenosine and adenine arabinoside during deoxycoformycin therapy. Proc Am Assoc Cancer Res 22:157.

33. Goldenberg DM, Bhan RD, Pavia RA (1971). In vivo human-hamster somatic cell fusion indicated by glucose 6-phosphate dehydrogenase and lactate dehydrogenase profiles. Cancer Res 31:1148.

34. Wiener F, Fenyo EM, Klein G, Harris H (1972). Fusion of tumor cells with host cells. Nature New Biology 238:155.

35. Sinkovics JG (1981). Early history of specific antibody-producing lymphocyte hybridomas. Cancer Res 41:1246.

36. Fox RM, Kefford RF (1982). Mechanism of action of deoxyadenosine/adenosine deaminase inhibitor combinations: lymphotoxicity in G1 and G0 phases of cell cycle. J Cellular Biochem Suppl 0, p. 301.

37. Durham JP, Ives DH (1969). Deoxycytidine kinase I. Distribution in normal and neoplastic tissues and interrelationships of deoxycytidine and 1-B-D-arabinofuranosyl cytidine phosphorylation. Mol Pharmacol 5:358.

38. Carson DA, Kaye J, Seegmiller JE (1977). Lymphospecific toxicity in adenosine deaminase deficiency and purine nucleoside phosphorylase deficiency:possible role of nucleoside kinase(s). Proc Natl Acad Sci USA 74:5677.

39. Siaw MFE, Mitchell BS, Koller CA, Coleman MS, Hutton JJ (1980). ATP depletion as a consequence of adenosine deaminase inhibition in man. Proc Natl Acad Sci USA 77:6157.

40. Yu AL, Bakay B, Kung FH, Nyhan WL (1981). Effects of 2'-deoxycoformycin on the metabolism of purines and the survival of malignant cells in a patient with T-cell leukemia. Cancer Res 41:2677.

41. Bagnara AS, Hershfield MS (1982). Mechanism of deoxyadenosine-induced catabolism of adenine ribonucleotides in adenosine deaminase-inhibited human T lymphoblastoid cells. Proc Natl Acad Sci USA 79:2673.

42. Tyrsted G, Gramulin V (1979). Cytidine 5'-diphosphate reductase activity in phytohemaglutinin stimulated human lymphocytes. Nucleic Acid Res 6:305.

43. Fox RM, Kefford RF, Tripp EH, Taylor IW (1981). G1-phase arrest of cultured human leukemic T-cells induced by deoxyadenosine. Cancer Res 41:5141.

44. Kefford RF, Fox RM (1982). Purine deoxynucleoside toxicity in nondividing human lymphoid cells. Cancer Res 42:324.

45. De La Haba G, Cantoni GL (1959). The enzymatic synthesis of S-adenosyl-L-homocysteine from adenosine and homocysteine. J Biol Chem 234:603.

46. Kredich NM, Martin DW Jr (1977). Role of S-adenosylhomocysteine in adenosine mediated toxicity in cultured mouse T lymphoma cells. 12:931.

47. Kredich NM, Hershfield MS (1979). S-adenosylhomocysteine toxicity in normal and adenosine kinase-deficient lymphoblasts of human origin. Proc Natl Acad Sci USA 76:2450.

48. Hershfield MS, Kredich NM (1978). S-adenosylhomocysteine hydrolase is an adenosine-binding protein: A target for adenosine toxicity. Science 202:757.

49. Hershfield MS (1979). Apparent suicide inactivation of human lymphoblast S-adenosylhomocysteine hydrolase by 2'-deoxyadenosine and adenine arabinoside:A basis for direct toxic effects of analogs of adenosine. J Biol Chem 254:22.

50. Hershfield MS, Kredich NM, Ownby DR, Ownby H, Buckley R (1979). In vivo inactivation of erythrocyte S-adenosylhomocysteine hydrolase by 2'-deoxyadenosine in adenosine deaminase-deficient patients. J Clin Invest 63:807

51. Hershfield MS, Small WC, Premakumar R, Bagnara AS, Fetter JE (1982). Inactivation of S-adenosylhomocysteine hydrolase: Mechanism and occurrence in vivo in disorders of purine nucleoside catabolism. In Borchardt RT, Usdin E, Creveling CR (eds): "The Biochemistry of S-Adenosylmethionine and Related Compounds," MacMillan, in Press.

Rational Basis for Chemotherapy, pages 291–294

WORKSHOP SUMMARY: BIOCHEMICAL TARGETTING -
THE T-LYMPHOCYTE MALIGNANCIES

Richard M. Fox

Ludwig Institute for Cancer Research (Sydney Branch)
Blackburn Building, University of Sydney
Sydney. N.S.W. 2006. Australia.

The basis of this workshop was discussion of the use and
mechanism of action of the adenosine deaminase (ADA)
inhibitor, Deoxycoformycin (DCF), in the treatment of T-
lymphocyte malignancies. The problems addressed included·
a) current status and results of its use in the clinic,
b) appropriate monitoring of the use of DCF,
c) biochemical consequences of inhibition of ADA with
emphasis on deoxyadenosine mediated lymphoid
toxicity.
A summary of the workshop discussion is given below. For
more details on each presentation, the authors abstracts
published in the Journal of Cellular Biochemistry, Supplement 6, 1982 could be consulted.
J. Smyth described his group's clinical experience with
DCF which produced a 72% objective response with 44% complete
remissions in patients with T-cell ALL who had failed previous treatment. These results suggested that there was no
cross-resistance to vincristine, prednisone, L-asparaginase,
adriamycin, daunorubicin, cyclophosphamide, methotrexate,
6-thioguanine, 6-mercaptopurine or cytosine arabinoside. It
was not possible to assess the duration of response as
responding patients proceeded to bone marrow transplantation.
The in vivo intracellular dATP accumulation in leukaemic
blasts correlated with clinical response. Interestingly, a
2-hour in vitro exposure of pre-treatment blasts to DCF
(10μM) plus deoxyadenosine (100μM) demonstrated a positive
correlation between the accumulation of dATP and subsequent
clinical response. Thus, it appears possible to predict
response in vitro. The major toxicity encountered was
renal (42%) with a 15% mortality. There was considerable

discussion regarding the mechanism of this toxicity, possibilities included:

a) direct renal toxicity by DCF; or
b) excessive tumour cell lysis products, including deoxyadenosine were toxic.

It was concluded that patients with high blast cell counts should have "tumour reduction" with conventional therapy, and then be treated with DCF. The use of intensive hydration and allopurinol to attempt to reduce potential renal toxicity was discussed.

M. S. Coleman discussed her results of biochemical monitoring of DCF therapy in T-cell and other lymphoid malignancies. She has developed a simple Enzyme Linked Immunoassay (ELISA) for human terminal deoxynucleotidyl transferase (TdT) which is also potentially applicable to ADA. The possible availability of these assays in simple kit form will simplify biochemical monitoring in clinical studies. In a study of 71 patients with CML, ADA was shown to exhibit a high correlation with disease course. Elevated ADA in the buffy coat occurred concurrently with acceleration of CML (24/31), and this may be useful in predicting the onset of blast crisis. Concurrent TdT assays in blast crisis identify those with a lymphoid type transformation (30% of patients). DCF had been used in some 60 patients with diagnosis including CLL, CML, ALL and mycosis fungoides. Biochemical parameters monitored have included ADA and S-Adenosylhomocysteine Hydrolase activities, serum and urinary Ado and dAdo levels, and nucleotide pools (ATP and dATP). The most important factors in predicting toxicity were the dATP/ATP ratios in patients' erythrocytes. However, ATP depletion was not seen in leukemic blasts from 14 patients and it was considered that ATP depletion was not the cause of the blast lysis.

Dr. J. Kurtzberg addressed the problem: why do T-lymphoblasts accumulate dATP from 2'dAdo (in the presence of an ADA inhibitor such as DCF)more efficiently than B lymphocytes. To gain more insight into the regulatory mechanisms in T and B cells, she constructed T x B cell hybrids. This was performed using a T cell parent (CCRF-CEM line, Oubain resistant and HGPRT-) and a B cell parent (WIL2 line, Oubain sensitive, HGPRT+). This T x B hybrid lymphoblast was characterised by its growth in various selective media, HLA phenotypes and enzyme activities. The dAdo kinases (Ado and dCyd kinase) were similar in parental lines and in the hybrid. The concentration of dAdo required for 50% growth inhibition of the CEM, WIL2 and the T x B hybrids were 0.3 - 0.6µM, 45µM and 25 - 27µM respectively. The capacity of the various cell lines to accumulate dATP after incubation with 2'dAdo (in the presence of DCF), as well as catabolise an expanded dATP pool was studied. Results indicated that "B-ness" was dominant over "T-ness", consistent with the operation in B cells of possible en- hanced nucleotidase activity diminishing their ability to accumulate dATP from dAdo.

V. L. Herhoef discussed the role of a soluble 5' nucleotidase in the differential sensitivity of human T and B lymphoblasts to nucleosides and analogs. He compared the cytotoxic effects of structurally related purine and pyrimidine analogs on cultured T and B lymphoblasts. The T cell selectivity of these agents and the substrate specificity of their phosphorylating and dephosphorylating pathways were also compared. Adenosine (in combination with DCF) 2'azido-2'deoxyara-A (with DCF), pyrazofurin and 5-fluoro-deoxyuridine were equally cytotoxic to T and B lymphoblasts and were termed "Type I" agents. In comparison ara-A (with DCF), 2-fluoro-ara-A, ara-C and 2'-O-nitro-ara-C were 2 - 6 fold more cytotoxic to T cells and were termed "Type II" agents. However, dAdo and thymidine were 28 - 50 fold more cytotoxic to T cells than B cells and were classed as "Type III" agents. All agents, except adenosine, required phosphorylation via one or more nucleoside kinases for cytotoxic activity; but there was no correlation bet- ween the route of phosphorylation of an agent and its selectivity for T cells. A partially purified soluble 5'nucleotidase from a CEM (T lymphoblast) line was charact- erosed. The 5' nucleotides of several of these various agents were tested as substrates for this enzyme. The sub- strate specificity of the soluble deoxynucleotidase for the 5' monophosphates of dAdo, thymidine, ara-A, ara-C and 2-fluoro-ara-A correlated with the T-cell selectivity of these agents.

R. M. Fox discussed the mechanisms by which elevated dATP pools (in response to incubation with dAdo in the pre- sence of an ADA inhibitor) is toxic to T cells. Studies were carried out using DNA flow cytometry, and dAdo, at cytostatic concentrations, was shown to induce a G_1 block. Using the G_2 -M phase specific inhibitor, ICRF-159 (Razoxane), it was shown that cells in S-phase, exposed to dAdo, were able to complete that S-phase and accumulate in G_2 -M. Using bromodeoxyuridine quenching of 33342 Hoechst fluorescence, it was possible to demonstrate that the cells in S-phase, exposed to dAdo, completed the S-phase, passed through G_2 +M and then returned to the G_1 phase. Cells were enriched for various phases of the cell cycle by centrifugal elutriation. dAdo was shown to elevate the dATP pool to a similar extent in the G_1, S and G_2 -M cell fractions, without an accompanying fall in the dCTP pool. It was concluded that dAdo induces a G_1 block, independent of ribonucleotide reductase inhibition. In contrast, B lymphoblasts, which required a 100-fold higher concentration of dAdo to induce cytostasis demonstrated a characteristic S-phase block. The exact biochemical mechanisms of the dATP mediated G_1 block was not known.

The workshop concluded that purine analogs, in particular ADA inhibitors, have a continuing role in the management of T cell and other malignancies. In particular, it was stressed that a great deal was understood about the biochemical rationale for the use of such drugs. Furthermore, studies of the biochemical pharmacology of purine analogs was producing fundamental information about molecular control mechanisms in the lymphoid system.

Rational Basis for Chemotherapy, pages 295–308
© 1983 Alan R. Liss, Inc., 150 Fifth Avenue, New York, NY 10011

MONOCLONAL ANTIBODY THERAPY IN A MOUSE MODEL[1]

Irwin D. Bernstein and Christopher C. Badger

Pediatric Oncology and Medical Oncology Programs
Fred Hutchinson Cancer Research Center
1124 Columbia Street and
Departments of Pediatrics and Medicine
University of Washington, Seattle, Washington 98104

ABSTRACT   Monoclonal antibodies are potentially useful in the treatment of cancer as therapeutic agents in unmodified form, or as carriers of a cytotoxic compound.   We have used monoclonal antibodies against a normal T cell differentiation antigen, Thy 1.1, to treat transplanted and spontaneous leukemia in AKR/J mice.   Anti-Thy 1.1 monoclonal antibody completely inhibited the growth of leukemia following implantation of up to 3×10^5 AKR/J SL2 leukemic cells.   Maximal effectiveness required a dose of 3200 ug of antibody per animal, which was the dose required to completely saturate cell surface antigenic sites on subcutaneous leukemic cells.   Failure to inhibit $>3 \times 10^5$ cells was a result of a limitation in the ability of the host to eliminate antibody-coated cells in the subcutaneous space.   The limiting factor was presumably an effector cell population.   In contrast, development of metastatic disease was the result of selection of stable antigen negative variant cells.
       Treatment of spontaneous leukemia in aged AKR/J mice with anti-Thy 1.1 antibody during a chemotherapy-induced remission led to a highly significant prolongation of disease-free survival in

[1] This work was supported by grants CA 26386 and CA 33477, awarded by the National Cancer Institute, DHEW.

a subgroup of animals. The implications of the results obtained with this system for future clinical trials and the possible use of antibody as a selective delivery agent are discussed.

INTRODUCTION

There is currently great interest in using monoclonal antibodies as therapeutic agents in the treatment of cancer either in unmodified form or as carriers to selectively deliver cytotoxic agents. While monoclonal antibodies against antigens uniquely expressed by tumors have not been generated, antibodies against a variety of normal differentiation antigens expressed by tumors have been produced (see reference 1). These antibodies, reactive with both malignant and normal cells, may be useful for therapeutic purposes if sufficient binding to malignant cells occurs in the absence of prohibitive toxicity. With this in mind, we have used monoclonal antibody against a normal murine T cell differentiation antigen, Thy 1.1, to treat transplanted and spontaneous leukemias in AKR/J mice (2-6). In this report, we review our studies evaluating the conditions leading to successful monoclonal antibody therapy of these tumors. Studies examining the localization of anti-Thy 1.1 antibodies to Thy 1.1-bearing target cells are also described.

RESULTS

Treatment of Transplantable Tumors

Our initial studies demonstrated that anti-Thy 1.1 antibody could prevent the growth of transplanted AKR/J SL2 leukemic cells (2, 3). These leukemic cells express high concentrations of Thy 1.1 antigen in vivo and in vitro. When inoculated subcutaneously, they give rise to a local tumor nodule at the subcutaneous inoculation site, and metastasize widely leading to death within a few weeks. In these initial studies, tumor cells were inoculated subcutaneously, and animals were treated with ascites fluid containing anti-Thy 1.1 monoclonal antibody (usually 100 ul i.v. given 1-2 hours after tumor inoculation, followed by 50 ul i.p. every 3-4 days for 3-5 doses). Two important conclusions could be drawn from those experiments. <u>First</u>, antibody against a widely expressed normal differentiation antigen was capable of mediating anti-tumor effects in vivo; and second, the antibody could do so without exerting significant toxic effects on the host.

Recently, we have performed a more detailed examination of antibody dose-effect relationships. In these experiments, mice were challenged with varying numbers of tumor cells, ranging from 3×10^5 to 3×10^6 cells. One to two hours later, the mice were treated with a single intravenous infusion of ascites fluid containing an IgG_{2a} monoclonal anti-Thy 1.1 antibody, 19-E12 (3), in doses of 400, 1200 or 3200 ug of antibody. A summary of the results (see Table 1) reveals that complete prevention of tumor outgrowth by antibody was achieved only in mice challenged with 3×10^5 cells. Consistent inhibition required a relatively high dose of 3200 ug per mouse of 19-E12 antibody. In other experiments, additional doses of antibody (half of the initial dose given every 3-4 days intraperitoneally for 4 doses) did not alter the outcome (Table 2). Thus, a high dose of antibody was needed to consistently achieve a maximal anti-leukemic cell kill of 3×10^5 cells.

TABLE 1
ANTIBODY THERAPY OF TRANSPLANTED LEUKEMIA

Antibody dose (ug)	3×10^5 cells	3×10^6 cells
0	0/19	0/10
400	7/15	0/10
1200	5/20	0/9
3200	15/18	0/11

AKR/J mice were subcutaneously implanted with single cell suspensions of 3×10^5 or 3×10^6 in vivo passaged syngeneic AKR/J SL2 leukemia cells in a volume of 0.1 ml. An infusion of antibody was given via the retro-orbital venous plexus one hour after tumor implantation. Antibody was given as unpurified ascites containing 4 mg/ml of the IgG_{2a} anti-Thy 1.1 monoclonal antibody 19-E12. The number of animals surviving tumor free at 120 days and considered cured (numerator) over the number of animals treated (denominator) is shown for the combined results of four experiments.

TABLE 2
ANTIBODY THERAPY OF TRANSPLANTED LEUKEMIA:
COMPARISON OF SINGLE VS MULTIPLE DOSES

Antibody dose (ug)	3×10^5 cells	3×10^6 cells
0	0/5	0/5
400/200	1/5	0/5
3600	4/5	0/5
3600/1800	4/5	0/5

Animals were implanted with AKR/J SL2 leukemia cells as in Table 1. Antibody treatment was started 1 hour later with either 400 ug i.v. followed by 200 ug i.p. days 3, 7, 11 and 14; 3600 ug i.v.; 3600 ug i.v. followed by 1800 ug days 3, 7, 11 and 14. A control group did not receive antibody. The number of mice cured (numerator) over the number treated (denominator) is shown.

The basis of the requirement for a high antibody dose to produce consistent inhibition of 3×10^5 cells was the need to achieve sufficient antibody coating of the target antigens on the tumor cell surface. This was demonstrated by examining the relationship of antibody dose to the amount of in vivo antibody coating of Thy 1.1 sites on the surface of the malignant cells in a subcutaneous tumor nodule. Mice with palpable subcutaneous leukemic nodules were treated intravenously with doses of antibody varying from 400 to 3200 ug, and the nodule excised 24 hours after infusion. Individual tumor cells were then examined for the presence of the infused antibody on their surfaces by indirect immunofluorescence using fluoresceinated anti-mouse IgG antibody (see Table 3 and reference 6 for details). In addition, the maximum amount of antibody that would bind to the cell surface was examined by first incubating the tumor cells in vitro with excess 19-E12 antibody before the incubation period with the fluoresceinated anti-mouse IgG reagent. In this manner, the level of cell surface Thy 1.1 expression, as indicated by the maximum amount of antibody bound, as well as the proportion of Thy 1.1 sites coated in vivo would be determined. The results demonstrated that increasing doses of antibody led to increasing amounts of antibody present on the tumor cell surfaces, with complete in vivo saturation of all the available Thy 1.1 sites achieved by the infusion of 3200 ug antibody (Table 3). There was no diminution in the amount of Thy 1.1 expression by the cells from treated mice as compared to those from untreated mice.

TABLE 3
IN VIVO SURFACE BINDING OF ANTIBODY

Antibody dose (ug)	% of Thy 1.1 sites coated with antibody
Control	0%
400	27%
1200	54%
3200	100%

AKR/J mice were implanted with 2 x 10^6 AKR/J SL2 leukemia cells. When a palpable nodule (5-10 mm diameter) developed, a single intravenous infusion of 19-E12 or control non-specific antibody of similar isotype was given. 24 hours after infusion the nodule was excised and a single cell suspension obtained. Aliquots were then tested by direct immunofluorescence with fluoresceinated rabbit anti-mouse IgG antibody to determine surface antibody bound in vivo, or by indirect immunofluorescence using excess 19-E12 followed by the fluoresceinated rabbit anti-mouse IgG antibody to determine the total amount of cell surface Thy 1.1. The percent of cell surface Thy 1.1 sites that were coated in vivo by antibody was estimated by dividing the amount of fluorescence obtained in the direct immunofluorescent test by that obtained in the indirect test. Background fluorescence was determined by direct immunofluorescence with fluoresceinated rabbit anti-mouse IgM antibody. Cell surface fluorescence was quantitated using the fluorescence activated cell sorter (see reference 6 for details). Mean saturation from 5-7 animals per group is shown.

Since the infused antibody can bind to and saturate all surface sites on tumor cells in vivo, the failure to eliminate $>3 \times 10^5$ leukemic cells must result either from failure of the host to eliminate larger numbers of antibody coated cells or, alternatively, from growth of cells lacking the target antigen. To examine this, mice were challenged with 3×10^6 AKR/J SL2 cells and treated with multiple high doses of antibody (3600 ug day 0, 1800 ul day 3, 7, 11 and 14). Immunofluorescence studies performed on cells from the subcutaneous nodules which had grown during antibody therapy showed nearly complete saturation of the cell surfaces by the infused antibody, and the surface expression of Thy 1.1 was maintained at levels comparable to control cells. Thus, the failure to eliminate leukemic cells was not due to the failure of antibody to saturate tumor cell surfaces, or the local escape of tumor cells that failed to express the target antigen. Rather, it was due to the inability of the host to eliminate antibody coated cells. This limiting host factor is presumably an effector cell population(s), rather than complement, because the anti-tumor effects described occurred in AKR/J mice which are known to be deficient for the fifth component of complement. In addition, we (3) and others (7, 8) have found that IgM antibody, which does not mediate cell dependent cytotoxicity in vitro, was much less effective in vivo than IgG antibodies which do mediate cell dependent cytotoxicity. The importance of host effector cells in the antibody-mediated elimination of tumor has also been suggested in studies using antisera (9, 10).

Another important observation was that antibody treatment, when it failed to cure the recipient mice (e.g., following inoculation of $>3 \times 10^5$ AKR/J SL-2 cells), delayed the occurrence of metastatic disease and death. Furthermore, lower or higher doses of antibody were equally effective in prolonging survival. When mice were challenged with 3×10^6 cells, a consistent 60% prolongation in median survival was seen whether the mice were treated with a single dose of either 400 or 3200 ug of 19-E12 antibody 1-2 hours after tumor inoculation or with multiple doses of antibody. Thus, antibody was more efficient in delaying metastatic growth than in preventing local growth at the subcutaneous inoculum site, and the time course for development of metastases was independent of the antibody dose. The reasons for these observations were investigated by examining the antigenic nature of the metastatic disease that occurred in antibody-treated mice. We determined whether the metastatic spleen cells eventually grew despite the presence of surface antibody, as found in the tumor nodule, or if they were variant cells that did not express the Thy 1.1 target antigen. For this purpose, mice were subcutaneously challenged with 3×10^6 AKR/J SL2 leukemic cells and treated 1-2 hours later with 19-E12 antibody. When metastatic growth was evident, the enlarged leukemic spleens were removed. Individual cells were examined by direct immunofluorescence for the presence of cell surface IgG antibody, and by indirect immunofluorescence for cell surface Thy 1.1 sites as described earlier. We found that the metastatic spleen cells from animals treated with either single doses of antibody or with multiple doses failed to react in either the direct or indirect immunofluorescent tests. This indicated that they were not coated with the infused anti-Thy 1.1 antibody, and did not express Thy 1.1. The lack of Thy 1.1 expression was shown to be due to the selection of stable antigen negative variant cells, since they maintained their antigen negative state upon serial in vivo passage (3, 6). Thus, even low doses of antibody effectively prevented metastasis of antigen-bearing cells, and prolongation of survival in antibody-treated animals was a result of the time necessary for the growth of antigen negative variants.

Treatment of Spontaneous AKR Leukemia

Although transplantable tumor models provide useful information about the principles of antibody therapy, only the treatment of naturally occurring malignancies provides an effective setting for determining ultimate clinical usefulness. The occurrence of spontaneous T-cell lymphomas in aged AKR mice has allowed us to evaluate the therapy of naturally occurring malignancies with anti-Thy 1.1 antibody. These spontaneous tumors occur in the majority of AKR/J mice between the ages of 6 and 13 months. They are primarily thymic in origin and metastasize to peripheral organs, including blood and bone marrow. The presence of leukemia can be assessed clinically by examining the mice for enlarged lymphoid organs including spleen, lymph node, and (visually) thymic size.

We have used anti-Thy 1.1 antibody to treat leukemic animals following the induction of a disease-free remission (lack of detectably enlarged lymphoid organs) with chemotherapy. This approach was used since the studies in transplanted leukemia suggested that antibody was unlikely to have a major impact on a large cell burden. Moreover, preliminary experiments had shown that treatment of frankly leukemic mice with antibody led to rapid death presumably from rapid cell lysis or agglutination.

In initial experiments, leukemic mice were treated with cyclophosphamide (100 mg/kg i.p. x 2). Mice in remission were then randomized between no further therapy and treatment with 19-E12 antibody (400 ug i.v. day 0, followed by 200 ug i.p. twice a week) (3, 4). Antibody treatment resulted in a modest increase in disease-free survival, but no increase in overall survival. There were, however, a significant number of deaths of mice during remission in the antibody-treated group. Preliminary evidence has indicated that infection, primarily pulmonary, was the cause.

More recent experiments have been aimed at increasing the influence of antibody therapy on survival by further reducing the tumor burden with more aggressive chemotherapy. We also examined the influence of tumor burden, as indicated by spleen and lymph node size and the peripheral white blood cell (wbc) count at diagnosis, on the outcome of the antibody treatment. Leukemic mice were first treated with an increased dose of cyclophosphamide (150 mg/kg days 1 and 4). Animals in remission on day 4 were randomized to receive antibody therapy (as in the previous experiment), or no further treatment. Antibody again produced a significant prolongation of disease-free survival in antibody-treated mice (Fig. 1A) (log rank, p = .005), but no difference in absolute survival was observed.

When the influence of lymphoid organ enlargement and white blood cell count was evaluated, the prolongation of disease-free survival was virtually restricted to animals with initial white cell counts of 10,000-20,000 (Figure 1B). Of particular importance, there was an absolute survival advantage for antibody-treated mice in this group (log rank, p = .01), with the majority of antibody treated animals dying in clinical remission. The causes of death in these mice are currently being investigated. In the small number of animals with <10,000 wbc at diagnosis,

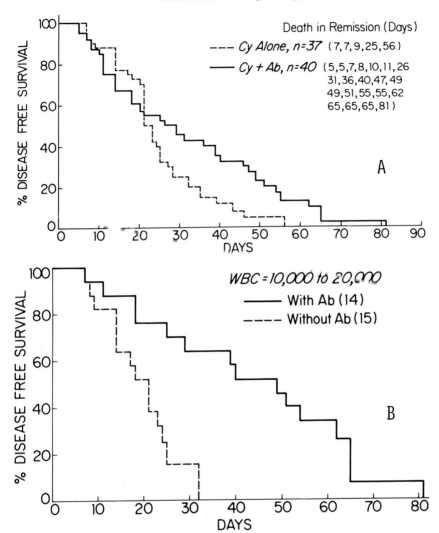

FIGURE 1.   Antibody therapy of spontaneous leukemia.
AKR/J mice with spontaneous leukemia were treated with
cyclophosphamide, 150 mg/kg i.p. on days 0 and 4.   Those
in remission on day 4 were randomized to no further
treatment or antibody therapy (400 ug day 0 then 200 ug
twice a week continuously, see text for details).   Time to
relapse or death in remission is shown in panel A.   Also
shown is day of death for animals dying in remission.
Results with animals that had pretreatment white blood
counts between 10,000 and 20,000 are shown in panel B.

there was a slight trend in favor of antibody therapy. Of significance, antibody therapy had no effect on either disease-free survival or absolute survival in animals with greater than 20,000 wbc. The failure of antibody treatment in these mice may have resulted from its ineffectiveness against larger numbers of tumor cells, or from a failure of the host to produce effector cells which eliminate antibody coated cells. The latter would be true if the white blood cell count reflected leukemia involvement of the marrow where such effector cells may arise (11, 12). These preliminary experiments offer the exciting possibility of defining conditions under which monoclonal antibody can be used effectively to treat a naturally occurring disease.

Antibody as a Selective Delivery Agent

While antibody can have a major effect on small numbers of malignant cells, the limitation imposed by the requirement for a host effector mechanism makes it unlikely that unmodified antibody will be very effective in the treatment of bulk disease. In this situation, antibody may be more useful as a carrier of a toxin or radio-isotope where the antibody-conjugate will be directly toxic to cells, and not require participating host effectors. The conjugate must bind to tumor cell surfaces while having minimal contact with critical populations of normal cells; e.g., bone marrow. Cytotoxic drugs (13), ricin or diptheria toxin (14-19), as well as radioisotopes (20) have been considered as potential candidates for selective delivery to tumors.

To this end, the ability of radiolabeled anti-Thy 1.1 antibody and antibody fragments to localize to lymphoid organs has been studied (21). Anti-Thy 1.1 antibody, labeled with ^{125}I, specifically localized to spleen and lymph nodes in animals whose T-cells expressed Thy 1.1 as compared to congenic animals expressing the Thy 1.2 antigen. A ratio of tissue to blood activity of 6.7 was obtained with whole antibody. Furthermore, antibody persisted in the lymphoid organs for up to 72 hours. F(ab')$_2$ fragments produced even better specific localization with lymph node activity up to 143 times that found in blood. The better localization of F(ab')$_2$ fragments presumably resulted from a decrease in nonspecific binding to Fc-receptors, as well as better diffusion out of the vascular system. Others have shown that radiolabeled monoclonal antibody can localize to tumor cells in vivo (22-24). These studies demonstrate the potential of antibody as a carrier. Further quantitative studies evaluating the relative distribution of antibody to tumor versus normal tissue targets will enable an improved assessment of the degree to which radioactivity or cytotoxic agents can be selectively delivered.

An alternative approach has been to achieve selective toxicity by using the A chain of ricin or diptheria toxin These molecules are toxic once inside the cell but cannot bind or enter in the absence of the B chain. By conjugation of the A chain with antibody, it is hoped that the conjugate will enter and kill cells bearing the target antigen. Results with antibody conjugates to date have shown selective toxicity both in vitro (14-19) and in vivo (14, 18-19). However, whether antibody-toxin conjugates are more effective in vivo than antibody alone is as yet uncertain (18). This approach is promising but awaits improved techniques to develop antibody conjugates which will be stable for a sufficient length of time to reach the extravascular space, and then enter and kill the tumor targets.

DISCUSSION

The studies described above have begun to elucidate the principals underlying antibody therapy. The collective results of these studies demonstrate that monoclonal antibody against a normal differentiation antigen can be used to eliminate up to 3×10^5 tumor cells at an extravascular site, and that it can be effectively used to prolong chemotherapy-induced remissions in spontaneous leukemia. Optimal therapy appears to require maximal amounts of antibody on the tumor cell surface. In spite of antibody saturation of cell surface antigenic sites, the effectiveness of antibody against bulk disease is limited, presumably by a host effector cell population(s). In contrast, antibody can be exquisitely effective in either preventing or eliminating metastatic disease due to leukemic cells expressing the target antigen. The failure of antibody to prevent metastatic growth results from the emergence of antigen-negative variants. Presumably this emergence could be further delayed, or prevented, by using combinations of antibodies against different cell surface antigens.

These results suggest that unmodified antibody will have its greatest value in situations of minimal residual disease, such as during a chemotherapy-induced remission. The effectiveness of antibody in preventing metastases of antigen bearing cells suggests its use for preventing metastatic spread during or following surgical removal of tumors. In these situations, effective therapy may require high doses of combinations of antibody against different tumor cell surface antigens. It seems unlikely that unmodified antibody will be effective in the treatment of larger numbers of tumor cells which will require the use of antibody to selectively deliver cytotoxic agents.

The great interest in monoclonal antibodies has led to rapid clinical trials. Although there have been a few responses to therapy, results have been for the most part disappointing (25). The application of principals learned from model systems should be an invaluable aid in improving these results.

REFERENCES

1. Mitchell MS, Oettgen HF (eds) (1982). "Hybridomas in Cancer Diagnosis and Treament," New York: Raven Press, 264 pp.
2. Bernstein ID, Tam MR, Nowinski RC (1980). Mouse leukemia: Therapy with monoclonal antibodies against a thymus differentiation antigen. Science 207:68.
3. Bernstein ID, Nowinski RC, Tam MR, McMaster B, Houston LL, Clark EA (1980). Monoclonal antibody therapy of mouse leukemia. In Kennett RH, McKearn TJ, Bechtol KB (eds): "Monoclonal Antibodies," New York: Plenum Publishing, p. 275.
4. Bernstein ID, Nowinski RC (1981). Monoclonal antibody treatment of transplanted and spontaneous murine leukemia. In Mitchell MS, Oettgen HF (eds): "Hybridomas in Cancer Diagnosis and Treatment," New York: Raven Press, p. 97.
5. Badger CC, Bernstein ID (In press). Monoclonal antibody therapy of murine leukemia. In August JT (ed): "Monoclonal Antibodies in Drug Development," Bethesda: Amer Soc Pharm & Exper Ther.
6. Badger CC, Bernstein ID. Therapy of murine leukemia with monoclonal antibody against a normal differentiation antigen. Submitted.

7. Young WW Jr, Hakomori S-I (1981). Therapy of mouse lymphoma with monoclonal antibodies to glycolipid: Selection of low antigenic variants in vivo. Science 211:487.

8. Kirch ME, Hammerling U (1981). Immunotherapy of murine leukemias by monoclonal antibody. I. Effect of passively administered antibody on growth of transplanted tumor cells. J Immunol 127:805.

9. Lanier LL, Babcock GF, Raybourne RB, Arnold LW, Warner NL, Haughton G (1980). Mechanism of B cell lymphoma immunotherapy with passive xenogeneic anti-idiotype serum. J Immunol 125:1730.

10. Shin HS, Mayden M, Langley S, Kaliss N, and Smith MR (1975). Antibody-mediated suppression of grafted lymphoma. III. Evaluation of the role of thymic function, non-thymus-derived lymphocytes, macrophages, platelets, and polymorphonuclear leukocytes in syngeneic and allogeneic hosts. J Immunol 114:1255.

11. Shin HS, Kaliss N, Borenstein D, Gately MK (1972). Antibody-mediated suppression of grafted lymphoma cells. II. Participation of macrophages. J Exp Med 136:375.

12. Volkman A, Gowans JL (1965). The origins of macrophages from bone marrow in the rat. Brit J Exp Pathol 46:62.

13. Ghose T, Blair AH (1978). Antibody-linked cytotoxic agents in the treatment of cancer. Current status and future prospects. J Natl Cancer Inst 61:657.

14. Blythman HE, Casellas P, Gros O, Gros P, Jansen FK, Paolucci F, Pau B, Vidal H (1981). Immunotoxins: Hybrid molecules of monoclonal antibodies and a toxin subunit specifically kill tumor cells. Nature 290:145.

15. Gilliland DG, Steplewski Z, Collier RJ, Mitchell KF, Chang TH, Koprowski H (1980). Antibody-directed cytotoxic agents: Use of monoclonal antibody to direct the action of toxin A chains to colorectal carcinoma cells. Proc Natl Acad Sci USA 77:4539.

16. Houston LL, Nowinski RC (1981). Cell-specific cytotoxicity expressed by a conjugate of ricin and murine monoclonal antibody directed against Thy 1.1 antigen. Cancer Res 41:3913.

17. Youle RJ, Neville DM Jr (1980). Anti-Thy 1.2 monoclonal antibody linked to ricin is a potent cell-type-specific toxin. Proc Natl Acad Sci USA 77:5483.

18. Trowbridge IS, Domingo DL (1981). Anti-transferrin receptor monoclonal antibody and toxin-antibody conjugates affect growth of human tumor cells. Nature 294:171.

19. Krolick KA, Uhr JW, Slavin S, Vitetta ES (1982). In vivo therapy of a murine B cell tumor (BCL_1) using antibody-ricin A chain immunotoxins. J Exp Med 155:1797.

20. Order SE (1976). The history and progress of serologic immunotherapy and radiodiagnosis. Radiol 118:219.

21. Houston LL, Nowinski RC, Bernstein ID (1980). Specific in vivo localization of monoclonal antibodies directed against the Thy 1.1 antigen. J Immunol 125:837.

22. Ballou B, Levine G, Hakala TR, Solter D (1979). Tumor location detected with radioactively labeled monoclonal antibody and external scintigraphy. Science 206:844.

23. Scheinberg DA, Strand M (1982). Leukemic cell targeting and therapy by monoclonal antibody in a mouse model system. Cancer Res 42:44.

24. Bernhard MI, Foon KA, Clarke GC, Christensen WL, Hoyer L, Key M, Hanna MG, Oldham RK (1982). Monoclonal antibody serotherapy of solid tumors: A guinea pig model. Proc Amer Assoc Cancer Res 23:256.

25. Ritz J, Schlossman SF (1982). Utilization of monoclonal antibodies in the treatment of leukemia and lymphoma. Blood 59:1.

Rational Basis for Chemotherapy, pages 309–314
© 1983 Alan R. Liss, Inc., 150 Fifth Avenue, New York, NY 10011

Binding of H59 and Other Monoclonal Antibodies to Human Breast Cancer[1]

Fred J. Hendler[2] and Dorothy Yuan

Departments of Internal Medicine and Microbiology
University of Texas Health Science Center
Southwestern Medical School
Dallas, TX   75235

ABSTRACT: Monoclonal antibodies which react with human
breast cancer have been developed using the human hormone
dependent breast cancer cell line, ZR-75-1 by hybridoma
techniques. The binding of three antibodies, H59, H71 and
H72 has been evaluated in breast cancer cell lines, non breast
cancer cells and tissue specimens from patients with breast
cancer, benign breast diseases, and other malignancies. All
three antibodies appear to recognize antigens which are
expressed predominately on human breast cells. Antibodies
bound 90% of breast cancers and almost all benign breast
disease specimens. H59 may be recognizing an estiogen
regulated cell surface antigen. H71 and H72 are probably
recognizing differentiation antigens. Future studies will
attempt to correlate antibody binding with the patients
prognosis and chemotherapy.

INTRODUCTION

Our research has centered on identifying biologic markers of
breast cancer and in particular, markers of steroid hormone dependence. We have endeavored to identify new tumor markers which

[1]This work was supported in part by NIH grant CA 23115
ACS grant #IN142, The Ira Kassanoff Fund, and The
Blanche Mary Taxis Foundation.
[2]FJH is a junior faculty fellow of the American Cancer
Society.

might be more closely associated with patient prognosis and response to therapy than those presently available such as the estrogen and progesterone receptor. Our most recent approach has been to generate a series of monoclonal antibodies using human breast cancer tissue culture cell lines as the source of antigens (1,2). One of our antibodies, H59, may be recognizing a hormone dependent cell surface protein. Two other antibodies, H71 and H72 appear to be binding differentiation antigens which are not hormone regulated. This report summarizes the tissue specificity of H59, H71 and H72 antibodies, the binding of the antibodies to breast biopsy specimens, and speculates as to the clinical potential of these monoclonal antibodies in breast cancer.

Schlom et al. have produced monoclonal antibodies to human breast cancer using B lymphocytes isolated from the draining axillary lymph nodes of patients with breast cancer (3) and using breast cancer antigens isolated from liver metastasis (4). We have chosen to use human breast cancer cells in continuous culture as the source of antigens because these cells are well characterized morphologically and biochemically. The cell lies are stable, cloned and an unlimited source of antigens. The cells in culture are a model system which can be explored to demonstrate the relationship of an antigen to hormone regulation or any other factors which might affect cell growth and viability. Cultured cells can also produce human tumors in athymic rodents; these are an excellent in vitro model to evaluate diagnostic reagents and specific immunotherapy.

RESULTS

Because of our selection techniques (1,2), the antibodies which we have generated predominately recognize cell surface antigens. It is our hypothesis that H59 antibody recognizes an estrogen regulated cell surface determinant and that H71 and H72 represent two distinct differentiation antigens.

H59

H59 binds only to hormone dependent human breast cancer cell lines (1,2). In addition, it does not bind R27 (5) and R3 (6), two tamoxifen resistant cell lines derived from the estrogen dependent, human breast cancer, MCF-7 cells. It has some weak cross reactivity with a neural line and three endometrial tumor cell lines (2). The antigen appears to be on the cell surface by immunofluorescent studies (2), and can be identified in the media of

MCF-7 and ZR-75-1 cell cultures. The antigen appears to be two peptides with a molecular weight of 28,000 and IEP of 5.5 and 6.0. Using a radioimmunoassay (1,2), H59 binds to a subset of estrogen receptor positive breast cancers and benign breast disease tissue specimens. The characteristics of this binding will be discussed below.

H71

H71 antibody binds predominately to well differentiated human breast cancer tissue culture cells but the binding does not correlate with the presence or absence of the estrogen receptor or the hormone dependence of the cell line. Similarly to H59, H71 binds MCF-7 and ZR-75-1 cells. However, H71 binds T47D cells which have progesterone receptor and are hormone independent, and BT-20, a cell line which has neither estrogen or progesterone receptor but retains glucocorticoid receptor. It also binds the two tamoxifen resistant cell lines, R27 and R3. The antibody does not react with the same non breast cancer cell lines which H59 weakly binds. H71 does weakly bind to a vaginal and a colon cell line carcimona. The antigen can be identified on the surface of breast cancer tissue culture cells and it is apparently secreted into the media. H71 antigen has also been isolated and purified by two dimensional gel electrophoresis. It consists of 4 peptides, the major two having molecular weights of 45,000 daltons and the minor two 28,000 daltons. Since the two smaller peptides are not isolated stoiche-metrically, it is unclear as to whether these peptides are part of the antigenic portion of the native protein. H71 also binds to both estrogen receptor positive and negative tumors and nonmalignant breast tissue.

H72

H72 binds the same breast cancer cell lines as H71. However, H72 binds to a cervical carcinoma cell line and binds more avidly the three endometrial carcinoma cell lines with which H59 reacts; H71 did not bind to any of these cell lines. The H72 antigen has not as yet been identified. Similarly to H71, H72 reacts with a subset of estrogen receptor positive and negative breast cancers and benign breast masses. Since H72 reacted with different cell lines than H59 and H71, we presume that the H72 antigen is not either H59 or H71 antigen.

TABLE 1
COMPARISON OF ANTIBODY BINDING TO
BREAST TISSUE SPECIMENS

	Total	H59	H71	None	
Breast Cancers	84	45	46	49	9
ER+ [a,b]	55	37	29	35	7
ER-	29	8	17	17	2
Benign Disease					
fa [a]	41	35	33	11	0
fcd [a]	67	48	53	45	0
others	4	0	0	2	2

[a] ER = estrogen receptor, fa = fibroadenoma, fcd = fibrocystic disease
[b] ER + > or = 7fM/mg cytosol protein

Clinical Studies

Using the direct radioimmunoassay technique (1,2), biopsy specimens from 84 patients with breast cancer and from 112 patients with benign breast lesions have been evaluated (Table 1). H59 bond to 53% of tumors and 75% of benign disease; H71 bound 54% and 77% respectively; and H72 bound 71% and 52% respectively. Only 10% of tumors and 2% of benign disease did not bind one of the antibodies. There were no differences observed when antibody binding was correlated with the size of the tumor, the presence of axillary nodes or the tumor histology. When antibody binding to tumors was correlated with the presence or absence of estrogen receptor, it appeared that H59 bound fewer estrogen receptor negative tumors while H71 and H72 bound a greater proportion of estrogen receptor negative tumors. All of the estrogen receptor negative patients who bound to H59 were either premenopausal or taking exogenous estrogenic compounds. All three antibodies bound extensively to benign breast disease. H59 and H71 bound fibroadenomas and fibrocystic disease equally. H72 bound fewer benign specimens and significantly fewer fibroadenomas.

To determine the degree of binding to other tissues, H59, H71, and H72 antibodies have been similarly reacted with non breast tumor specimens. These have included lung, liver, stomach, pancreas, colon, ovarian, endometrial, prostate, renal, adrenal, lymphomas, and sarcomas. Those few non breast tumor to which the antibodies reacted are shown in Table 2. All three antibodies bound to the same ovarian tumor, one of four which was studied. H59 reacted with no other tumor. H71 bound a renal cell carcinoma and H72 bound a pancreatic tumor.

TABLE 2
ANTIBODY BINDING TO NON BREAST TUMORS

Antibody Binding		All	Tumors Tested Ovarian	Renal	Pancreas
H59	+	1	1	0	0
	-	29	3	1	∠
H71	+	2	1	1	0
	-	28	3	0	2
H72	+	2	1	0	1
	-	28	3	1	1

DISCUSSION

Our purpose in producing the H59 antibody has been to develop an antibody which would recognize an estrogen regulated breast cancer antigen. We have begun to develop data which suggests that H59 antigen is hormone regulated: the binding of the antibody cancer cell lines which are estrogen regulated and the binding of the antibody estrogen receptor positive breast cancer specimens. The estrogen receptor negative specimens to which H59 bound were obtained either from premenopausal patients or post menopausal patients taking exogenens estrogens. In these patients, it is probable that the dextran coated charcoal assay for estrogen receptor is invalid. Thus, it is possible that the estrogen receptor negative specimens which bind H59 may be hormone regulated tumors. Studies are underway to verify this hypothesis. The binding results with H59 are clearly different from those attained with H71 and H72 which bind breast tissue considerably more indiscriminately. Since H71 and H72 bind benign and malignant breast tissue, these are probably binding breast differentiation antigens. If indeed H59 is recognizing an estrogen regulated protein, one would presume that tumors which bound H59 would be hormone responsive having retained the ability to synthesize this protein during the malignant transformation. Future studies will correlate various prognostic factors, the response to hormones, and antibody binding in patients with breast cancer. The minimum cross reactivity observed with other tissues may indicate that these antibodies will be useful for immunodiagnostics and specific immunotherapy.

ACKNOWLEDGMENTS

We thank the Breast Cancer Task Force of the National Cancer Institute and Dr. M.E. Lippman for providing cell lines. We also thank Ms. L. Frank, Ms. L. Brettell, and Ms. E. Carlton for technical assistance. We are grateful for Dr. William Kingsley, Department of Pathology, Baylor University Medical Center for review of the scientific data. And we are especially indebted to Dr. Ellen S. Vitetta for constant support and advice.

REFERENCES

1. Hendler FJ, Yuan D, Vitetta ES (1981). Characterization of a monoclonal antibody to human breast cancer cells. Trans Assoc Am Phys 84:217.
2. Yuan D, Hendler FJ, Vitetta ES (1982). Characterization of a monoclonal antibody reactive with a subset of human breast tumors. J Natl Canc Inst 68:719.
3. Schlom J, Wunderlich D, Teramoto YA (1980). Generation of human monoclonal antibodies reactive with human mammary carcinoma cells. Proc Natl Acad Sci 77:6841.
4. Colcher D, Horan Hand P, Nuti M, Schlom J (1981). A spectrum of monoclonal antibodies reactive with human mammary tumor cells. Proc Natl Acad Sci 78:3199.
5. Nawata H, Bronzert D, Lippman ME (1981). Isolation and characterization of a tamoxifen-resistant cell line derived from human MCF-7 breast cancer cells. J Biol Chem 256:5016.
6. Nawata H, Chong MT, Bronzert D, Lippman ME (1981). Estradiol-independent growth of a subline of MCF-7 human breast cancer cells in culture. J Biol Chem 256:6895.
7. Horowitz KB, Mockus MP, Lessey BA (1982). Variant T47D human breast cancer cells with high progesterone-receptor levels despite estrogen and antiestrogen resistance. Cell 28:633.

Rational Basis for Chemotherapy, pages 315–358
© 1983 Alan R. Liss, Inc., 150 Fifth Avenue, New York, NY 10011

RATIONAL BASIS FOR THE DIAGNOSTIC, PROGNOSTIC, AND
THERAPEUTIC UTILITY OF MONOCLONAL ANTIBODIES IN THE
MANAGEMENT OF HUMAN BREAST CANCER

P. Horan Hand, D. Colcher, D. Wunderlich
M. Nuti, Y.A. Teramoto, D. Kufe, and J. Schlom

National Cancer Institute
National Institutes of Health
Bethesda, Maryland 20205

ABSTRACT Murine monoclonal antibodies reactive with
human mammary tumor associated antigens have been
Generated and characterized. The immunogens used in
these studies were membrane-enriched fractions of
human metastatic mammary carcinoma lesions. The
thirteen monoclonal antibodies characterized could be
divided into five major groups based on differential
reactivity to various mammary carcinoma lesions,
binding to the surface of carcinoma cell lines, and the
molecular weight of the reactive antigen precipitated.
Two monoclonals (B1.1 and F5.5) were reactive with
purified carcinoembryonic antigen, and showed
differential binding to the surface of various
non-breast tumor cells. Monoclonals B6.2 and B72.3
were extensively characterized as to their range of
reactivities, and were shown to immunoprecipitate a
90,000d protein, and a 220,000d-400,000d high molecular
weight protein complex, respectively. The monoclonals
were used to demonstrate a wide range of differential
expression of several tumor associated antigens among
various mammary carcinomas, and even within a given
tumor mass. Purified immunoglobulin, $F(ab')_2$, and
Fab' fragments of monoclonal B6.2 were radiolabeled and
used in gamma scanning studies to successfully localize
human mammary tumor transplants in athymic mice. The
utility of the monoclonal antibodies generated in
developing a firm understanding of the dynamics of
mammary carcinoma cell populations, as well as several
potential clinical applications are discussed.

INTRODUCTION

Numerous investigators have reported the existence of human mammary tumor associated antigens (1-9). These studies, all conducted with conventional hyperimmune poly-clonal sera, however, were hampered with regard to the heterogeneity of the antibody populations employed, and the amount of specific immunoglobulin that could be generated. Since the advent of hybridoma technology, monoclonal antibodies of predefined specificity and virtually unlimited quantity, can now be generated against a variety of anti-genic determinants present on normal and/or neoplastic cells.

Monoclonal antibodies reactive with human mammary tissues have been generated by a number of laboratories using a variety of immunogens. Several groups have generated monoclonal antibodies against human milk fat globule membranes (10-14). These antibodies react strongly with lactating breast tissues and to a lesser extent with normal resting breast. Monoclonal antibodies have also been generated to estrogen receptors from the MCF-7 human breast tumor cell line (15). These antibodies bind to a variety of estrogen receptors, including those purified from monkey endometrium, and can be used to detect estrogen receptor positive human mammary tumors by immunofluorescence of frozen sections and immunoperoxidase of fixed sections. Human mammary tumor cell lines have been used as immunogens by several laboratories (16-18). The antibody generated against the ZR-75-1 cell line reacts with approximately half of the malignant mammary tumors tested and to greater than 80% of the benign mammary tumors tested (18). Monoclonal antibodies have also been generated against human breast fibroblasts with some reported reactivity to the MCF-7 cell line (19).

Studies previously reported from our laboratory have demonstrated that lymphocytes, obtained from lymph nodes of mastectomy patients, may be fused with murine nonimmuno-globulin secreting myeloma cells to generate human-mouse hybridomas secreting human monoclonal antibodies (20, 21). One of these monoclonals (22) has been shown to be selectively reactive with human breast carcinoma and selected non-breast carcinoma cells, but is of the IgM isotype. Further studies to generate human monoclonals of the IgG isotype are in progress.

A number of laboratories have also generated monoclonal antibodies to a variety of tumors that cross react with breast tumors. Antibodies prepared using melanomas (23-25), lung carcinomas (26, 27), renal carcinomas (28), and prostate carcinomas (29) as immunogens bind to a variety of breast tumor cell lines or sections of breast tumors. Antibodies to antigens found on normal human cells have shown reactivity with human breast carcinomas (30).

The rationale of the studies overviewed here was to utilize membrane-enriched extracts of human metastatic mammary tumor cells as immunogens in an attempt to generate and characterize monoclonal antibodies reactive with determinants that would be maintained on metastatic, as well as primary, human mammary carcinoma cells. Multiple assays using tumor cell extracts, tissue sections, and live cells in culture have been employed to reveal the diversity of the monoclonal antibodies generated (31-36).

RESULTS AND DISCUSSION

Generation of Monoclonal Antibodies.

Mice were immunized with membrane-enriched fractions of human metastatic mammary carcinoma cells from either of two involved livers (designated Met 1 and Met 2)of two different patients. Spleens of immunized mice were fused with non-immunoglobulin secreting NS-1 murine myeloma cells to generate 4,250 primary hybridoma cultures. All hybridoma methodology and assay methods employed have been described previously (37, 38). Supernatant fluids from hybridoma cultures were first screened in solid phase radioimmuno-assays (RIAs) for the presence of immunoglobulin reactive with extracts of metastatic mammary tumor cells from involved livers and not reactive with extracts of apparently normal human liver. Following passage and double-cloning by endpoint dilution of cultures secreting immunoglobulins demonstrating preferential reactivity with breast carcinoma cells, the monoclonal antibodies from eleven hybridoma cell lines were chosen for further study. The isotypes of all eleven antibodies were determined; ten were IgG of various subclasses and one was an IgM (Table 1).

The eleven monoclonal antibodies could immediately be divided into three major groups based on their differential reactivity to Met 1 vs. Met 2 in solid phase RIA (Fig. 1). It is interesting to note that the immunogen used in the generation of monoclonal B72.3 was Met 1, while the immunogen used for the generation of monoclonal B25.2 was

TABLE 1

REACTIVITY OF MONOCLONAL ANTIBODIES IN SOLID PHASE RIAS

MONOCLONAL ANTIBODY	ISOTYPE	CELL EXTRACTS[a]			LIVE CELLS[b]				
		Met 1	Met 2	LIVER	MAMMARY CARCINOMA			MELANOMA SARCOMA[c]	NORMAL[d]
					BT-20	MCF-7	ZR-75-1		
B6.2	IgG$_1$	+++	++	NEG	++	+++	++	NEG	NEG
B14.2	IgG$_1$	+++	++	NEG	+	++	+	NEG	NEG
B39.1	IgG$_1$	+++	++	NEG	++	++	++	NEG	NEG
F64.5	IgG$_{2a}$	+++	++	NEG	++	++	+	NEG	NEG
F25.2	IgG$_1$	+++	++	NEG	+	+	+	NEG	NEG
B84.1	IgG$_1$	++	+	NEG	+	+	+	NEG	NEG
B50.4	IgG$_1$	++	+	NEG	NEG	+	NEG	NEG	NEG
B50.1	IgG$_1$			NEG	NEG	+	NEG	NEG	NEG
B25.2	IgM	NEG	+++	NEG	NEG	NEG	NEG	NEG	NEG
B72.3	IgG$_1$	+++	NEG	NEG	NEG	+	NEG	NEG	NEG
B38.1	IgG$_1$	+	+	NEG	+++	++	+++	NEG	NEG
W6/32	IgG$_{2a}$	NEG	NEG	NEG	+	+	NEG	++	++
B139	IgG$_1$	+++	NEG	++	++	++	++	++	++

[a] Solid-phase RIAs. NEG, <500; +, 500-2000cpm; ++, 2001-5000cpm; +++, >5000cpm.

[b] The live cell immunoassay was performed on human cells. NEG, <300cpm; +, 300-1000cpm; ++, 1001-2000cpm; +++, >2000cpm.

[c] Rhabdomyosarcoma (A204), Fibrosarcoma (HT-1080), and Melanoma (A375, A101D, A875, A3875).

[d] Human cell lines were derived from apparently normal breast (HSo584Bst, HSo578Bst), embryonic skin (Detroit 550, 551), fetal lung (WI-38, MRC-5), fetal testis (HSo181Tes), fetal thymus (HSo208Th), fetal bone marrow (HSo074BM), embryonic kidney (FLOW-4,000), fetal spleen (HSo203Sp), and uterus (HSo769Ut).

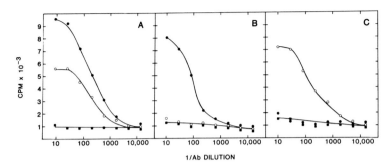

Fig. 1.   Reactivity of monoclonal antibodies with extracts of metastatic breast tumors to the liver, and normal liver, in solid phase RIA.   Metastases from patient 1 (closed circle) and patient 2 (open circle); normal liver (square). Panel A, monoclonal B6.2; Panel B, monoclonal B72.3; Panel C, monoclonal B25.2.

Met 2.   All eleven antibodies were negative when tested against similar extracts from normal human liver, a rhabdomyosarcoma cell line, the HBL100 cell line derived from cultures of human milk, mouse mammary tumor and fibroblast cell lines, disrupted mouse mammary tumor virus and mouse leukemia virus, purified carcinoembryonic antigen (CEA) and ferritin.   Two monoclonal antibodies were used as positive controls in all these studies: (a) W6/32, an anti-human histocompatibility antigen (39) and (b) B139, which was generated against a human breast tumor metastasis, but which showed reactivity to all human cells tested (Table 1).
    To determine if the monoclonals bind cell surface determinants, each antibody was tested for binding to live cells in culture, i.e., established cell lines of human mammary carcinomas.   The nine monoclonals grouped together on the basis of their binding to both metastatic cell extracts could be further separated into three different groups on the basis of their differential binding to cell surface determinants (Table 1).   Some of the monoclonals bound to the surface of selected non-breast carcinoma cell lines.   None of the eleven monoclonal antibodies, however, bound to the surface of sarcoma or melanoma cell lines, nor to the surface of a variety of cell lines derived from apparently normal human tissues (Table 1).   Control monoclonals W6/32 or B139, however, did bind all of these cells (Table 1).

Monoclonal antibody B6.2 was further analyzed by Kufe, et al. (40) for surface binding to a panel of human cell lines using fluorescent activated cell sorter analyses. Antibody B6.2 was reactive with five of six breast carcinoma cell lines, but was unreactive with most other carcinomas. Cell lines derived from melanomas, sarcomas and lymphoid tumors were uniformly unreactive. There was complete agreement in assay results when the same cell lines were tested in live cell RIA and by cell sorter analysis. A variety of tissues obtained directly from biopsy were also evaluated via fluorescence activated cell sorter analyses. Breast carcinoma cells were examined from patients with malignant pleural effusions. Tumor cells from three of six were positive with B6.2. Single cell suspension derived from normal lymphoid tissue including bone marrow, lymph node, spleen and tonsil demonstrated no reactivity.

To further define specificity and range of reactivity of each of the eleven monoclonal antibodies, the immuno-peroxidase technique was employed on tissue sections. All the monoclonals reacted with mammary carcinoma cells of primary mammary carcinomas, both infiltrating ductal (Fig. 2A,B) and lobular (Fig. 2D). Formalin fixed and frozen section tissue preparations gave comparable results. The percentage of primary mammary tumors that were reactive varied for the different monoclonals; this point will be discussed in detail later on. In many of the positive primary and metastatic mammary carcinomas, not all tumor cells stained. In certain tumor masses, furthermore, heterogeneity of tumor cell staining was observed in different areas of a tumor, and even within a given area, as will be discussed in detail below. A high degree of selective reactivity with mammary tumor cells, and not with apparently normal mammary epithelium, stroma, blood vessels, or lymphocytes of the breast was also observed. This is exemplified with monoclonal B6.2 in Fig. 2A and C. A dark reddish-brown stain (the result of the immunoperoxidase reaction with the diaminobenzidine substrate) was observed only on mammary carcinoma cells, whereas only the light blue hematoxylin counterstain was observed on adjacent normal mammary epithelium, stroma, and lymphocytes. Occasionally, a few of the apparently normal mammary epithelial cells immediately adjacent to the mammary tumor did stain weakly with the same pattern of staining seen in the tumor cells. The polymorphonuclear leukocytes and histiocytes in the stroma only in the area of mammary tumor also showed positive cytoplasmic staining. This would suggest that this

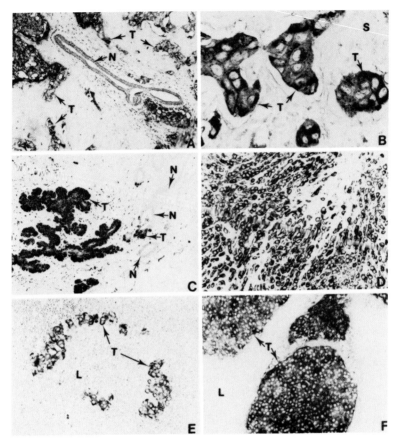

Fig. 2.   Immunoperoxidase staining of fixed tissue
sections of primary and metastatic mammary carcinomas with
monoclonal antibody B6.2. (A) Infiltrating duct carcinoma:
at the center of the field is a negative normal duct (N)
surrounded by positive stained tumor cells (T). 130x; (B)
Higher magnification of tumor cells (T) and stroma (S) from
same tissue section shown in panel A. 540x; (C)
Cancerization of a mammary lobule: note the positive
stained tumor cells (T) and the unstained normal mammary
cells (N). 130x; (D) Infiltrating lobular carcinoma. 220x;
(E) Breast tumor metastasis of the lymph node: tumor cells
(T), lymphocytes (L). 220x; (F) Breast tumor metastasis of
the lymph node from another patient: tumor cells (T),
lymphocytes (L). 220x.

reactivity may be due to antigen shed by the tumor and phagocytized by reactive cells in the immediate proximity.

Experiments were then carried out to determine if the eleven monoclonals could detect mammary carcinoma cell populations at distal sites, i.e., in metastases. Since the monoclonals were all generated using metastatic mammary carcinoma cells as antigens, it was not unexpected that the monoclonals all reacted, but with different degrees, to various metastases (Fig. 2E, F; Fig. 3D). As exemplified in Fig. 2E and F, none of the monoclonals reacted with normal lymphocytes or stroma from any involved or uninvolved nodes. The monoclonals were then tested for reactivity to normal and neoplastic non-mammary tissues. Some of the monoclonals showed reactivity with selected non-breast carcinomas such as adenocarcinoma of the colon. These observations are currently being extended. Other neoplasms tested, which showed no staining, were sarcomas, lymphomas, glioblastomas, and melanomas. All 11 monoclonals were negative for cellular reactivity with apparently normal tissues of the following organs: thyroid, intestine, kidney, liver, bladder, tonsils, and prostate.

A factor in the potential utility of any monoclonal antibody is its selective reactivity. The immunoperoxidase method of staining of fixed tissue sections with antibody has the advantage of screening large amounts of tissues in a relatively short period of time. Moreover, it permits the testing of antibody reactivity with tissues that would otherwise be inaccessible. For example, to date there are no cell lines available from in situ breast carcinoma. A major drawback of using fixed tissue sections in the immuno-peroxidase technique, however, is that this procedure makes it extremely difficult to define cell surface reactivities; one must therefore employ techniques using live cells to determine surface binding. One example of this is the observation that antibody B6.2 has shown some reactivity with subpopulations of polymorphonuclear leukocytes in fixed tissue sections of spleens of some patients using the immunoperoxidase technique. Antibody B6.2, however, has shown no binding to the surface of unfixed bone marrow, spleen, lymph node, and tonsil cell preparations from a variety of patients using fluorescent activated cell sorter analyses (40). This antibody is unreactive with the surface of all normal cells tested thus far. Since it is cell sur-face binding which is of clinical importance, one must dis-tinguish between potential reactivity of an antibody with a cross-reactive internal antigen, versus cell surface binding.

Of the eleven monoclonals described above, B72.3 (an IgG$_1$) displayed the most restricted range of reactivity for human mammary tumor versus normal cells. Monoclonal B72.3 was used at various concentrations in immunoperoxidase assays of tissue sections to determine the effect of antibody dose on the staining intensity and the percent of tumor cells stained. Since one cannot titrate antigen in the fixed tissue section, an antibody dilution experiment was performed to give an indication of the relative titer of reactive antigen within a given tissue. A range of antibody concentrations, varying from 0.02 ug to 10 ug of purified immunoglobulin (per 200 ul) per tissue section, was used on each of four mammary carcinomas from different patients. The results (Table 2) demonstrate that: (a) different mammary tumors may vary in the amount of the antigen detected by B72.3, (b) a given mammary tumor may contain tumor cell populations which vary in antigen density, and (c) some mammary tumors may score positive or negative depending on the dose of antibody employed.

TABLE 2

DOSE OF MONOCLONAL ANTIBODY B72.3 VS. REACTIVITY OF HUMAN
MAMMARY CARCINOMA CELLS IN IMMUNOPEROXIDASE ASSAY

	Tumor Staining Intensity (% Reactive Tumor Cells)			
ug B72.3	Tumor 1	Tumor 2	Tumor 3	Tumor 4
10	1+(90) 2+(10)	3+(100)	3+(80)	NEG
4	1+(5)	2+(100)	3+(80)	NEG
2	NEG	1+(80)	3+(70)	NEG
1	NEG	NEG	3+(70)	NEG
0.2	NEG	NEG	2+(50)	NEG
0.02	NEG	NEG	2+(30)	NEG

Staining intensity: 1+ weak, 2+ moderate, 3+ strong.
0.02 ug of B72.3 is equivalent to a 1:100,000 dilution
of B72.3 produced in mouse ascites fluid.

To further characterize the range of reactivity of B72.3, the immunoperoxidase technique was used to test a variety of malignant, benign and normal mammary tissues.

Using 4 ug of monoclonal per slide the percent of positive
primary breast tumors was 46% (19/41); 62% (13/21) of the
metastatic lesions scored positive. Several histologic
types of primary mammary tumors scored positive: these were
infiltrating duct (Fig. 3A and B), infiltrating lobular, and
comedo carcinomas. Many of the in situ elements present in
the above lesions also stained (Fig. 3C). None of the six
medullary carcinomas tested were positive. Approximately two
thirds of the tumors that showed a positive reactivity
demonstrated a cell associated membrane and/or diffuse
cytoplasmic staining (Fig. 3B), approximately five percent
showed discrete focal staining of the cytoplasm (Fig. 3D),
and approximately one-fourth of the reactive tumors showed
an apical or marginal staining pattern. Metastatic breast
carcinoma lesions that were positive were in axillary lymph
nodes, and at the distal sites of skin, liver, lung, pleura
(Fig. 3D) and mesentery. Fifteen benign breast lesions were
also tested; these included fibrocystic disease, fibroadenomas and sclerosing adenosis. Two specimens showed
positive staining: one case of fibrocystic disease where a
few cells in some ducts were faintly positive, and a case of
intraductal papillomatosis and sclerosing adenosis with the
majority of cells staining strongly. Monoclonal B72.3 was
also tested against normal breast tissue and normal
lactating breast from non-cancer patients and showed no
reactivity. A variety of non-breast cells and tissues were
tested and were negative; these included two uteruses, two
livers, two spleens, three lungs, two bone marrows, five
colons, one stomach, one salivary gland, five lymph nodes
and one kidney.

Differential Binding to Human Mammary and Non-Mammary Tumors
of Monoclonal Antibodies Reactive with Carcinoembryonic
Antigen.

The presence of high plasma levels of CEA (41) has been
reported to be an indicator of the possible presence of
metastatic disease in patients with cancers of the digestive
system, breast, lung, as well as other sites (42-44). Using
assays based on antibodies to colonic CEA, elevated plasma
levels of CEA (above 2.5 ng/ml) have been reported in 38-79%
of patients with mammary carcinomas (42, 45-51). There have
been several reports (52-56), however, indicating that "CEA"
is a heterogeneous family of glycoproteins, some of which
demonstrate cross-reactivity with each other as well as with
so called "CEA-related" proteins. One issue that has not

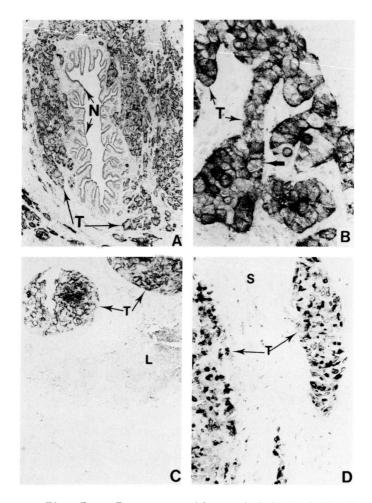

Fig. 3.   Immunoperoxidase staining of fixed
tissue sections of primary and metastatic mammary carcinomas
of four different patients with monoclonal antibody B72.3:
(A) Infiltrating duct carcinoma: at the center of the field
is a negative large normal duct (N) surrounded by positively
staining infiltrating tumor cells (T). 54x; (B) Infiltrating duct carcinoma; note the intense membrane and faint
cytoplasmic staining of the tumor cells (T). The broad
arrow indicates a negative tumor cell flanked by positive
tumor cells. 540x; (C) In situ element (T) of an infiltrating duct carcinoma: note the stroma and lymphocytes (L)
which are negative. 130x; (D) Breast tumor metastasis in the

Fig. 3 (cont.) pleura. This is an example of the focal pattern of staining: intense stain is concentrated in the cytoplasm of tumor cells (T). The stroma (S) is negative. 330X

---

yet been clearly resolved is the possibility that different tumor cell types may produce, or maintain on their cell surface, a CEA that is only partially related to CEAs associated with other malignancies. Monoclonal antibodies should be a valuable reagent toward resolving this point. To date, several monoclonal antibodies have been generated and characterized using CEA from colon carcinomas as the immunogen (57-62). In the studies reported here, monoclonal antibodies were generated to membrane-enriched fractions of human mammary carcinoma metastases and screened for reactivity with purified CEA. The differential binding properties of two of these antibodies (B1.1 and F 5.5) to CEA and to breast and non-breast tumors was investigated. Monoclonal B1.1 is an IgG_{2a} while F5.5 is an IgG_1.

Both B1.1 and F5.5 precipitated iodinated CEA, resulting in a radiolabeled peak at approximately 180,000d. No precipitation of purified CEA was obtained using monoclonal antibody B6.2 nor with any of the monoclonals described above. Cross reactivities have been reported (63) between determinants on CEA and an antigen expressed in normal spleens termed normal cross-reacting antigen (NCA). Monoclonals B1.1 and F5.5 did not react however with a normal spleen extract rich in NCA. Purified immunoglobulin preparations of monoclonals Bl.l and F5.5 were then titered for binding to five CEAs purified from five different patients with colon cancer. As can be seen in Fig 4, significant binding was observed with both antibodies to all five CEAs. Monoclonals Bl.l and F5.5 are clearly reactive with different epitopes on the CEA molecule, however, as evidenced by their differential binding to the various CEA preparations. Specifically, monoclonal F5.5 reacted similarly with all five CEA preparations, whereas Bl.l exhibited preferential binding to different CEA preparations. Monoclonals Bl.l and F5.5 were tested for binding to live cells in culture to further define their range of reactivities, and to ascertain if they bind to antigenic determinants that are present on the cell surface. As seen in Table 3, both monoclonals bound to the same three of six established human mammary carcinoma cell lines and to the two colon carcinoma cell lines, but not to the lung carcinoma or vulva carcinoma cell lines. No surface binding

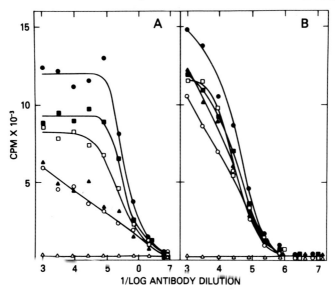

Fig. 4.   Titration of monoclonal antibodies B1.1 and
F5.5 against five preparations of CEA from different
patients.   Thirty nanograms of purified CEA from five
different patients were utilized in a solid phase RIA.   CEA
DH3B (closed circle); CEA BP160 (open circle); CEA DH2-3
(closed square); CEA HCA3B (open square); CEA JFII (closed
triangle); bovine serum albumin (open triangle).   Ascitic
fluid from mice containing monoclonal antibodies B1.1 (Panel
A) or F5.5 (Panel B) were titered against the different CEAs
in a solid phase RIA as described (34).

was observed with either antibody to normal breast cell
lines nor to a variety of cell lines derived from apparently
normal human tissues (Table 3).   The two monoclonals could
be distinguished, however, by their differential reactivity
to the surface of melanoma cell lines.   B1.1 bound to three
of four melanoma cell lines tested, while F5.5 did not bind
to any of the four (Table 3).   Reactivity with B1.1 was
repeatedly observed with late passages (greater than passage
80) of the A204 rhabdomyosarcoma cell line (Table 3).   These
findings are further substantiated by a comparative titration of monoclonals B1.1 and F5.5 against breast carcinoma,
colon carcinoma and melanoma cell lines.   As seen in Fig.
5A, B1.1 binds the melanoma, colon, and breast tumor cell
lines comparably.   There is a clear preferential binding of

TABLE 3
REACTIVITY OF MONOCLONAL ANTIBODIES IN LIVE CELL RIAs[a]

CELL TYPE	CELL LINE	B1.1	F5.5	B139[b]
MAMMARY CARCINOMA	MCF-7	2,391	2,239	1,343
	ZR-75-1	1,350	1,331	605
	BT-20	1,899	1,563	1,818
	MDA-MB-231	NEG	NEG	2,800
	ZR-75-31A	NEG	NEG	3,219
	T47D	NEG	NEG	2,501
CARCINOMA				
Colon	WIDR	1,959	506	2,110
Colon	HT-29	2,683	1,463	2,646
Lung	A549	NEG	NEG	3,060
Vulva	A431	NEG	NEG	2,250
MELANOMA	A3827	2,840	NEG	3,780
	A101D	1,453	NEG	4,482
	A875	876	NEG	3,747
	A375	NEG	NEG	4,813
SARCOMA				
Rhabdomyo-	A204,P18-79[c]	NEG	NEG	4,456
	P80-90	1,024	NEG	4,673
Fibro-	HT-1080	NEG	NEG	3,688
NORMAL				
Breast	HSo584Bst	NEG	NEG	1,481
Breast	HSo578Bst	NEG	NEG	1,360
Embryonic Skin	D550	NEG	NEG	2,100
Embryonic Skin	D551	NEG	NEG	2,296
Embryonic Kidney	Flow-4,000	NEG	NEG	2,256
Fetal Lung	MRC-5	NEG	NEG	3,210
Fetal Lung	WI-38	NEG	NEG	2,331
Fetal Testis	HSo181Tes	NEG	NEG	2,298
Fetal Thymus	HSo208Th	NEG	NEG	3,391
Fetal Bone Marrow	HSo074BM	NEG	NEG	1,062
Fetal Spleen	HSo203Sp	NEG	NEG	2,500
Fetal Kidney	HSo807K	NEG	NEG	3,682
Uterus	HSo769Ut	NEG	NEG	1,647

[a]Live cell immunoassays were performed as described (31).
Negative (NEG) indicates less than 300 cpm above background
(approximately 200 cpm).
[b]B139 is a monoclonal antibody that binds to all human cell lines
tested.
[c]At different passage (P) levels within our laboratory the
reactivity with B1.1 was altered. At passage levels below 80,
B1.1 was negative; at passage levels above 80 there was
significant binding of B1.1.

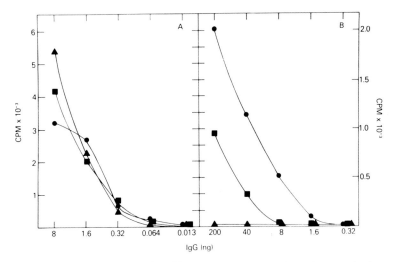

Fig. 5.   Reactivity of monoclonal antibodies B1.1 and
F5.5 in live cell RIA. Increasing amounts of purified IgG
of B1.1 (Panel A) and F5.5 (Panel B) were reacted in a live
cell RIA with 5×10^4 cells of the following established human
cell lines: MCF-7, mammary adenocarcinoma, (closed circle);
HT-29, colon adenocarcinoma, (closed square); and A3827,
melanoma, (closed triangle).

monoclonal F5.5, however, with the mammary tumor line as
compared to the colon tumor or melanoma cell lines (Fig.5B).
     To further identify the range of reactivities of mono-
clonals B1.1 and F5.5 with human mammary carcinomas, the
immunoperoxidase technique was used on formalin-fixed tumor
sections. Positive staining with both B1.1 and F5.5 was
observed with three colon carcinomas and three lung carcinomas. Monoclonals F5.5 and B1.1 reacted positively with 55
and 66 percent, respectively, of the mammary carcinomas
tested. The positive mammary tumors included infiltrating
ductal, in-situ, and medullary carcinomas. Monoclonals B1.1
and F5.5 also reacted positively with metastatic mammary
tumor cells in lymph nodes and at distal sites.
     It is anticipated that studies can now be undertaken to
determine if the presence of, the intensity of, or the
cellular localization of these reactions, using either or
both of these monoclonals with tissue sections of primary
breast lesions, is of any prognostic value. A previous
study (64), performed using heterologous antisera and small

cell carcinomas of the lung, has indicated that CEA
reactivity of tissue sections may have prognostic significance. Since radiolabeled immunoglobulin preparations of
heterologous sera to CEA (derived from colon carcinoma) have
already been used (65, 66) for binding metastatic breast
carcinoma lesions in-situ, appropriately labeled immunoglobulin or antibody fragment preparations of monoclonals
F5.5 and B1.1 may also eventually prove useful toward this
end.

Identification and Purification of Mammary Tumor Associated
Antigens.

     As a first step in the identification of the best source
of antigens reactive with the monoclonal antibodies
described, monoclonal antibodies were screened by solid
phase RIA for reactivity with a variety of mammary tumor
extracts including primary and metastatic tumors and
established cell lines. Monoclonals B1.1 and B6.2 reacted
similarly with tissue extracts and extracts of cell lines.
Antibody B72.3, however, showed very strong reactivity with
some human tumor extracts, but reacted poorly with mammary
tumor cell lines. Two breast tumor metastases to the liver
were chosen as the prime sources for antigen identification
and purification on the basis of their broad immunoreactivity to all the monoclonal antibodies, and the quantity of
tumor tissue available.
     Immunoprecipitation studies were initiated to determine
the molecular weights of the tumor associated antigens
(TAAs) reactive with the monoclonal antibodies described.
Purified CEA was iodinated and was used as antigen source
for the binding of B1.1 and F5.5. SDS-polyacrylamide gel
electrophoresis (SDS-PAGE) of the immunoprecipitates showed
that the polypeptide precipitated by both monoclonal antibodies is a heterogenous protein with an average molecular
weight of 180,000. An extract of a breast tumor metastasis
to the liver was used as the antigen source for the other
monoclonal antibodies described. Initial attempts to
identify the various reactive antigens in radioiodinated
extracts of the metastasis were unsuccessful. The limiting
factor appeared to be either an inability to label the
desired antigen, and/or an inability to detect an antigen
which may constitute a very small percentage of the total
tumor mass. To determine which hypothesis was correct,
experiments were undertaken to determine if CEA could be
immunoprecipitated in "CEA-spiked" extracts of the mammary

tumor metastasis. Purified CEA was iodinated and added to
an extract of the breast tumor metastasis at a final
concentration of 0.2%; monoclonal antibody B1.1 was able to
precipitate the CEA in this extract. However, a similar
amount of unlabeled CEA added to the extract prior to
labeling was not detected by similar immunoprecipitation
procedures. It appeared, therefore, that there was a
preferential labeling of proteins other than CEA in this

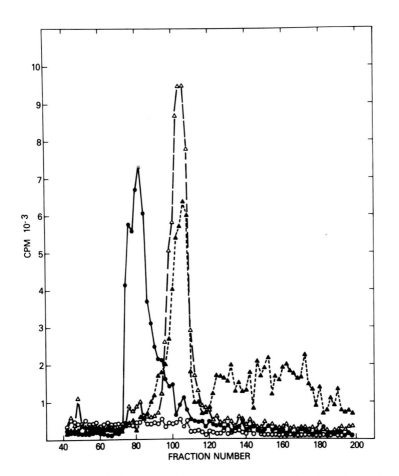

Fig. 6.   Gel filtration of an extract of a breast
tumor on Ultrogel AcA34. Immunoreactivity of fractions was
determined in a solid phase RIA. B72.3, (closed circle);
B6.2, (open triangle); B1.1 (closed triangle); PBS, (open
circle).

extract. In order to overcome this problem, experiments were undertaken to increase the relative antigen concentration by partial purification of the extract. The metastatic liver extract was detergent-disrupted and separated using molecular sieving on Ultrogel AcA34. The column fractions were assayed for reactivity with monoclonals B1.1, B6.2, and B72.3 by solid phase RIA (Fig. 6). The appropriate immunoreactive fractions were then pooled and labeled with ^{125}I. SDS-PAGE analyses of the immunoprecipitates generated are seen in Fig. 7. B72.3 immunoprecipitated a complex of four bands with estimated molecular weights of approximately 220,000, 250,000, 285,000, and 340,000. B1.1 immunoprecipitated a heterogenous component with an average estimated molecular weight of 180,000. B6.2 immunoprecipitated a 90,000d component as did several other monoclonal antibodies.

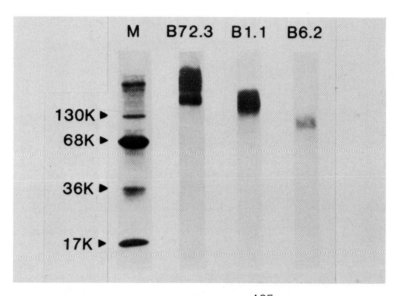

Fig. 7.   Immunoprecipitation of ^{125}I-labeled partially-purified extract of a human breast tumor. Lane a: markers (M), immunoprecipitation by monoclonal antibodies B72.3 (lane b), B1.1 (lane c) and B6.2 (lane d).

Extracts of a breast tumor metastasis to the liver, normal liver, and the MCF-7 breast tumor cell line, were disrupted and run on an SDS-polyacrylamide gel. The

polypeptides were electrophoretically transferred to nitro-
cellulose filters, and the filters were incubated with IgG
from B1.1, B6.2 or B72.3. The filters were washed, and the
remaining antibodies were detected with rabbit anti-murine
IgG and ^{125}I-Protein A. B72.3 bound to a high molecular
weight complex of approximately 220,000d-400,000d in the
extract from the metastasis. B1.1 bound to a 180,000d
polypeptide and B6.2 bound to a 90,000d polypeptide in
extracts of both the breast tumor metastasis and the MCF-7
cell line. These data demonstrate that the immunoreactivity
of the antigenic determinants are not destroyed by SDS and
mercaptoethanol, and that molecular weights of the polypeptides in the crude extracts are consistent with those
obtained by the immunoprecipitations from semipurified
extracts as described above.

Five of the monoclonal antibodies, including B6.2, were
reactive with an antigen of approximately 90,000d. To
determine whether these antibodies reacted with the same
determinants, a competitive binding assay was established.
Purified monoclonal antibody B6.2 was labeled with ^{125}I.
Increasing amounts of unlabeled monoclonal antibodies were
added to a breast tumor extract followed by the addition of
^{125}I-labeled B6.2 IgG. As little as 10ng of B6.2 IgG was
able to inhibit the binding of the labeled antibody by
greater than 90 percent. Various degrees of competition
were also observed with other antibodies (B39.1, B14.2,
B50.4, F25.2, B84.1). The ability of some of these other
monoclonal antibodies to compete for the binding of B6.2 to
the breast tumor metastasis extract indicates that these
antibodies react to the same antigen. Differences in the
slope of the competition curve and the amount of antibody
needed to achieve the competition may be due to differences
in the antibodies affinities to the same epitope. Another
possibility may be the existence of spacially close epitopes, which may result in steric inhibition of the binding
of ^{125}I-labeled B6.2 to a nearby epitope.

Purification of the 220,000d high molecular weight
complex. Monoclonal antibody B72.3 has been shown to have
highly selective reactivity to tumor versus normal tissues.
We thus attempted to purify the antigen reactive with B72.3
first, so that further immunological and biochemical
characterization could be made. An extract of a breast
tumor metastasis to the liver, which contained the highest
immunoreactivity with B72.3, was used as the starting
material for purification of the 220,000d high molecular
weight complex. Following detergent disruption and high

speed centrifugation, the supernatant was subjected to
molecular sieving using Ultrogel AcA34. Immunoreactive
fractions were then passed though a B72.3 antibody affinity
column and eluted with 3M KSCN. Radiolabeled aliquots from
the various purification steps were analysed by SDS-PAGE
(Fig. 8). Only minimal radioactivity in the high molecular
weight range was seen in gel patterns of the AcA34 pool,
whereas the affinity column eluant demonstrated the four
distinct bands of the 220,000d complex. ^{125}I-labeled B72.3
affinity purified antigen was tested for immunoreactivity by
solid phase RIA. Approximately 70 percent of the purified
^{125}I-labeled antigen was bound in B72.3 antibody excess.
The identical method of purification was used with a normal
human liver extract, and at no step within the purification
scheme was any reactivity with B72.3 detected.

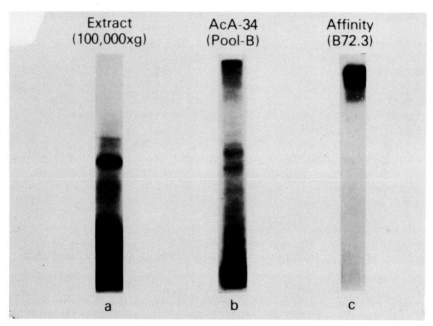

Fig. 8. Purification of mammary tumor associated
antigen reactive with monoclonal B72.3. SDS-PAGE of
^{125}I-labeled extract from a breast tumor metastasis at
various purification steps. An equal number of counts was
loaded onto each lane. Lane: (a) crude extract; (b) pool of
AcA-34 fractions reactive with B72.3; (c) pool of affinity
column fractions reactive with B72.3.

Heterogeneity Among Human Mammary Carcinoma Cell
Populations.

In 1954, Foulds documented the existence of distinct
morphologies in different areas of a single mammary tumor
(67). Since then, several investigators have reported the
occurrence of heterogeneity in a variety of tumor cell
populations (68, 69). Using a variety of methods and
reagents including heterologous antisera, heterogeneity has
also been observed with respect to the antigenic properties
of tumor cell populations (69-73). Consistent with this
finding, we have observed antigenic heterogeneity, as
defined by the expression of TAAs detected by monoclonal
antibodies, among and within murine mammary tumor masses
(37). The objectives of the studies described below were to
use the monoclonal antibodies to: (a) determine the extent
of antigenic heterogeneity of specific TAAs that exist among
human mammary tumors as well as within a given mammary tumor
population; (b) determine some of the parameters which
mediate the expression of various antigenic phenotypes; and
(c) develop model systems in which to study and perhaps
eventually control these phenomena.

Formalin-fixed tissue sections of human mammary tumors
were examined, using the immunoperoxidase method, in an
attempt to determine the range of expression of TAAs
reactive with monoclonal antibodies (31). Although some
mammary tumors reacted with all monoclonal antibodies
tested, other mammary tumors reacted with none. Both fixed
and frozen sections gave similar results. Some mammary
tumors showed a differential expression of one antigen
versus another. As shown in Fig. 9, an infiltrating duct
mammary carcinoma contains the 90,000d TAA reactive with
monoclonal antibody B6.2 (Fig. 9A), but not the 220,000d TAA
reactive with monoclonal B72.3 (Fig. 9B). Conversely, an
infiltrating duct mammary carcinoma from another patient,
expresses the TAA detected only by B72.3 (Fig. 9 C-D). To
exclude the possibility of variation due to location of
tissue within the tumor, several alternate serial sections
of the tumors were used in these experiments with identical
results.

The immunoperoxidase method was then used to test the
reactivity of fixed sections of primary infiltrating duct
mammary carcinomas from 45 different patients to a panel of
5 monoclonal antibodies (Table 4). What emerges is a
variety of antigenic phenotypes of the 45 mammary tumors
that can be placed into several distinct groups. Reactivity

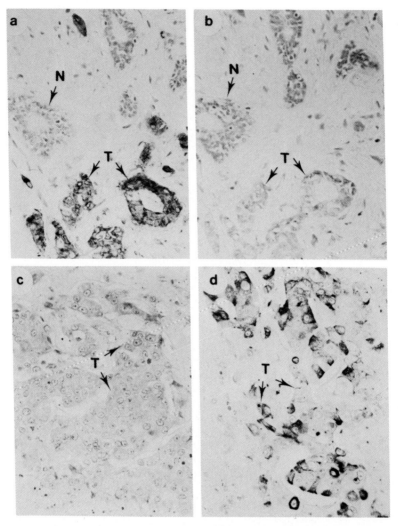

Fig. 9.   Differential reactivity of monoclonal antibodies B72.3 and B6.2 with two different human mammary
adenocarcinomas using the immunoperoxidase technique.
Serial tissue sections in panel A and B are from an
infiltrating duct carcinoma; in panel C and D serial
sections are from an infiltrating duct carcinoma from
another patient.   Panel A and C are reacted with monoclonal
antibody B6.2.   Panel B and D are stained with monoclonal
antibody B72.3.   Note the stained tumor cells (T) and
unstained normal mammary cells (N).   (A-C, 220x; D, 330x).

Table 4

DIFFERENTIAL REACTIVITY OF MONOCLONAL ANTIBODIES WITH
DIFFERENT HUMAN MAMMARY TUMORS[a]

Tumor Phenotype	No. Patients[a]	Monoclonal Antibody				
		B72.3	B1.1	B6.2	F25.2	B38.1
Group A	6	+	+	+	+	+
Group B	1	+	NEG	+	+	+
Group C	2	+	+	+	+	NEG
Group D	10	NEG	+	+	+	+
Group E	4	NEG	+	+	+	NEG
Group F	3	+	NEG	+	NEG	NEG
Group G	1	NEG	+	NEG	+	NEG
Group H	2	NEG	NEG	NEG	+	+
Group I	1	NEG	+	+	NEG	NEG
Group J	1	NEG	+	NEG	NEG	NEG
Group K	2	NEG	NEG	+	NEG	NEG
Group L	3	NEG	NEG	NEG	NEG	+
Group M	9	NEG	NEG	NEG	NEG	NEG
Total:	45					

[a]Serial sections of formalin-fixed mammary tumors were
tested for expression of TAAs detected by monoclonal
antibodies using the immunoperoxidase method. Tumors
were scored positive if antigen was present on 5% or
more of carcinoma cells.
[b]Number of patients with tumor specimens displaying
the indicated pattern of reactivity with the
monoclonal antibodies.

to all 5 monoclonal antibodies, including B1.1 which is
directed against CEA, was demonstrated by the presence of
antigens in 6/45 (13.3%) of the mammary tumors, while 9/45
(20.0%) contained none of these TAAs (Table 4). The
remaining 30 tumors displayed a variety of immunologic
phenotypes with the 5 monoclonal antibodies. What emerges
from these studies is a demonstration of the wide range of
antigenic phenotypes present in human mammary tumors.
Different tumors also differed in their pattern of staining
with a given monoclonal antibody. These patterns included
focal staining (representing dense foci of TAA in the
cytoplasm), diffuse cytoplasmic staining, membrane staining,
and apical or luminal staining (representing a concentration

of TAA on the luminal borders of cells).

Phenotypic variation was also observed in the expression of TAAs within a given mammary tumor. One pattern observed repeatedly was that one area of a mammary tumor contained TAAs reactive with a particular monoclonal antibody, while another area of the same tumor was not reactive with the identical antibody (Fig. 10A). Another type of antigenic heterogeneity was observed among cells in a given area of a tumor mass. This type of antigenic diversity, termed "patchwork," is demonstrated by the presence of tumor cells expressing a specific TAA directly adjacent to tumor cells negative for the same antigen (Fig. 9B). Patterns of reactivity with a specific monoclonal antibody were also observed to vary within a given tumor mass, i.e., antigen was detected in the cytoplasm of cells in one part of the tumor mass, and on the luminal edge of differentiated structures in a different part of the same mass.

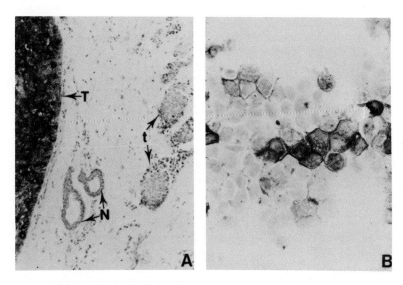

Fig. 10. Heterogeneity of antigenic expression of TAAs. In panel A, an infiltrating duct mammary carcinoma was reacted with monoclonal antibody B6.2 using the immunoperoxidase technique. Note the stained (T) and unstained (t) tumor cells. Normal mammary cells (N) do not react with the antibody (130x). In panel B, using the cytospin/immunoperoxidase technique as described (32, 36), MCF-7 cells were stained with monoclonal antibody B6.2 (540x).

Heterogeneity of TAA Expression in Human Mammary Tumor Cell Lines. In an attempt to elucidate the phenomenon of variation of antigenic phenotypes in primary human mammary tumors, model systems were examined. Human mammary tumor cell lines, transplanted in athymic mice, demonstrated antigenic heterogeneity. To determine if this phenomenon also exists in human mammary tumor cell lines grown in vitro, MCF-7 cells were tested for the presence of TAAs using the cytospin/immunoperoxidase method (32, 36). As seen in Fig. 10B, the MCF-7 cell line contained various subpopulations of cells as defined by variability in expression of TAA reactive with monoclonal antibody B6.2. Positive MCF-7 cells are seen adjacent to cells which scored negative.

Antigenic Drift of Mammary Tumor Cell Populations. Studies were then undertaken to determine if any change in antigenic phenotype occurs during extended passage of cells in culture. The BT-20 cell line, obtained at passage 288 was serially passaged and assayed at each passage level during logarithmic growth. As seen in Table 5, a cell surface HLA antigen, detected by monoclonal antibody W6/32 (39), was present at all passage levels, as was the antigen detected by monoclonal antibody B38.1. The antigen detected by monoclonal antibody B6.2 was expressed on the BT-20 cell surface up to passage 319, but was not evident after this passage level. Similarly, monoclonal B14.2 reacted with BT-20 cells only up to passage 317. This phenomenon was repeatedly observed in several separate experiments, at approximately the same passage levels. Antigenic drift was also observed with the MCF-7 cell line.

As a result of the phenotypic changes observed after passage in culture, MCF-7 cell lines obtained from four sources were examined for the presence of several cell surface TAAs. Karyotype profiles of the four cell lines were tested and were all identical and characteristic of the MCF-7 cell line. A single LDH band, characteristic of only a few breast tumor cell lines including MCF-7, was also supportive evidence that these cell lines were indeed MCF-7. Using a live cell RIA, which detects the reactivity of antigens at the cell surface, antigenic profiles of the four MCF-7 cell lines were determined. Using three monoclonal antibodies (B1.1, B6.2, and B50.4), four different antigenic phenotypes emerged.

To further understand the nature of antigenic hetero-geneity of human mammary tumor cell populations, MCF-7 cells were cloned by end-point dilution and ten different clones

Table 5

DIFFERENTIAL EXPRESSION OF TUMOR ASSOCIATED
ANTIGENS IN BT-20 CELLS UPON PASSAGE[a]

MCL AB	PASSAGE NUMBER					
	316	317	318	319	320	323
W6/32	690[b]	1,620	750	620	700	500
B38.1	2,560	2,280	1,380	1,640	1,550	1,320
B6.2	1,620	2,910	560	710	NEG[c]	NEG
B14.2	1,600	1,380	NEG	NEG	NEG	NEG

[a]Monoclonal antibodies were tested for binding to the surface of BT-20 mammary tumor cells in a live cell RIA.
[b]Values are expressed as cpm above background.
[c]Neg=<200 cpm.

were obtained and assayed for cell surface TAAs. As seen in Fig. 11, the parent MCF-7 culture reacts most strongly with monoclonal antibody B1.1 and least with monoclonal B72.3. Clone 6F1 (Fig. 11B)exhibits a similar phenotype to that of the parent. At least three additional major phenotypes were observed among the other clones. For example, clone 10B5 is devoid of detectable expression of any of the antigens assayed (Fig. 11C), although it does contain HLA and human antigens detected by monoclonal antibodies W6/32 and B139, respectively.

Studies were then undertaken to determine the stability of the cell surface phenotype of the MCF-7 clones. These cell lines have been monitored through a four month period, and assayed during log phase at approximately every other passage. A dramatic change in antigenic phenotype was observed in some of the clones, while other MCF-7 clones maintained a stable antigenic phenotype throughout the same observation period.

Antigenic variability of TAAs among and within human mammary tumor cell populations presents a potential problem in the development and optimization of immunodiagnostic and therapeutic procedures for breast cancer. Knowledge about the nature of this antigenic heterogeneity may be helpful in

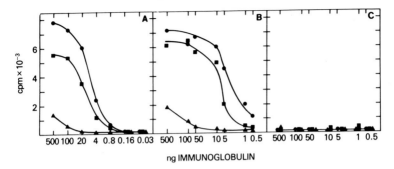

Fig. 11. Reactivity of monoclonal antibodies with the surface of the parent MCF-7 mammary adenocarcinoma cell line and cloned MCF-7 cell populations. Using a live cell radioimmunoassay, increasing amounts of monoclonal antibodies B1.1 (closed circle), B6.2 (closed square), and B72.3 (closed triangle), were tested for binding to the parent MCF-7 cell line (Panel A), MCF-7 clone 6F1 (Panel B), and MCF-7 clone 10B5 (Panel C).

the prediction or control of the expression of specific antigenic phenotypes. The studies described have enabled us to demonstrate the extent of specific antigenic variability in vivo among and within human mammary tumor cell populations. Heterogeneity was not only observed within a given mammary tumor cell line, but also among the "same" mammary tumor cell line obtained from four different laboratories. This observation should serve as a caveat to investigators who are utilizing established cell lines in their studies and attempting to correlate their results with those of other laboratories.

In collaboration with Dr. D. Kufe and colleagues (Sidney Farber Cancer Institute, Boston, MA), other studies, using fluorescent activated cell sorter analyses, have shown that at least two of the monoclonal antibodies developed (B6.2 and B38.1) are most reactive with the surface of MCF-7 cells during S-phase of the cell cycle (40). For this reason, all the experiments using cell lines described above were performed with cells in log phase of growth.

Using model systems, including the monoclonal antibodies and the cloned human mammary tumor cell lines described here, determinations of the parameters associated with a distinct change in antigenic phenotype are now feasible. Studies may now be undertaken to examine the relationship between the expression of specific antigenic phenotypes and such variables as morphology, tumorigenicity, drug susceptibility, growth rate, and the presence of specific hormone receptors in cloned mammary tumor cell lines. In view of the wide spread variation of antigenic phenotypes among and within human mammary tumors and its implications for the immunodiagnosis and therapy of breast cancer, it would also be of importance to determine which compounds, that could potentially be used clinically, will enhance the expression of specific TAAs on the surface of human mammary tumor cells.

Radiolocalization of Human Mammary Tumors in Athymic Mice by a Monoclonal Antibody.

Radioactively labeled antibodies to a variety of TAAs have been used to detect the presence of tumors in both experimental animals and humans by gamma scintigraphy. The majority of the antibodies used for clinical trials were constituents of goat or rabbit antisera, and were directed against antigens such as CEA (65, 66, 74) alpha-fetoprotein (75-77) ferritin (78) and human chorionic gonadatropin (79, 80); the studies using anti-CEA demonstrated the localization of malignant breast tumors (65, 66). In some of these studies (65, 66, 79, 80, 81, 74) the immunoglobulins have been partially purified using affinity chromotography with an increase in immunoreactivity of the IgG (81). With the development of the hybridoma technology, homogenous populations of monoclonal antibodies (82, 83) to TAAs can now be utilized to this end. In the studies described below, monoclonal B6.2 IgG was purified and $F(ab')_2$ and Fab' fragments were generated by pepsin digestion. These three forms of the antibody were radiolabeled and used to determine their utility in the radioimmunolocalization of human mammary tumor masses.

Monoclonal antibody B6.2 IgG, obtained from ascitic fluid, was precipitated with ammonium sulfate, dialyzed and purified by ion exchange chromatography. The IgG was further purified by molecular sieving using an Ultrogel AcA 44 column to remove low molecular weight contaminants with a similar charge as the IgG. Some of the purified IgG was used to generate $F(ab')_2$ and Fab' fragments. The fragments were purified by molecular sieving and retained all their immunoreactivity to mammary tumor extracts and not normal liver in solid phase RIAs when compared on a molar basis to the intact IgG. The IgG and its fragments were labeled with

^{125}I using the iodogen method, and specific activities of 15-50 uCi/ug of protein were easily obtained. The labeled antibody was shown to bind to the surface of live MCF-7 cells and retained the same specificity as the unlabeled antibody. Better than 70 percent of the antibody remained immunoreactive in sequential saturation solid phase RIAs after labeling.

Athymic mice were implanted with 1-2 mm^3 pieces of the transplantable Clouser human mammary tumor. After approximately 10-20 days the tumors grew to detectable nodules and continued to grow until they obtained diameters of 2.5 cm or more. Some tumors grew rapidly while others, from the same inoculum, stopped growing at various times yielding stable tumors as small as 0.6 cm in diameter. This variation in growth rate and ultimate tumor size, even arising from different aliquots of the same mammary tumor, is important in view of subsequent variations observed among different tumors in the amount of radiolabeled antibody bound per mg of tumor tissue. Athymic mice bearing the Clouser human mammary tumor were injected with 0.1 ug of B6.2 IgG labeled with ^{125}I to a specific activity of approximately 15 uCi per ug. The ratio of radioactivity/mg in the tumor compared to that of various tissues rose over a 4 day period (Fig. 12 A-E) and then fell at 7 days. The tumor to tissue ratios were 10:1 or greater in the liver, spleen and kidney at day 4. Ratios of the counts in the tumor to that found in the brain and muscle were greater than 50:1 and as high as 110:1. Lower tumor to tissue ratios were obtained when compared to blood and the lungs with their large blood pool. The activity found in the lungs was probably not a consequence of trapping of particulates, as evidenced by the low uptake in the liver and spleen.

When the Clouser mammary tumor bearing mice were injected with ^{125}I-F(ab')$_2$ fragments of B6.2, higher tumor to tissue ratios were obtained (Fig. 12 F-J). The tumor to tissue ratios in the liver and spleen were 15-20:1 at 96 hours. The tumor to tissue ratios were somewhat lower with blood and lungs, but were still higher than those obtained using IgG. This is probably due to the faster clearance of the F(ab')$_2$ fragments as compared to the IgG. The tumor to kidney ratio was relatively low and was probably due to the more rapid clearance of Fab' fragments, which may have been generated from the F(ab')$_2$ _in vivo_ by the breakage of the cross linking disulfide bonds.

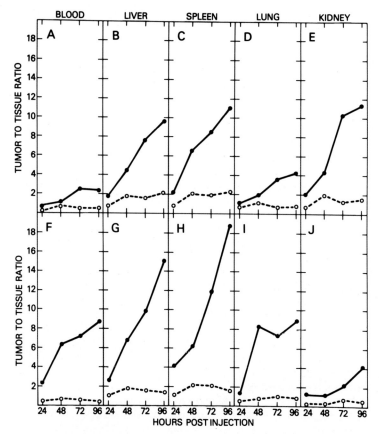

Fig. 12.   Tissue distribution of ^{125}I-B6.2 IgG and
F(ab')$_2$ in athymic mice bearing human tumor transplants.
Athymic mice bearing a transplantable human mammary tumor
(Clouser, closed circles) or a human melanoma (A375, open
circles) were inoculated with ^{125}I-B6.2.   Approximately 1.5
uCi of IgG (Panels A-E) or F(ab')$_2$ (Panels F-J) were
injected i.v. and the mice were sacrificed at daily
intervals.   The radioactivity per mg of tumor was determined
and compared to that of various tissues, the averages of
2-20 mice per group are shown.

Athymic mice bearing a human melanoma (A375), a tumor
that shows no surface reactivity with B6.2 in live cell
RIAs, were used as controls for non-specific binding of the
labeled antibody or antibody fragments to tumor tissue.   As

shown in Fig. 12 (open circles), no preferential localization of the monoclonal antibody was observed in the tumor; in fact, the counts per mg in the tumor were lower than that found in many organs resulting in ratios of less than 1. Similarly, no localization was observed when either normal murine IgG or MOPC-21 IgG$_1$ (the same isotype as B6.2) from a murine myeloma, or their F(ab')$_2$ fragments, were inoculated into athymic mice bearing Clouser mammary tumors or melanomas, with tumor to blood ratios of less than or equal to 0.5:1. Athymic mice bearing human mammary tumors derived from tissue culture cell lines were also injected with labeled B6.2 antibody and fragments. Tumor to spleen and liver ratios of 6-8:1 were obtained using B6.2 F(ab')$_2$ in mice bearing tumors derived from MCF-7 cells and BT-20 cells.

Athymic mice bearing Clouser mammary tumors were also injected with ^{125}I-labeled B6.2 Fab'. The clearance rate of the Fab' fragment was considerably faster than the larger F(ab')$_2$ fragment and the intact IgG. Acceptable tumor to tissue ratios were obtained, but the fast clearance rate resulted in a large amount of the labeled Fab' being found in the kidney and bladder, resulting in low tumor to kidney ratios. These studies therefore indicate that F(ab')$_2$ fragments are superior to Fab' or intact IgG in the radiolocalization studies in mice with monoclonal antibody B6.2.

Scanning of athymic mice bearing human tumors. Studies were undertaken to determine whether the localization of the ^{125}I-labeled antibody and fragments in the tumors was sufficient to detect using a gamma camera. The scanning studies were performed in collaboration with Drs. M. Zalutsky and W. Kaplan of the Harvard Medical School (35). Athymic mice bearing the Clouser mammary tumor or the A375 melanoma were injected i.v. with approximately 30 uCi of ^{125}I-B6.2 IgG. The mice were scanned and then sacrificed at 24 hour intervals. The Clouser tumors were easily detected at 24 hours (Fig. 13A) using radiolabeled B6.2 IgG, with a small amount of activity detectable in the blood pool. The tumor remained strongly positive over the 4 day period with the background activity decreasing to the point where it was barely detectable at 96 hours (Fig. 13B). The 0.5cm diameter tumors localized in Figures 13A and B appear bigger than their actual size; this may be due to the dispersion of rays through the pinhole collimeter. No tumor localization was observed using radiolabeled B6.2 IgG in mice bearing the control human melanoma transplants (Fig. 13C).

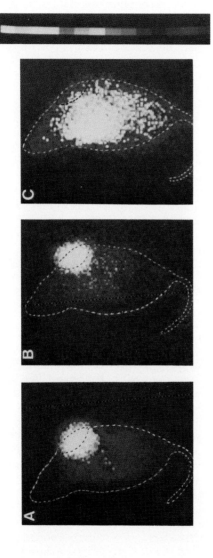

Fig. 13. Gamma camera scanning with B6.2 IgG of athymic mice bearing transplanted human tumors. Athymic mice bearing a transplantable human mammary tumor (Clouser, Panels A and B) or a human melanoma (A375, Panel C) were inoculated with approximately 30 uCi of ^{125}I-B6.2 IgG. The mice were scanned after various time intervals (24 hours, Panel A, C; 96 hrs., Panel B) until an equal number of counts were detected in each field. The color bar denotes the relative amounts of activity with the highest levels at the top of the bar.

Mice were also injected with ^{125}I-B6.2 F(ab')$_2$ fragments. The mice cleared the fragments faster than the intact IgG and a significant amount of activity was observed in the two kidneys and bladder at 24 hours (Fig. 14A), but tumors were clearly positive for localization of the ^{125}I-B6.2 F(ab')$_2$ fragments. The activity was cleared from the kidneys and bladder by 48 hours and the tumor to background ratio increased over the 4 day period of scanning, with little background, and good tumor localization observed at 96 hours (Fig. 14B). No localization of activity was observed with the radiolabeled B6.2 F(ab')$_2$ fragments in the athymic mice bearing the A375 melanoma (Fig. 14C).

The utility of radiolabeled antibodies for the in vivo localization of tumors in humans has been shown with heterologous polyclonal antibodies to a number of different antigens. Human mammary tumors have been localized using antibodies to CEA (65, 66) that have been affinity purified. Murine mammary tumors have been localized using antibodies to murine mammary epithelial antigens generated in rabbits (84). These studies required computer aided background subtraction (employing a second radiolabeled Ig or other protein) and are thus limited in use to institutions with such sophisticated equipment. The use of monoclonal antibodies with defined specificities should eliminate such additional manipulations, and should also thus reduce radiation dose to the patients.

Monoclonal antibodies to murine Thy 1.1 antigens (85) Rauscher leukemia virus gp70 (using ^{111}In; 86) and to a stage-specific embryonic antigen (87), have been used to show localization of tissues in mice. The study by Houston et al. (85) using ^{125}I-labeled anti-Thy 1.1 showed selective localization of the antibody to lymphatic tissues in mice containing the antigen. Scheinberg, et al. (86) were able to show the localization of radioactivity in leukemic spleens of mice injected with the Rauscher leukemia virus. This work has been extended with the successful localization of human colon carcinomas in athymic mice and in patients with monoclonal antibodies to CEA (88) and in athymic mice bearing a human germ cell tumor using monoclonal antibodies generated against the tumor (89). Attempts to localize human tumors in mice with monoclonal antibodies to HLA were unsuccessful (90).

The studies described here demonstrate the ability of radiolabeled monoclonal antibody to detect human breast tumor xenografts in athymic mice. The ^{125}I-labeled antibody and fragments all successfully localized tumors with the

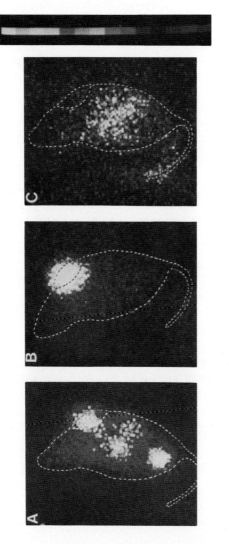

Fig. 14. Gamma camera scanning with B6.2 F(ab')$_2$ of athymic mice bearing transplanted human tumors. Athymic mice bearing a transplantable human mammary tumor (Clouser, Panels A and B) or a human melanoma (A375, Panel C) were inoculated with approximately 30 uCi of ^{125}I-B6.2 F(ab')$_2$. The mice were scanned after various time intervals (24 hrs., Panel A; 96 hrs., Panels B and C) until an equal number of counts were detected in each field. The color bar denotes the relative amount of activity with the highest levels at the top of the bar.

F(ab')$_2$ fragment giving the overall highest tumor to tissue ratios. The F(ab')$_2$ fragments may be the best form of the antibody to use because of the potential problem of Fc receptors on a variety of cells binding the labeled IgG and yielding a higher non-specific distribution of the antibody. The use of an antibody without the Fc portion should also reduce its immunoreactivity in patients and thus minimize an immune response. The smaller fragments also clear the body faster than intact immunoglobulin and should thus result in a lower whole body radiation absorbed dose to the host.

Radiolabeled monoclonal antibodies that are reactive with the surface of human mammary carcinoma cells may eventually prove useful in several areas in the management of human breast cancer. The detection of occult metastatic lesions at distal sites via gamma scanning could serve as an adjunct in determining which patients should receive adjuvant therapy, and subsequent scanning may reveal which tumors are responding to therapy. At present, only axillary lymph nodes, removed at mastectomy, are examined for tumor involvement for use in staging; the extent of nodal tumor involvement in the internal mammary chain is not determined. The use of radiolabeled monoclonal antibodies in lymphangiography of the internal mammary chain may thus eventually increase the reliability of staging of nodal involvement (both axillary and internal chain) as a prognostic indicator. Along with their potential in the diagnosis and prognosis of breast cancer, monoclonal antibodies coupled with isotopes decaying via high energy transfer with short range radiation may eventually prove useful as radiotherapeutic agents. This approach, however, is obviously quite complex and would require extensive studies in an experimental model. The system described here, of a radiolabeled monoclonal antibody that is selectively reactive with the surface of human mammary tumor cells <u>in vivo</u> may provide an excellent experimental system for such therapy studies.

ACKNOWLEDGEMENTS

We wish to thank D. Poole, D. Simpson, J. Howell, J. Collins, J. Crowley, R. Fitzgerald, and A. Sloan for expert technical assistance in these studies. We also thank Dr. D. Stramignoni for many helpful discussions. Some of these studies were supported, in part, by a contract from the National Cancer Institute, National Institutes of Health, Bethesda, Maryland.

REFERENCES

1.   Hollinshead AC, Jaffurs WT, Alpert LK, Harris JE, Herberman RB (1974). Isolation and identification of soluble skin-reactive membrane antigens and normal breast cells. Cancer Res 34:2961.

2.   Avis F, Avis I, Newsome JF, Haughton G (1976). Antigenic cross-reactivity between adenocarcinoma of the breast and fibrocystic disease of the breast. J Natl Cancer Inst 56:17.

3.   Mesa-Tejada R, Keydar I, Ramanarayanan M, Ohno T, Feoglio C, Spiegelman S (1978). Detection in human breast carcinomas of an antigen immunologically related to a group-specific antigen of mouse mammary tumor virus. Proc Natl Acad Sci (USA) 75:1529.

4.   Black MM, Zachrau RE, Shore B, Dion AS, Leis HP (1978). Cellular immunity to autologous breast cancer and RIII-murine mammary tumor virus preparations. Cancer Res 38:2068.

5.   Springer, GF, Desai PR, Murthy MS, Scanlon EF (1979). Human carcinoma-associated precursor antigens of the NM blood group system. J Surg Oncol 11:95.

6.   Leung, JP, Borden GM, Nakamura RM, Delteer DH, Edgington TS (1979). Frequency of association of mammary tumor glycoprotein antigen and other markers with human breast tumors. Cancer Res 39:2057.

7.   Howard DR, Taylor CR (1979). A method for distinguishing benign from malignant breast lesions utilizing antibody present in normal human sera. Cancer 43:2279.

8.   Sheikh KMA, Quismorio FA, Friou GJ, Lee Y (1979). Ductular carcinoma of the breast. Serum antibodies to tumor-associated antigens. Cancer 44:2083.

9.   Yu, GSM, Kadish AS, Johnson AB, Marcus DM (1980). Breast carcinoma associated antigen: An immunocytochemical study. A brief scientific report. Amer J Clin Path 74:453.

10. Arklie J, Taylor-Papadimitriou J, Bodmer W, Egan M, Millis R (1981). Differentiation antigens expressed by epithethial cells in the lactating breast are also detectable in breast cancers. Int J Cancer 28:23.

11. Hilgers J, Hilkens J, Buijis F, Hageman P, Sonnenberg A, Koldovsky U, Karande K, van Hoeven RP, Feltkamp C, van de Rijn JM (1981). Monoclonal antibodies against human milk fat globule membranes detecting

differentiation antigens of the mammary gland.
Monoclonal Antibodies and Breast Cancer, Breast Cancer
Task Force Committee.

12. Taylor-Papadimitriou J, Peterson JA, Arklie J, Burchell
J, Ceriani RL (1981). Monoclonal antibodies to
epithelium-specific components of the human milk fat
globule membrane: Production and reaction with cells
in culture. Int J Cancer 28:17.

13. Foster CS, Dinsdale EA, Edwards PAW, Neville AM (1982).
Monoclonal antibodies to the human mammary gland: II.
Distribution of determinants in breast carcinomas.
Virchows Arch [Pathol Anat] 394:295.

14. Foster CS, Edwards PAW, Dinsdale EA, Neville AM (1982).
Monoclonal antibodies to the human mammary gland: I.
Distribution of determinants in non-neoplastic mammary
and extra mammary tissues. Virchows Arch [Pathol Anat]
394:279.

15. Greene GL, Nolan C, Engler JP, Jensen EV (1980).
Monoclonal antibodies to human estrogen receptor. Proc
Natl Acad Sci (USA) 77:5115.

16. Grzyb K, Ciocca DR, Murthy SR, Bjercke RJ, McGuire WL
(1981). Monoclonal antibodies to human breast cancer
cells. Monoclonal Antibodies and Breast Cancer, Breast
Cancer Task Force Committee.

17. Krolick KA, Yuan D, Vitetta ES (1981). Specific
killing of a human breast carcinoma cell line by a
monoclonal antibody coupled to the A-chain of ricin.
Cancer Immunol Immunother 12:39.

18. Yuan D, Hendler FJ, Vitetta ES (1982).
Characterization of a monoclonal antibody reactive with
a subset of human breast tumors. J Natl Cancer Inst
68:719.

19. Edwards PAW, Foster CS, McIlhinney RAJ (1980).
Monoclonal antibodies to teratomas and breast.
Transplantation Proceedings 12:398.

20. Schlom J, Wunderlich D, Teramoto YA (1980). Generation
of human monoclonal antibodies reactive with human
mammary carcinoma cells. Proc Natl Acad Sci (USA)
77:6841.

21. Wunderlich, D, Teramoto, YA, Alford C, Schlom J (1981).
The use of lymphocytes from axillary lymph nodes of
mastectomy patients to generate human monoclonal
antibodies. Eur J Cancer Clin Oncol 17:719.

22. Teramoto YA, Mariani R, Wunderlich D, Schlom J (1982).
The immunohistochemical reactivity of a human
monoclonal antibody with tissue sections of human

mammary tumors. Cancer 50:241.

23. Woodbury RG, Brown JP, Yeh MY, Hellstrom I, Hellstron KE (1980). Identification of a cell surface protein, p97, in human melanomas and certain other neoplasms. Proc Natl Acad Sci (USA) 77:2183.

24. Loop SM, Nishiyama K, Hellstrom I, Woodbury RG, Brown JP, Hellstrom, KE (1981). Two human tumor-associated antigens, p155 and p210, detected by monoclonal antibodies, Int J Cancer 27:775.

25. Natali PG, Wilson BS, Imai K, Bigotti A, Ferrone S (1982). Tissue distribution, molecular profile, and shedding of a cytoplasmic antigen identified by the monoclonal antibody 465.125 to human melanoma cells. Cancer Research 42:583.

26. Cuttitta F, Rosen S, Gazdar AF, Minna, JD (1981). Monoclonal antibodies that demonstrate specificity for several types of human lung cancer. Proc Natl Acad Sci (USA) 78:4591.

27. Mazauric T, Mitchell KF, Letchworth III GJ, Koprowski H, Steplewski Z (1982). Monoclonal antibody-defined human lung cell surface protein antigens. Cancer Research 42:150.

28. Ueda R, Ogata S, Morrissey DM, Finstad CL, Szkudlarek J, Whitmore WF, Oettgen HF, Lloyd KO, Old LJ (1981). Cell surface antigens of human renal cancer defined by mouse monoclonal antibodies: Identification of tissue-specific kidney glycoproteins. Proc Natl Acad Sci (USA) 78:5122.

29. Frankel AE, Rouse RV, Herzenberg LA (1982). Human prostate specific and shared differentiation antigens defined by monoclonal antibodies. Proc Natl Acad Sci (USA) 79:903.

30. Daar AS, Fabre JW (1981). Demonstration with monoclonal antibodies of an unusual mononuclear cell infiltrate and loss of normal epithelial membrane antigens in human breast carcinomas. Lancet Aug 29:434.

31. Colcher D, Horan Hand P, Nuti M, Schlom J (1981). A spectrum of monoclonal antibodies reactive with human mammary tumor cells. Proc Natl Acad Sci (USA) 73:3199.

32. Nuti M, Teramoto YA, Mariani-Costantini R, Horan Hand P, Colcher D, Schlom J (1982). A monoclonal antibody (B72.3) defines patterns of distribution of a novel tumor associated antigen in human mammary carcinoma cell populations. Int J Cancer 29:539.

33. Nuti M, Colcher D, Horan Hand P, Austin F, Schlom J (1981). Generation and characterization of monoclonal antibodies reactive with human primary and metastatic mammary tumor cells. In Albertini A, Ekins R (ed): "Monoclonal Antibodies and Development in Immunoassay," North Holland: Elsevier/North Holland Biomedical Press, p 87.

34. Colcher D, Horan Hand P, Nuti M, Schlom J (1982). Differential binding to human mammary and non-mammary tumors of monoclonal antibodies reactive with carcinoembryonic antigen. Cancer Invest (in press).

35. Colcher D, Zalutsky M, Kaplan W, Kufe D, Austin F, Schlom J (submitted for publication). Radiolocalization of human mammary tumors in athymic mice by a monoclonal antibody.

36. Horan Hand P, Nuti M, Colcher D, Schlom J (submitted for publication). Monoclonal antibodies to tumor associated antigens define antigenic heterogeneity among human mammary carcinoma cell populations.

37. Colcher D, Horan Hand P, Teramoto YA, Wunderlich D, Schlom J (1981). Monoclonal antibodies define diversity of mammary tumor viral gene products in virions and mammary tumors of the genus Mus. Cancer Res 41:1451.

38. Herzenberg LA, Herzenberg LA, Milstein C (1979). Cell hybrids of myelomas with antibody forming cells and T lymphocytes with T cells. In Weir DM (ed): "Handbook of Experimental Immunology," London: Blackwell Scientific, p 25.1.

39. Barnstable CJ, Bodmer WF, Brown G, Galfre G, Milstein C, Williams AF, Ziegler A (1978). Production of monoclonal antibodies to group A erthrocytes, HLA and other human cell surface antigens - New tools for genetic analysis. Cell 14:9.

40. Kufe DW, Nadler L, Sargent L, Shapiro H, Horan Hand P, Austin F, Colcher D, Schlom J (submitted for publication). Cell surface binding properties of monoclonal antibodies reactive with human mammary carcinoma cells.

41. Gold P, Freedman SO (1964). Demonstration of tumor-specific antigens in human colonic carcinomata by immunological tolerance and absorption techniques. J of Experimental Med 121:439.

42. Hansen HJ, Snyder JJ, Miller E, Vandevoorde JP, Miller ON, Hines LR, Burns JJ (1974). Carcinoembryonic antigen (CEA) assay. Human Pathology 5:139..

43. Krebs BP, Lalanne CM, Schneider M (1978). Clinical application of carcinoembryonic antigen assay: Proc. of a Symposium, Nice, France, Amsterdam, Excerpta Medica.

44. Gold P, Freedman SO, Shuster J (1979). Carcinoembryonic antigen: Historical perspective, experimental data. In Herberman RB, McIntire KR (eds): "Immunodiagnosis of Cancer," New York: Marcel Dekker, Inc, p 147.

45. Chu TM, Nemoto T (1973). Evaluation of carcinoembryonic antigen in human mammary carcinoma. J Natl Cancer Inst 51:1119.

46. Steward AM, Nixon D, Zamcheck N, Aisenberg A (1974). Carcinoembryonic antigen in breast cancer patients: Serum levels and disease progress. Cancer 33:1246.

47. Menendez-Botet CJ, Nisselbaum JS, Fleisher M, Rosen PP, Fracchia A, Robbins G, Urban JA, Schwartz MK (1976). Correlation between estrogen receptor protein and carcinoembryonic antigen in normal and carcinomatous human breast tissue. Clin Chem 22:1366.

48. Lokich JJ, Zamcheck N, Lowenstein, M (1978). Sequential carcinoembryonic antigen levels in the therapy of metastatic breast cancer: A predictor and monitor of response and relapse. Annals of Internal Med 89:902.

49. Waalkes TP, Gehrke CW, Tormey DC, Woo KB, Kuo KC, Snyder J, Hansen H (1978). Biologic markers in breast carcinoma: IV. Serum fucose-protein ratio, comparisons with carcinoembryonic antigen and human chorionic gonadotrophin. Cancer 41:1871.

50. Wilkinson, EJ, Hause LL, Sasse EA, Pattillo RA, Milbrath JR, Lewis JD (1980). Carcinoembryonic antigen and L-fucose in malignant and benign mammary disease. Amer J Clin Pathol 73:669.

51. Chatal JF, Chupin F, Ricolleau G, Tellier JL, le Mevel A, Fumoleau P, Godin O, le Mevel BP (1980). Use of serial carcinoembryonic antigen assays in detecting relapses in breast cancer involving high risk of metastasis. Europ J Cancer 17:233.

52. Vrba R, Alpert E, Isselbacher KJ (1975). Carcinoembryonic antigen: Evidence for multiple antigenic determinants and isoantigens. Proc Natl Acad Sci (USA) 72:4602.

53. Chism SE, Noel LW, Wells JV, Crewther P, Hunt S, Marchalonis JJ, Fudenberg HH (1977). Evidence for common and distinct determinants of colon

carcinoembryonic antigen, colon carcinoma antigen-III, and molecules with carcinoembryonic antigen activity isolated from breast and ovarian cancer. Cancer Res 37:3100.

54. Pusztaszeri G, Mach JP (1973). Carcinoembryonic antigen (CEA) in non-digestive cancerous and normal tissues. Immunochemistry 10:197.

55. Dent PB, Carrel S, Mach JP (1980). Detection of new cross-reacting carcinoembryonic antigen(s) on cultured tumor cells by mixed hemadsorption assay. J Natl Cancer Inst 64:309.

56. Rogers GT, Rawlins GA, Keep PA, Cooper EH, Bagshawe KD (1981). Application of monoclonal antibodies to purified CEA in clinical radioimmunoassay of human serum. Br J Cancer 44:371.

57. Koprowski H, Steplewski Z, Mitchell K, Herlyn M, Herlyn D, Fuhrer P (1979). Colorectal carcinoma antigens detected by hybridoma antibodies. Somatic Cell Genet 5:957.

58. Miggiano V, Stahli C, Haring P, Schmidt J, LoDein M, Glatthaar B, Staehelin T (1979). Monoclonal antibodies to three tumor markers: Human chorionic gonadotropin (hCG), prostatic acid phosphatase (PAP) and carcinoembryonic antigen (CEA). In Peeters H (ed): "Proc. of the Twenty-Eighth Colloquium," Oxford: Pergamon Press, p 501.

59. Accolla RS, Carrel S, Mach JP (1980). Monoclonal antibodies specific for carcinoembryonic antigen and produced by two hybrid cell lines. Proc Natl Acad Sci (USA) 77:563.

60. Mitchell KF (1980). A carcinoembryonic antigen (CEA) specific monoclonal hybridoma antibody that reacts only with high-molecular-weight CEA. Cancer Immunol Immunother 10:1.

61. Kupcik HZ, Zurawski Jr VR, Hurrell JGR, Zamcheck N, Black PH (1981). Monoclonal antibodies to carcinoembryonic antigen produced by somatic cell fusion. Cancer Res 41:3306.

62. Rogers GT, Rawlins GA, Bagshawe KD (1981). Somatic-cell hybrids producing antibodies against CEA. Br J Cancer 43:1.

63. von Kleist S, Burtin P (1979). Antigens cross-reacting with CEA. In Herberman RB, McIntire KR (eds): "Immunodiagnosis of Cancer," New York: Marcel-Dekker, Inc, p 322.

64. Sehested, M, Hirsch FR, Hou-Jensen K (1981).
Immunoperoxidase staining for carcinoembryonic antigen
in small cell carcinoma of the lung. Eur J Cancer Clin
Oncol 17:1125.

65. DeLand FH, Kim EE, Corgan RL, Casper S, Primus FJ,
Spremulli E, Estes N, Goldenberg DM (1979). Axillary
lymphoscintigraphy by radioimmunodetection of
carcinoembryonic antigen in breast cancer. J Nucl Med
20:1243.

66. Goldenberg DM, Kim EE, DeLand FH, Bennett S, Primus FJ
(1980). Radioimmunodetection of cancer with
radioactive antibodies to °carcinoembryonic antigen.
Cancer Res 40:2984.

67. Foulds L (1954). The experimental study of tumor
progression: A review. Cancer Res 14:327.

68. Hart IR, Fidler IJ (1981). The implications of tumor
heterogeneity for studies on the biology and therapy of
cancer metastasis. Biochem Biophys Acta 651:37.

69. Kerbel RS (1979). Implications of immunological
heterogeneity of tumors. Nature 280:358.

70. Miller FR, Heppner GH (1979). Immunologic
heterogeneity of tumor cell subpopulations from a
single mouse mammary tumor. J Natl Cancer Inst
63:1457.

71. Pimm MV, Baldwin RW (1977). Antigenic differences
between primary methylcholanthrene-induced rat sarcomas
and post-surgical recurrences. Int J Cancer 20:37.

72. Poste G, Doll J, Fidler IJ (1981). Interactions among
clonal subpopulations affect stability of the
metastatic phenotype in polyclonal populations of B16
melanoma cells. Proc Natl Acad Sci (USA) 78:6226.

73. Prehn, RT (1970). Analysis of antigenic heterogeneity
within individual 3-methylcholanthrene-induced mouse
sarcomas. J Natl Cancer Inst 45:1039.

74. Mach JP, Carrel S, Forni M, Ritschard J, Donath A,
Alberto P (1981). Tumor localization of radiolabeled
antibodies against carcinoembryonic antigen in patients
with carcinoma. New England Journal of Medicine 303:5.

75. Goldenberg DM, DeLand FH, Kim EE, Primus FJ (1980).
Xenogeneic antitumor antibodies in cancer
radioimmunodetection. Transplant Proc 12:188.

76. Goldenberg DM, Kim EE, DeLand FH, Spremulli E, Nelson
MO, Gockerman JP, Primus, FJ, Corgan RL, Alpert E
(1980). Clinical studies on the radioimmunodetection
of tumors containing alpha-fetoprotein. Cancer
45:2500.

77. Kim EE, DeLand FH, Nelson MO, Bennett S, Simmons G, Alpert E, Goldenberg DM (1980). Radioimmunodetection of cancer with radiolabeled antibodies to a-fetoprotein. Cancer Res 40:3008.

78. Order SE, Klein JL, Leichner PK (1981). Antiferritin IgG antibody for isotopic cancer therapy. Oncology 38:154.

79. Goldenberg DM, Kim EE, DeLand FH, vanNagell Jr JR, Iavadpour N (1980). Clinical radioimmunodetection of cancer with radioactive antibodies to human chorionic gonadotropin. Science 208:1284.

80. Goldenberg DM, Kim EE, DeLand FH (1981). Human chorionic gonadotropin radioantibodies in the radioimmunodetection of cancer and for disclosure of occult metastases. Proc Natl Acad Sci (USA) 78:7754.

81. Primus FJ, Goldenberg DM (1980). Immunological considerations in the use of goat antibodies to carcinoembryonic antigen for the radioimmunodetection of cancer. Cancer Res 40:2079

82. Kohler G, Milstein C (1975). Continuous cultures of fused cells secreting antibody of predefined specificity. Nature 256:494.

83. Kohler G, Milstein C (1976). Derivation of specific antibody producing tissue culture and tumor lines by cell fusion. Eur J Immunol 6:511.

84. Wilbanks T, Peterson JA, Miller S, Kaufman L, Ortendahl D, Ceriani RL, (1981). Localization of mammary tumors in vivo with ^{131}I-labeled Fab fragments of antibodies against mouse mammary epithelial (MME) antigens. Cancer 48:1768.

85. Houston LL, Nowinski RC, Bernstein ID (1980). Specific in vivo localization of monoclonal antibodies directed against the Thy 1.1 antigen. J Immunology 125:837.

86. Scheinberg DA, Strand M, Gansow O (1982). Tumor imaging with radioactive metal chelates conjugated to monoclonal antibodies. Science 215:1511.

87. Ballou B, Levine G, Hakala TR, Solter D (1979). Tumor location detected with radioactively labeled monoclonal antibody and external scintigraphy. Science 206:844.

88. Mach JP, Buchegger F, Forni M, Ritschard J, Berche L, Lumbroso JD, Schreyer M, Girardet C, Acolla RS, Carrel S (1981). Use of radiolabeled monoclonal anti-CEA antibodies for the detection of human carcinomas by external photoscanning and tomoscintigraphy. Immunology Today:239.

89. Moshakis V, McIlhinney RAJ, Raghavan D, Neville AM (1981). Localization of human tumor xenografts after i.v. administration of radiolabeled monoclonal antibodies. Br J Cancer 44:91.

90. Warenius HM, Galfre G, Bleehen NM, Milstein C (1981). Attempted targeting of a monoclonal antibody in a human tumor xenograft system. Eur J Cancer Clin Oncol 17:1009.

Rational Basis for Chemotherapy, pages 359–377
© 1983 Alan R. Liss, Inc., 150 Fifth Avenue, New York, NY 10011

LYSIS OF FRESH HUMAN SOLID TUMORS BY ACTIVATED AUTOLOGOUS
LYMPHOCYTES: POTENTIAL APPLICATIONS TO TUMOR IMMUNOTHERAPY

Amitabha Mazumder and Steven A. Rosenberg

Surgery Branch, Division of Cancer Treatment, National
Cancer Institute, Bethesda, Maryland 20205

ABSTRACT   Human peripheral blood lymphocytes (PBL),
obtained from patients with a variety of malignancies,
when incubated in vitro with phytohemagglutinin (PHA),
lymphokines or allogeneic lymphocytes, lysed fresh autologous NK-insensitive tumor cells during a short term
^{51}Cr release assay. Metastases and allogeneic tumors
but not autologous PBL or lymphoblasts were lysed by
these activated cells. Some adherent cells were necessary for activation, but higher numbers were suppressive. The precursor and effector cells were found to be
distinct from NK cells. The phenotype of the effector
cells was found to be similar to that of conventional
cytotoxic T lymphocytes (CTL) (OKT3+, OKT8+), although
the kinetics of appearance of the activated cells was
more rapid than that of CTL. Activated T cells thus
represent a population of non-NK cells with broad lytic
specificity for tumor cells. A phase I clinical trial
has been completed demonstrating that large numbers of
autologous PHA activated PBL can be safely obtained and
infused into humans. These infusions resulted in an
increase in the number of circulating activated cells
with evidence of migration of cells to tumor, lungs,
liver and spleen. The biologic and therapeutic significance of these activated cells are being investigated.

INTRODUCTION

We and others have demonstrated that lymphoid cells expanded in vitro in Interleukin-2 (IL-2) maintain specific cytotoxic reactivity after prolonged growth (1,2,3). In the

murine system, we have developed models for studying the in
vivo efficacy of cells grown and expanded in IL-2. Rosenstein
et al.(4) have shown that highly sensitized cytotoxic lymphoid
cells grown in IL-2 can mediate the accelerated rejection
of allogeneic skin grafts. Eberlein et al. (5,6), using
the FBL-3 lymphoma model of Fefer and his coworkers, have
cured C57Bl/6 mice of disseminated tumor by the adoptive
transfer of syngeneic lymphocytes sensitized either in vivo
or in vitro to the tumor and then expanded in IL-2.

These approaches, however, rely on the repeated immunization of syngeneic donors and the ready availability
of purified, highly antigenic tumors for sensitization, procedures not usually feasible for the treatment of human
cancer. Despite the extensive effort that has been devoted
to develop methods for the generation of human PBL cytotoxic
for human tumor (7,8), most available techniques lead to
poor induction of cells lytic for fresh autologous tumor
cells (9,10,11,12).

Our laboratory has, therefore, adopted an alternative
approach -- the activation of PBL in culture without tumor
to generate cells cytotoxic for fresh human tumor.

Lymphoid cells that lyse fresh autologous human tumor
can be generated by lectin activation (13,14), allosensitization (15,16) and lymphokine activation (17,18). This review will discuss these systems and our preliminary use of
such activated cells in the treatment of human cancer.

Lectin Activation

We have demonstrated (13), in over 30 experiments to
date, that PBL from patients with a variety of malignancies,
when incubated with lectins (Concanavalin A or PHA) for 2-3
days in human AB or autologous serum, lyse fresh autologous
tumor but not lymphocytes or lymphoblasts in a 4-hour ^{51}Cr
release assay. Tumor cells are obtained fresh (without
tissue culture) by mincing and enzymatic treatment of surgical specimens. Results of studies in 3 representative
patients are shown in Figure 1 (13).

FIGURE 1

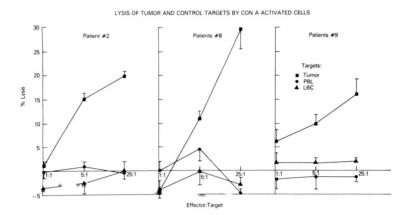

LYSIS OF TUMOR AND CONTROL TARGETS BY CON A ACTIVATED CELLS

FIGURE 1. Lysis of fresh autologous tumor, PBL and Con A-induced lymphoblasts (LBC) in 3 patients by PBL incubated for 3 days in Con A 10 μg/ml (13). Points and bars represent means and standard errors of triplicate measurements in a 4-hour ^{51}Cr release assay.

Using fresh cells obtained individually from autologous tumor at several different metastatic sites, we have further demonstrated the lysis of fresh autologous metastases but not of autologous lymphocytes or lymphoblasts (Fig. 2, left panel). The lysability of each of the target cells, determined by using as effectors allogeneic PBL allosensitized to the patieint's PBL, were approximately equal (Fig. 2, right panel).

FIGURE 2

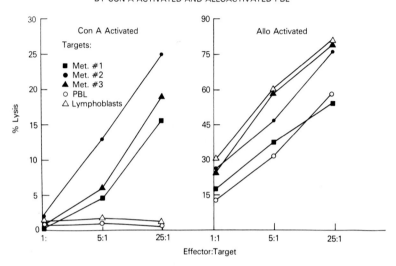

FIGURE 2. **Left:** Lysis of cells from 3 different fresh autologous metastases (met) (in this case of melanoma, s.c. nodules), PBL and LBC by Con A activated PBL. **Right:** Lysis of the various targets by allogeneic normal PBL sensitized in vitro to the patient PBL. Percentage lysis of each target shown is that determined by triplicates in a 4-hour ^{51}Cr release assay.

Allogeneic tumors are lysed equally well as autologous tumors. In fact, as shown in Figure 3, cold (unlabelled) fresh allogeneic tumors of various histologic types but not autologous PBL were capable of decreasing the lysis of labelled fresh autologous tumor cells in a dose-dependent manner, when added to the effectors in the assay. Thus, the same subset of activated cells lyses fresh autologous and allogeneic tumor cells.

FIGURE 3

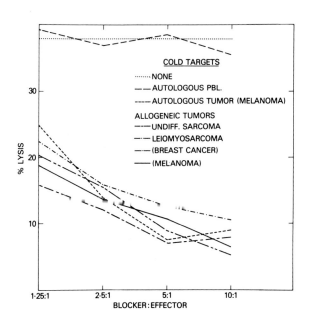

FIGURE 3. Cold target inhibition by fresh allogeneic
tumors or autologous PBL of the lysis of fresh autologous
tumor cells by PHA activated PBL. Points shown are those obtained in a 4-hour ^{51}Cr release assay by the addition of 10,
5, 2.5 or 0 (none) cold (unlabelled) targets per labelled target in triplicate wells containing a 20:1 ratio of effectors
to labelled target cells.

The lysis is not merely a lectin dependent cellular
cytotoxicity effect since inhibitors of the lectin (e.g.
α -methylmannoside for Concanavalin A) do not decrease the
lysis when present in the assay (13).

Activation by allosensitization

Zarling et al. have previously demonstrated that allogeneic sensitization of human PBL was capable of generating cells cytotoxic for fresh autologous leukemic cells (19). We have extended these observations to a variety of human solid tumors (15,16) and have demonstrated that the lysis of fresh autologous tumor cells but not of autologous PBL or lymphoblasts is mediated by PBL from cancer patients allosensitized in vitro to a pool of or single allogeneic normal donor PBL (Fig. 4).

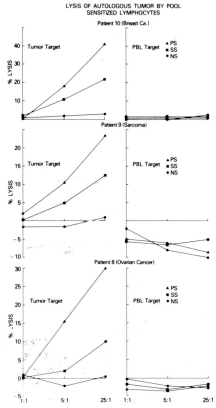

FIGURE 4. Lysis of fresh autologous tumor and PBL in 3 patients by PBL sensitized for 7 days to pooled (PS) or single (SS) allogeneic normal donor PBL or incubated for 7 days without stimulators (nonsensitized--NS) (15). Responder to stimulator ratios during sensitizations were 1:1.5. Percent lysis was determined in a 4-hour ^{51}Cr release assay at the effector to target ratios shown.

Here, as with lectin activation, fresh autologous metastases and allogeneic tumors are lysed. The alloactivation
appears to be enhanced by the presence of IL-2 containing
preparations during the in vitro sensitization.

Lymphokine Activation

Lotze et al. and Grimm et al. have demonstrated that
human PBL, in media containing IL-2, can develop the a-
bility to lyse fresh autologous tumor, but not autologous
PBL or lymphoblasts (17,18). In this system, as well as
in the lectin and allo-activations, the NK-sensitive target
K562 and NK-insensitive target Daudi (20) are also lysed
(Fig. 5).

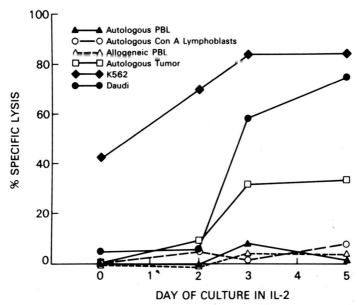

FIGURE 5. PBL from a patient, incubated with Inter-
leukin-2 (IL-2) were tested for the development of lysis
of autologous tumor, autologous Con A induced lymphoblasts,
autologous and allogeneic PBL and NK-sensitive (K562) and
NK-insensitive (Daudi) tissue cultured tumor lines. The
IL-2 was used at a titer shown to be optimal by short term
proliferation assays. All tests were performed in parallel
in a 4-hour ^{51}Cr release assay and the data shown is for
an effector to target ratio of 50:1.

This activation does not appear to be interferon induced
(18).

There are several similarities of note between the three types of activation of PBL that result in lysis of fresh autologous tumor cells but normal cells. NK cells do not appear to be involved in the generation of these activated PBL, since the precursors are negative for OKM1 (14,16, Grimm – unpublished observations), which is present on NK cells (21). Also, lytic cells can be generated from thoracic duct lymphocytes, a population devoid of NK cells (14,16,18). Adherent cells are necessary for activation, but can be suppressive. The effector cells are radioresistent and nonadherent. They have the phenotype of CTL (OKT3+, OKT8+, OKM1-, OKT4-), but can be seen to appear in culture more rapidly than CTL. For example, cells lytic for tumor can be seen by day 3 of pool sensitization whereas 7-8 days are required for the appearance of CTL-induced allogeneic PBL lysis (Fig. 6).

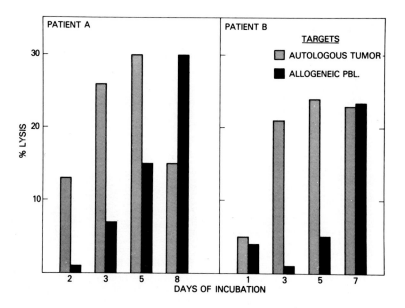

FIGURE 6. Kinetics of the development of lysis of fresh autologous tumor by pool-sensitized PBL (shaded bars) and of the lysis of allogeneic PBL by the patient PBL sensitized in vitro to the allogeneic PBL (solid a bars). Percentage lysis of each target shown was measured in parallel in a 4-hour ^{51}Cr release assay at effector to target ratios of 25:1. Two different patients are shown (16).

The effector cells also appear not to be NK cells based on their phenotype (OKT3+, OKM1-). In fact, they can lyse fresh tumor cells which are NK-insensitive targets (Fig. 7).

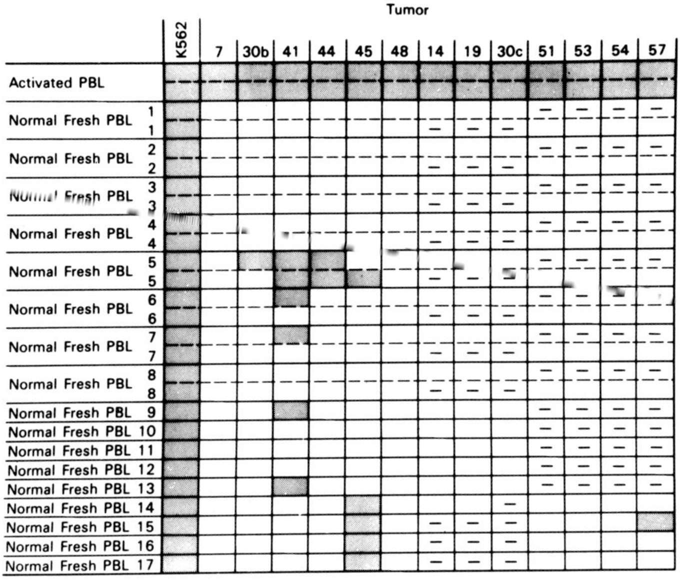

FIGURE 7. Fresh solid tumor cells are resistant to NK cells but sensitive to lymphokine activated cells. 13 fresh solid tumor samples were tested as targets for their susceptibility to lysis by NK-containing PBL of 17 normal individuals, at an effector to target ratio of 150:1. PBL from the first 8 individuals were tested in both experiments. Lysis was considered positive when the % specific lysis was statistically significant at the $p \leqslant 0.01$ level using the student's T test. Activated PBL are cancer patient PBL cultures in media containing IL-2 at the optimum titer for 5 days or allo-activated for 7 days. ■ = positive lysis, □ = negative lysis, ⊟ = not tested. (From Grimm et al. (18).

These activated cells can be expanded in IL-2 containing media without loss of cytotoxicity for fresh tumor.

There are, however, differences between our three activation systems. In PHA activation, the precursor is radioresistant, while the lymphokine and alloactivation precursors are radiosensitive. Also, an OKT3+ cell appears to be required only in the PHA and alloactivation systems. However, it's possible that the generation of killer cells by alloactivation or lectin incubation is mediated by the production of lymphokines by an OKT3+ cell and that this is the same final pathway to the generation of human lymphoid cells capable of lysing fresh autologous tumor in all three systems.

In vivo infusion of lectin activated cells

We instituted a phase I protocol in cancer patients who had failed all other therapies to determine the toxicity and effects in vivo of the infusion of PHA activated autologous PBL. We have studied 10 patients, 7 with sarcoma, 1 with melanoma and 2 with colorectal cancer. Up to 1.7×10^{11} PBL were obtained from 7-15 successive leukaphereses and incubated in vitro in medium containing PHA and human AB serum for 2 days and then reinfused following the next leukapheresis. Toxicity of the infusions included fever and chills in all, with headaches, nausea and vomiting and a transfusion requirement in only a few patients. Autoimmune workup was also negative.

In 9/9 patients tested, there was evidence for activated PBL in the circulation by the sixth leukapheresis (Fig. 8). The background incorporation of ^{3}HTdr into fresh PBL from the leukaphereses increased from 3-8 fold with successive elukaphereses and could be enhanced in vitro by the addition of lectin-free IL-2.

FIGURE 8

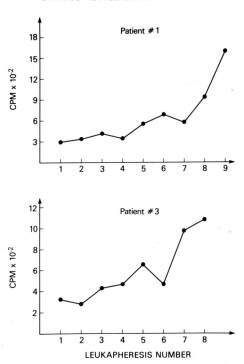

FIGURE 8. Proliferation in medium alone of fresh lymphocytes from successive leukaphereses. Points represent the means of duplicate measurements of ^{3}H incorporation in a 2 day assay (22). Two different patient results are shown.

Furthermore, the lysis of fresh tumor cells by such fresh PBL increased from a mean of 2% initially to a mean of 31% on successive collections in 7/8 tested (Fig. 9).

FIGURE 9

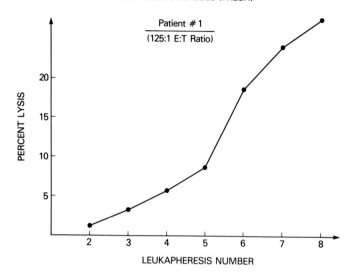

LYSIS OF FRESH AUTOLOGOUS TUMOR BY CELLS
FROM LEUKAPHERESES (FRESH)

FIGURE 9.   Lysis of fresh tumor cells (autologous in
this case) by fresh PBL from successive leukaphereses. Points
represent means of triplicate measurements of ^{51}Cr release
in a 4-hour assay.

In vivo distribution studies of these activated cells
showed that the PBL remained in the circulation for up to
two weeks, with large percentages trafficking to the spleen,
liver and lungs. Labelled PBL also appeared to migrate more
to the lungs and tumor (right thigh in Fig. 10) and less to
the liver in the last infusion than seen in the first infusion, implying some saturation of the clearance mechanism
of activated cells (Fig. 10).

FIGURE 10

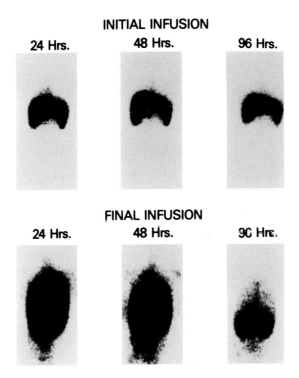

FIGURE 10. Whole body rectilinear scanning 24, 48 and 96 hours after the initial and final infusions of [111]Indium labelled PHA activated PBL. Tumor was in right thigh. Trafficking is greater to the lungs and tumor after the final infusion.

No reduction in tumor size was seen in any of the 10 patients entered thus far into our protocol. It should be emphasized that all of the patients treated had tumor burdens of several kilograms. Also, there is increasing evidence in the mouse (23) of the significance of cytoxan-sensitive suppressor cells in the host counteracting the effect of adoptively transferred cells. There is evidence also for activation of suppressor cells in vitro by PHA. In our future protocols, we are attempting to overcome these problems.

DISCUSSION

We have shown that activation by lectins, alloantigens or lymphokines of PBL, from cancer patients with a variety of malignancies, can lead to the generation of cells lytic for fresh autologous tumor but not for autologous lymphocytes or lymphoblasts. The determinant recognized is unknown, but does not appear to be on normal cells. In preliminary experiments, fresh liver cells (in addition to lymphocytes and lymphoblasts) are not lysed. Xenogeneic serum components or neoantigens arising in tissue culture are not involved in this tumor recognition and lysis since all of our experiments were performed solely in human AB or autologous serum with fresh, uncultured tumor cells as targets. While the tumor cells were usually obtained through mechanical or enzymatic treatments, these manipulations are not involved in the expression of the antigenic determinants since untreated tumor cells from ascites and effusions are lysed equally well (13,15,17). The lysis of a variety of tumors but not normal cells by the activated PBL may involve membrane components that differ from classical specific antigen recognition systems of CTL and are more akin to NK determinants (24).

A variety of other phenomena producing human cells lytic for tumor cells have been described including natural killing (NK) (25,26), mixed lymphocyte-tumor reactions, some with conventional CTL-type cytotoxicity (10,11,27,28,29), anomalous cytotoxicity (30), activated cell killing (20), activation by BCG, tuberculin or staphylococcus filtrates (31,32), N-cell activation (33), activation by xenogeneic serum (34) and activated macrophage killing (35). Most of these activations were tested using only tissue cultured tumor target cells often using xenogeneic serum.

We have shown that our activated cells appear to be distinct from NK cells and conventional CTL. Our systems also differ from the mixed lymphocyte-tumor or mixed lymphocyte cultures (MLTC, MLC) used as activations by Klein et al. (27). Our data shows that autologous and allogeneic tumors are lysed equally well, and in fact, by the same subset of effector cells. Furthermore, the ability of PBL from normal donors to lyse allogeneic tumors but not the corresponding PBL after our short activation cultures (13-18) suggests that these activated cells are not an anamnestic response against autologous tumor antigen awakened in cancer patient PBL by the activation.

Though there are numerous and varied methods for PBL activation cited in the literature, there are similarities in mechanism between them. IL-2 and other lymphokines are produced by the stimulated population in most and possibly all of the activation systems (e.g. MLC or lectin incubation). These lymphokines may include killer helper factors (such as those already found in certain human T cell hybridoma supernatants (36)), activating responses against poor immunogens. These factors could then activate killers of autologous tumor, thus requiring much shorter periods of activation than those required to generate conventional CTL responses. This rapid response with lymphokines would be similar to that seen after an MLC, where just a 5-hour pulse of antigen can be sufficient to render the responder cells reactive to IL-2 (37). The lymphokine may act through proliferation, with its effect thus being radiosensitive, as in our alloantigen and lymphokine activation systems (16,18). Alternatively, it may act as a direct, nonproliferative (i.e. radioresistant) activation signal, as in our lectin incubation system (14), thus accounting for the different radiosensitivity of the three systems.

The broad tumor lytic specificity of these activated PBL may involve nonconventional membrane interactions with protection by self recognition rather than lysis by allo-recognition. This would explain the vast diversity of 'altered self' targets lysed by a single subset of effectors.

Thus, all these activations may ultimately have the common mechanism of transformation to the membrane configuration of a killer cell, as shown for the effector cells generated by membrane oxidation (38). In fact, we have found in preliminary experiments that periodic oxidation can lead to the generation of cells lytic for autologous tumor.

In conclusion, it appears that activation of PBL by various stimuli can lead to the generation of cells lytic for fresh human tumor. These activated cells may play a biologically important role in natural antitumor immune surveillance. In our phase I protocol using these activated cells, we have found that large numbers of autologous PHA activated cells can be safely obtained and infused into humans, achieving an increase in the number of circulating activated cells with evidence of migration of cells to tumor, lungs, liver and spleen. The therapeutic value of these cells is being investigated.

REFERENCES

1. Lotze MT, Strausser JL, Rosenberg SA (1980). In vitro growth of cytotoxic human lymphocytes. II. Use of T cell growth factor (TCGF) to clone human T cells. J Immunol 124:2972.
2. Rosenberg SA, Schwarz S, Spiess PJ (1978). In vitro growth of murine T cells. II. Growth of in vitro sensitized cells cytotoxic for alloantigens. J Immunol 121:1951.
3. Gillis S, Smith KA (1977). Long term culture of tumor specific cytotoxic T cells. Nature 268:154.
4. Rosenstein M, Eberlein TJ, Kemeny MM, Sugarbaker PH, Rosenberg SA (1981). In vitro growth of murine T cells. VI. Accelerated skin graft rejection caused by adoptively transferred cells expanded in T cell growth factor. J Immunol 127:566.
5. Eberlein TJ, Rosenstein M, Spiess P, Wesley R, Rosenberg SA (1982). Adoptive chemoimmunotherapy of a syngeneic murine lymphoma using long term lymphoid cell lines expanded in T cell growth factor. Ca Immunol and Immunother, in press.

6. Eberlein TJ, Rosenstein M, Rosenberg, SA (1982). Regression of a disseminated syngeneic solid tumor by systemic transfer of lymphoid cells expanded in interleukin-2. J Exp Med, in press.

7. Kedar E, Raanan Z, Kafka I, Holland JF, Bekesi GF, Weiss DW (1979). In vitro induction of cytotoxic effector cells against human neoplasms. I. Sensitization conditions and effect of cryopreservation on the induction and expression of cytotoxic responses to allogeneic leukemia cells. J Immunol Meth 28:303.

8. Rosenberg SA and Terry WD (1977). Passive immunotherapy of cancer in animals and man. Adv Cancer Res 25:323.

9. Golub SH, Golightly MG, Zielske JV (1979). NK-like cytotoxicity of human lymphocytes cultured in media containing fetal bovine serum. Int J Cancer 24:273.

10. Martin-Chandon MR, Vanky F, Carnand C, Klein E (1975). In vitro 'education' on autologous human sarcoma generates nonspecific killer cells. Int J Cancer 15:342.

11. Treves AJ, Heidelberger E, Feldman M, Kaplan HA (1978). In vitro sensitization of human lymphocytes against histiocytolymphoma lines. II. Characterization of two different effector activities and of suppressor cells. J Immunol 121:86.

12. Sharma B, Terasaki PI (1974). In vitro immunization to cultured human tumor cells. Cancer Res 34:115.

13. Mazumder A, Grimm EA, Zhang HA, Rosenberg SA (1982). Lysis of fresh human solid tumors by autologous lymphocytes activated in vitro with lectins. Cancer Res 42:913.

14. Mazumder A, Grimm EA, Rosenberg SA. Characterization of the lysis of fresh human solid tumors by autologous lymphocytes activated in vitro with lectins. J Immunol, submitted for publication.

15. Strausser JL, Mazumder A, Grimm EA, Lotze MT, Rosenberg SA (1981). Lysis of fresh human solid tumors by autologous cells sensitized in vitro to alloantigens. J Immunol 127:266.

16. Mazumder A, Grimm EA, Rosenberg SA. The lysis of fresh human solid tumors by autologous lymphocytes activated in vitro by allosensitization. J Exp Med, submitted for publication.

17. Lotze MT, Grimm EA, Mazumder A, Strausser JL, Rosenberg SA (1981). Lysis of fresh and cultured autologous tumor by human lymphocytes cultured in T-cell growth factor. Cancer Res 41:4420.

18. Grimm EA, Mazumder A, Zhang HZ, Rosenberg SA (1982). The lymphokine activated killer cell phenomenon: Lysis of NK resistant fresh solid tumor cells by IL-2 activated autologous human peripheral blood lymphocytes. J Exp Med 155:1823.

19. Zarling JM, Robins HI, Raich PC, Bach FH, Bach ML (1978). Generation of cytotoxic T lymphocytes to human leukemia cells by sensitization to pooled allogeneic normal cells. Nature 274:269.

20. Masucci MG, Klein E, Argov S (1980). Disappearance of the NK effect after explantation of lymphocytes and generation of similar non-specific cytotoxicity correlated to the level of blastogenesis in activated cultures. J Immunol 124:2458.

21. Ortaldo JR, Sharrow SO, Timonen T, Herberman RB (1981). Determinations of surface antigens on highly purified human NK cells by flow cytometry with monoclonal antibodies. J Immunol 127:2401.

22. Mazumder A, Eberlein TJ, Wilson DJ, Grimm EA, Aamodt R, Keenan AW, Rosenberg SA. Phase I study of the adoptive immunotherapy of cancer with lectin activated autologous mononuclear cells. Cancer, submitted for publication.

23. Berendt MJ, North RJ (1980). T cell-mediated suppression of anti-tumor immunity: An explanation for progressive growth of an immunogenic tumor. J Exp Med 151:69.

24. Klein E, Vanky F (1981). Natural and activated cytotoxic lymphocytes which act on autologous and allogeneic tumor cells. Cancer Immunol Immunother 11:183.

25. Bolhuis RL, Shunt ARE, Nooy AM, Ronteltap CPM (1976). Characterization of natural killer (NK) and killer (K) cells in human blood: Discrimination between NK and K cell activities. Eur J Immunol 8:731.

26. Mukherji B, Flowers A, Rothman L, Nathanson L (1980). Spontaneous in vitro cytotoxicity against autochthonous human melanoma cells. J Immunol 124:412.

27. Vanky F, Gorsky T, Gorsky Y, Masucci MG, Klein E (1982). Lysis of tumor biopsy cells by autologous T lymphocytes activated in mixed cultures and propagated with T cell growth factor. J Exp Med 155:83.

28. Poros A, Klein E (1979). Culture with K562 leads to blastogenesis and increased cytotoxicity with changed properties of active cells when compared to fresh lymphocytes. Cell Immunol 41:240.

29. Golub SH (1977). In vitro sensitization of human lymphoid cells to antigens on cultured melanoma cells. II. Sensitization against melanoma associated antigens. Cell Immunol 28:379.
30. Seeley JK, Golub SH (1978). Studies on cytotoxicity generated in human mixed lymphocyte cultures. I. Time course and target spectrum of several distinct concomitant cytotoxic activities. J Immunol 124:2458.
31. Sharma B, Odom LF (1979). Generation of killer lymphocytes in vitro against human autologous leukemia cells with leukemic blasts and BCG extract. Cancer Immunol Immunother 7:99.
32. Stejskal V, Holm G, Perlmann P (1973). Differential cytotoxicity of activated lymphocytes on allogeneic and xenogenic target cells. I. Activation by tuberculin and staphylococcus filtrate. Cell Immunol 8:71.
33. Koide YS, Takasugi M (1978). Augmenation of human natural cell-mediated cytotoxicity by a soluble factor. I. Production of N-cell-activating factor (NAF). J Immunol 121: 872.
34. Zielske JV, Golub SH (1976). Fetal calf serum induced blastogenic and cytotoxic response of human lymphocytes. Cancer Res 36:3842.
35. Sone S, Fidler IJ (1980). In vitro activation of tumoricidal properties in alveolar macrophages by synthetic muramyl dipeptide encapsulated in liposomes. Cell Immunol 57:42.
36. Okada M, Yoshimura N, Kaieda T, Yamamura Y, Kishimoto T (1981). Establishment and characterization of human T hybrid cells secreting immunoregulatory molecules. Proc Natl Acad Sci 78:7717.
37. Larsson EL (1981). Mechanisms of T cell activation. II. Antigen and lectindependent acquisition of responsiveness to TCGF is a non-mitogenic, active response of resting T cells. J Immunol 126:1323.
38. Suthanthiram M, Rubin AL, Novogrodsky A, Stenzel KH (1981). Biological effects of activation of peripheral blood mononuclear cells by mitogenic oxidizing agents. Cell Immunol 59:26.

Rational Basis for Chemotherapy, pages 379–387
© 1983 Alan R. Liss, Inc., 150 Fifth Avenue, New York, NY 10011

THE EVALUATION OF RADIOLABELED MONOCLONAL ANTIBODY
PARAMETERS NECESSARY FOR CANCER IMMUNORADIOTHERAPY[1]

S.J. DeNardo,[2] H.H.Hines,
K.L. Erickson,[3] and G.L. DeNardo

Division of Nuclear Medicine
University of California, Davis Medical Center
Sacramento, California 95817

ABSTRACT Development of effective immunoradiotherapy
for cancer requires specific monoclonal antibody fragments to tumor membrane molecules, radionuclides with
appropriate energies and half lives, and an effective
selection and combination of these entities. The final
radiolabeled antibody fragment must be evaluated for
tumor extraction rate, tumor dose delivery, tumor uptake uniformity and whole body dosimetry.

Information derived from the study of specific monoclonal antibodies to P-51 murine melanoma in the C-57
black mouse has been used to address these questions,
to deliver in vivo radiation therapy to these tumored
mice, and to develop parameters for improving the tumor
to whole body radiation dosimetry. Preliminary computer
analysis has been performed demonstrating the effect of
varying the physical decay, renal clearance and tumor
extraction. At realistic tumor extraction rates, blood
clearance of the radiolabeled antibody fragment, renal
clearance of the total body radiation, and T½ of the radionuclide, become important in achieving the necessary
radiation dosimetry for effective human therapy.

[1]This work was supported by DOE #DE-AT03, ACS #PDT-45D
and CRCC.
[2]Division of Nuclear Medicine, UCD Medical Center
[3]Department of Anatomy, UCD School of Medicine

INTRODUCTION

Fifteen years ago, Spar et al. (1) demonstrated that radiolabeled antibodies could be made, which would concentrate at the site of tumors. Since that time, several investigators, working with polyclonal antibodies from a variety of animals, have demonstrated that a significant tumor uptake of radiolabeled antibodies could be achieved, even with non-homogeneous immunoglobulins. Goldenberg and Deland et al., working with the anti CEA system, have demonstrated surprising tumor uptake, in spite of the circulating antigen. (2) Order et al. (3)(4), using I-131 labeled antibodies against ferritin from several species, have described the delivery of tumorcidal doses of radiation to hepatoma.

However, before this approach can be applied to the treatment of human cancer in an effective and widespread manner, it is necessary to understand and solve certain fundamental problems. These deal with the optimization of target (tumor) radiation dose while delivering minimal radiation doses to the rest of the body. The selected production of monoclonal antibodies by the cell hybridization techniques demonstrated by Köhler and Milstein (5) makes possible the development of a much more specific carrier for the radioactivity. Judicious choice of tumor antigens for targets must be made and well characterized; avid antibody fragment carriers must be produced; radionuclides appropriate to the biokinetics must be selected; and radiochemical attachment of the nuclide and antibody carrier performed in a manner that will assure a stable, safe and dependable radiopharmaceutical.

METHODS AND RESULTS

Carrier Antibody.

The feasibility of radiation therapy with radiolabeled monoclonal antibody compared to polyclonal antibodies was assessed by a study with the P-51 mouse melanoma in cell culture and in tumor-bearing mice. Antibodies from rabbits immunized with radiated P-51 melanoma cells were compared in tissue culture to antibodies from hybrid clones developed from NS-1 myeloma and fused with spleen cells from C-57 black mice, which had been immunized with irradiated P-51 melanoma cells. P-51 melanoma cells grown as a monolayer in

MEM media were given varied numbers of antibody molecules from 4×10^{12} to 2×10^{14} of either I-131 rabbit absorbed specific immune globulin, I-131 absorbed non-immune globulin and I-131 specific monoclonal A-12.

There was no significant binding of the non-immune globulin. After 24 hours the media containing unattached radiolabeled antibodies was removed, the cells washed, and new media added. The monoclonal antibodies to the P-51 melanoma cells were bound greater than 10 times more frequently for the added immunoglobulin concentration than the absorbed rabbit anti-mouse melanoma specific immunoglobulin. (6)

In cell cultures binding an average of 5×10^4 I-131 antibody per cell of either rabbit immune or specific monoclonal (0.075μCi/10^6 cells), death significantly exceeded cell division by 3 days postradiation. Figure 1.

In vivo distribution studies performed with radioiodinated monoclonal antibodies to the P-51 melanoma tumor demonstrated that the radiolabeled monoclonal immunoglobulin (one I-131 per molecule) had a blood clearance and tissue distribution expected from a normal mouse immunoglobulin. (6)(7)(8) Tumor-bearing animals demonstrated two differences from the normal: the early uptake in the tumor, and a slow and delayed uptake in the spleen and liver. (7)(8)(9)

In order to enhance the blood clearance of radiolabeled antibodies, radiolabeled active fragments are being produced by carefully controled enzymatic digestion under the appropriate conditions for each monoclonal antibody. (9) These conditions vary significantly between immunoglobulin subclasses in the murine-produced monoclonal antibody.

Antigen Selection.

Antigen selection for radioimmunotherapy must not only deal with the uniqueness of the antigen, its frequency on the tumor cell, and how uniformly it is expressed, but also the time that the target antigen molecule resides in available form on the neoplastic cell membrane. This "residence time" provides the opportunity for the radiolabeled antibody in the antigen/antibody complex to deliver radiation to the tumor, rather than be released to radiate the rest of the body.

In cell culture studies of monoclonal antibodies to the P-51 tumor, an antigen was targeted which was expressed in excess of 5×10^4 times on the available half of each melanoma cell in the cultures. This suggests that it is expressed in

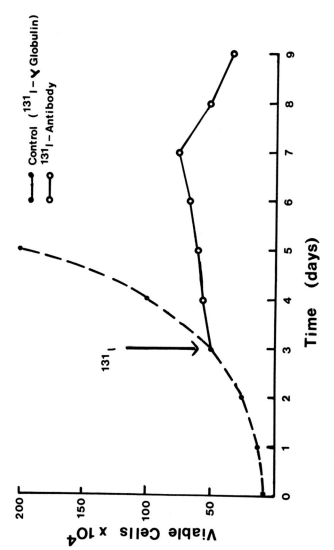

FIGURE 1. Normal growth curve for P-51 murine melanoma monolayer cell culture is demonstrated (---). Culture cells to which non-immune (control) I-131 immunoglobulin or non-radiolabeled monoclonal antibody was added and removed follows the same curve (·--·). Cell cultures binding 5 x 10⁴ I-131 antibodies (monoclonal or specific immune absorbed antisera) demonstrated the marked change in growth curve (○——○)

excess of 10^5 times on the entire cell.

Evaluation of tumor uptake and residence time <u>in vivo</u> of the radiolabeled monoclonal antibody developed in our laboratory against the P-51 tumor can be seen in Figure 2. The radiolabeled antibodies were present on the tumor several times longer than other tumor-seeking radiopharmaceuticals. The average peak tumor uptake percent injected dose per gram was 15% with a range of 30-7%.

As previously reported, 5 tumored mice were given intravenous doses of I-131 labeled monoclonal antibody calculated to deliver tumorcidal radiation (approximately 10,000 rads). The tumors in these animals regressed from 0.4cm to nonpalpable in 5 days and the animals had no recurrence. (7) (8)

Computer Analysis.

Preliminary computer evaluation of the interaction of variable parameters on tumor and whole body dosimetry was performed with a simple three-compartment system. This enabled us to explore the effect of varied levels of renal clearance, tumor uptake and radioactive decay.

The method of formulation of this type of computer model is described by Welch et al. (10) The concentration of radiopharmaceutical in the whole body is described by

$$C_2 = C_2^o \left[\frac{k_{32}-\lambda_2}{\lambda_3-\lambda_2} \, e^{-\lambda_2 t} - \frac{k_{32}-\lambda_3}{\lambda_3-\lambda_2} \, e^{-\lambda_3 t} \right]$$

The concentration in the tumor is described by

$$C_3 = C_2^o \left[\frac{k_{23}e^{-\lambda_2 t}}{\lambda_3 - \lambda_2} - \frac{k_{23}e^{\lambda_3 t}}{\lambda_3 - \lambda_2} \right]$$

If flow of antibody is allowed into and out of the tumor, the absorbed radiation dose to the tumor compared to the whole body is directly related to the cumulated concentration in each, and does not depend on the rate of radioactive decay. Thus, the radiation dose to the tumor can be maximized if the resident antibody antigen complex has maximum resident time on the tumor.

When antibody residence time was maximized in this

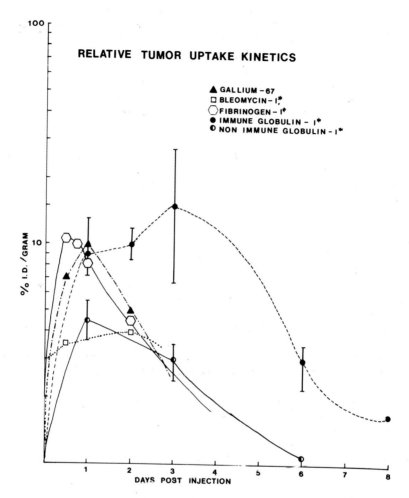

FIGURE 2.   P-51 mouse melanoma tumor uptake of I-131 monoclonal antibody compared to murine tumor kinetics of other radiopharmaceuticals.   Extended radiolabeled antibody residence time on the tumor allows for a significant increase in tumor radiation dose.

computer model by allowing no flow out of the tumor, a marked effect was demonstrated on whole body dose by decreased radionuclide physical half time and increased renal clearance. (Figure 3)

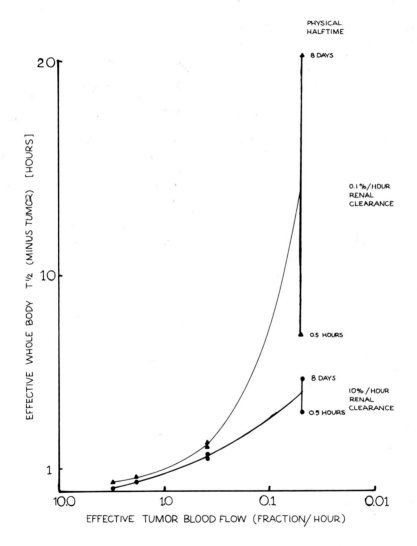

FIGURE 3.   At realistic tumor blood flow, the effect of variation in physical $T\frac{1}{2}$ and renal clearance on whole body dose is demonstrated.

DISCUSSION

Monoclonal antibodies can now be produced against well-characterized tumor-associated or tumor specific molecules which reside in an available form on the tumor membrane. To apply this system to delivering radiation therapy to human cancer requires the appropriate selection of antigen/antibody fragment, radionuclide, and dose schedule. The most effective antigen to use as a target on tumor cell membranes would be one which is not shed in an antigenic form from the tumor cell, and is available for antibody interaction for an extended period of days. The work described in this communication demonstrates that finding such antigens in biologic systems is feasible.

Monoclonal antibodies against the appropriate chosen antigens now allow specific and pure carriers of radioactivity to the chosen target. The technical problem relating to production of the necessary monoclonal antibodies, and the careful choice and production of active selected fragments of these antibodies, are being addressed and resolved. Since the distribution kinetics and renal excretion of the radiolabeled antibody fragment or its metabolic products dictates the degree of total body radiation dose for any particular radionuclide label, it is extremely useful to use computer modeling techniques to balance and compare the effects of varying fragment size and radionuclide. Furthermore, tumor uptake and therefore tumor dose is related to a balance between the time significant concentration of the radiolabeled antibody fragment is in the circulation, and its ability to move from the intravascular space to the extravascular compartment bathing the tumor.

The feasibility studies in the murine P-51 melanoma model described here, suggest that cancer cells can be given most effective radiation therapy by the use of radionuclides with half-times of 1-4 days and energy deposition of a few cell diameters. These nuclides are and can be made available, and the radiochemistry for attaching them to the appropriate antibody fragments is within present-day techniques.

This approach to cancer therapy holds great promise and its feasibility has been demonstrated in animals. Effective clinical use of radiation therapy with radiolabeled antibody fragments in many types of cancer awaits the careful work of optimizing methods already in our grasp.

REFERENCES

1. Spar IL, Bale WF, Marrack D, Dewey WC, McCardle RJ,
    Harper PV (1967). I-131-labeled antibodies to human
    fibrinogen: diagnostic studies and therapeutic trials.
    Cancer 20:865.
2. Goldenberg DM, Deland F, Kim E, Bennett S, Primus FJ,
    Nagel JR van, Estes N, DeSimone P, Rayburn P (1978).
    Use of radiolabeled antibodies to carcinoembryonic
    antigen for the detection and localization of diverse
    cancers by external photoscanning. New Engl J Med
    298:1384-1388.
3. Order SE, Klein JL, Leichner PK (1981). Antiferritin
    IgG antibody for isotopic cancer therapy. Oncology
    38:154-160.
4. Order SE, Klein JL, Ettinger D, Alderson P, Siegelman
    S, Leichner P (1980). Phase I-II study of radiolabeled
    antibody integrated in the treatment of primary hepatic
    malignancies. Int J Radiation Oncology Biol Phys 6:
    703-710.
5. Kohler G, Milstein C (1976). Continuous cultures of
    fused cells secreting antibody-producing tissue culture
    and tumor lines by cell fusion. European J of Immunology
    6:511.
6. DeNardo SJ, Erickson KL, Benjamini E, Hines H, Scibienski
    R (1981). I-131 monoclonal antibodies for radioimmuno-
    therapy to melanoma. Journal of Nuclear Medicine. In
    Press.
7. DeNardo SJ, Erickson K, Benjamini E, Hines H, Scibienski
    R, DeNardo G (1982). Monoclonal antibodies for radiation
    therapy of melanoma. Proceedings of the Third World Con-
    gress World Federation of Nuclear Medicine and Biology.
8. DeNardo SJ, Erickson KL, Benjamini E, Hines H, Scibienski
    R (1981). Radioimmunotherapy for melanoma. Clinical
    Research 29(2).
9. Peng J-S, DeNardo SJ, DeNardo GL (1982). Development of
    pure, homogeneous monoclonal antibody fragments as a
    resource for radiopharmaceuticals. Journal of Nuclear
    Medicine 23(5).
10. Welch, Potchen, Welch (1972). "Fundamentals of the
    Tracer Method." Philadelphia: Saunders, p 178-183.

Rational Basis for Chemotherapy, pages 389–405
© 1983 Alan R. Liss, Inc., 150 Fifth Avenue, New York, NY 10011

DEVELOPMENT OF IMPROVED HYPOXIC CELL RADIATION SENSITIZERS

G.E. Adams and I.J. Stratford

Radiobiology Unit, Institute of Cancer Research,
Sutton, Surrey, England

ABSTRACT The neurotoxicological problems encountered
in the use of misonidazole in radiotherapy indicate
that it is most unlikely that this drug can be used
clinically at doses sufficient to achieve maximum
radiosensitization of hypoxic cells.   Methods aimed at
improving therapeutic ratio include protection against
neurotoxicity, exploitation of the thiol-suppressing
activity of misonidazole and other radiation sensitizers,
and the synthesis and development of more effective compounds.   This paper discusses approaches in the development of new drugs and emphasizes some of the physical,
chemical and biological properties that are important in
determining drug activity.

INTRODUCTION

The possibility that hypoxic cells, probably present in
most solid tumors, may limit the successful local control of
some of these tumors by radiotherapy, has long been recognized by radiation oncologists.   Hypoxic cells develop as a
consequence of tumor growth essentially outstripping its own
vascular system and hence the supply of essential nutrients,
particularly oxygen.   Tumor cells near to a microcapillary
are fairly well oxygenated and are the source of tumor growth.
However, the oxygen tension falls off with distance from the
capillary and gradually falls to a level insufficient to sustain cell division.   Eventually the cells deficient in
oxygen will die and this causes the necrosis often seen
developing about 150-200 μm from the nearest blood vessel.

It is believed that viable hypoxic cells occur in the inter-face regions between the well-oxygenated tissue and the necrotic regions.

In general, hypoxic cells are radiation-resistant relative to oxic cells and it is now well established, in experimental murine tumor systems, that their radiation resistance is the largest factor influencing local tumor control by radiation. In an untreated tumor, hypoxic cells will eventually die, but in the event of tumor regression, i.e. during or after radiation treatment, some of these hypoxic cells may be reoxygenated, enter cycle and cause tumor regrowth.

Several methods aimed at overcoming hypoxic cell radiation resistance have been explored clinically. These include the use of unconventional fractionation regimes aimed at optimising reoxygenation, radiotherapy in hyper-baric oxygen chambers, high LET radiotherapy and, most recently, chemical radiation sensitizers. Many types of chemical compounds, including particularly the nitro-imidazoles, act as hypoxic cell sensitizers in experimental systems. One of these, misonidazole, has been shown to be highly effective in many laboratory tumor systems and in recent years has been undergoing clinical trial. However, it is now clear from the numerous clinical studies, that the dose-limitations imposed by the neurotoxic properties of this drug will seriously limit its use in clinical radiotherapy. This is because the acceptable dose levels that can be used with fractionated radiation fall well below those theoreti-cally required to achieve maximum sensitization. There are a number of approaches that can be employed to improve on the therapeutic ratio achievable with misonidazole. These are discussed in the next section.

INCREASE IN THERAPEUTIC RATIO

Therapeutic ratio can be increased either by protecting against the neurotoxic properties of misonidazole itself, the development of new sensitizers with lower neurotoxic potential or by the development of compounds with higher sensitizing efficiencies.

Protection against Neurotoxicity.

The incidence of peripheral neuropathy in patients
receiving misonidazole is lower if the patients also receive
phenytoin (1,2). It has been proposed that this is due to
the enzyme-inducing properties of this drug, since the half-
life of misonidazole is reduced in man (3) and in dogs (4)
if phenytoin is also administered. Clinical brain tumor
studies have also provided evidence that neuropathies have
a much lower incidence in patients receiving the anti-
inflammatory agent dexamethasone (1). Here, the mechanism
does not involve changes in the pharmacokinetics of misonidazole.

Development of Less Neurotoxic Sensitizers.

The synthesis and development of new sensitizers has
been guided by structure-activity studies on both the neurotoxic potentials and the sensitizing efficiencies of new
sensitizers. There is evidence, from rodent models, that
the lipophilicities of sensitizing compounds may play a role
in their toxic properties in vivo (5-7). The development
of new sensitizers partly reflects this lead. Table 1
shows some of the second generation sensitizers structurally
related to misonidazole.

TABLE 1
SOME SECOND GENERATION RADIATION SENSITIZERS

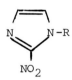

Name	Substituent R
Misonidazole	$CH_2CH(OH)CH_2OCH_3$
Desmethylmisonidazole	$CH_2CH(OH)CH_2(OH)$
SR 2508	$CH_2CONHCH_2CH_2OH$
Ro 03-8799	$CH_2CH(OH)CH_2N$ ⬠
RSU 1047	$CH_2CH(OH)CH_2CH_2N$ ⬡O

Desmethylmisonidazole is the major metabolite of misonidazole in both rodents and humans. Its sensitizing
efficiency is comparable to misonidazole both in vitro and
in vivo. It has a lower octanol-water partition
coefficient and it less toxic in experimental animal systems.
Accordingly, Phase 1 clinical studies with desmethylmisonidazole have been carried out (8,9). However, despite its
substantially lower half-life in man compared with misonidazole, the incidence of peripheral neuropathy is not much
different from that with misonidazole at comparable doses.
Significantly, though, no central neurotoxicities have so
far been reported.

The drug SR 2508, developed at the Stanford Research
Institute, is also being considered. This compound has an
octanol-water partition coefficient lower than both misonidazole and desmethylmisonidazole, it shows less uptake into
brain than the previous drugs (5) and it is substantially
less neurotoxic than misonidazole (6). Since its sensitizing efficiency is comparable to that of misonidazole, there
are good grounds for expecting an improved therapeutic ratio
in man. Clinical studies with this drug are expected to
commence shortly.

The 1-alkanolamine derivatives, Ro 03-8799 and RSU 1047,
arose out of studies of the effect of chain length and the
effect of a basic group in that side-chain (10,11). The
presence of an ionizable group means that the lipophilicities
of the compounds are highly pH-dependent. This is likely
to confer selective tissue uptake and as a result modify
both sensitizing and cytotoxic properties. Both Ro 03-8799
and RSU 1047 are at least as efficient sensitizers as misonidazole and both appear less neurotoxic than misonidazole
in mice (Clarke, Sheldon, Dawson, unpublished observations).
Studies in primates have also shown Ro 03-8799 to be substantially less toxic than misonidazole (C.E. Smithen,
private communication) and clinical studies with this compound have commenced.

Mechanistic Considerations in Sensitizer Development.

The electron affinity relationship. Many compounds
now exist that sensitize hypoxic cells to radiation in vitro.
Virtually all of these show no activity against oxic cells
and this differential activity remains the sole rationale
for developing suitable compounds that will sensitize tumor
response to radiation without increasing the radiation

morbidity of normal tissues.   Several factors contribute to
the sensitizing properties of such compounds but by far the
most important are their electron affinic properties.   The
proposal that the sensitizing efficiencies of compounds of
diverse chemical structure relate directly to their redox
properties has now been substantiated by many studies involving both mammalian and bacterial cells (e.g. 12).   Specifically, sensitization efficiency, defined as the concentration
required for a given dose enhancement ratio in vitro,
correlates with the thermodynamic one-electron reduction
potential (E_7^1).   The mechanism involves enhancement of
radiation-induced damage in cellular DNA and application of
cellular fast-mixing processes are involved.   Space
limitations, however, preclude further discussion of these
aspects of the mechanism other than to comment that, for
sensitization to operate by this mechanism it is only
necessary for the drug to be present at the instant of
irradiation.

Thiol suppression.   There is evidence that slow non-
radical processes can also contribute to overall radiation
sensitization.   Depending on the conditions, this additional
sensitization can appear as a reduction, or removal of the
shoulder on the survival curve (13), or increase in the slope
(14) of the survival curve, or both.   Figure 1 summarises
some published data on this aspect of sensitization (15,16).

Hypoxic cells incubated in the presence of misonidazole
for 5 hours and subsequently irradiated in N_2 after removal
of the drug show the shoulder suppression phenomenon first
described by Wong et al. (13).   If the irradiation is
delayed several hours after removal of the sensitizer, the
shoulder suppression is lost.   Also shown in Figure 1 is
the increased sensitization seen when the cells are
irradiated in the presence of misonidazole after prolonged
incubation with this drug (i.e. compare the curves after 1
hour and 3 hours incubation).   It has been suggested that
these additional sensitization effects of prolonged incubation
are due to reduction of intracellular thiol levels (14).
Some aspects of the influence of thiol depletion on overall
radiation sensitization is discussed later in this paper.

Clinical implications.   The existence of the "slow"
non-radical component of sensitization may be of value in
clinical studies with radiation sensitizers of this type.
In radiotherapy studies, misonidazole is usually administered
3-4 hours before radiotherapy in order to allow adequate
access of the drug to hypoxic cells in poorly-vascularized

PRE-INCUBATION OF HYPOXIC CELLS IN 2mM MISONIDAZOLE IN N₂

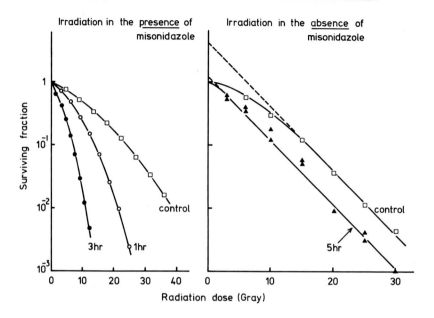

FIGURE 1. Radiosensitization of hypoxic Chinese
Hamster cells pre-incubated with 2 mM misonidazole in N₂ at
37°C for various periods of time prior to irradiation (15,16).

regions of the tumor.   At clinical dose levels of the drug
this period is too short to permit any additional sensitization brought about by reduction of intracellular thiol levels.
It is worthwhile to consider the value of clinical protocols
in which misonidazole (or other sensitizers) is administered
much earlier, say 10-12 hours before radiotherapy.   This
would allow sufficient time to reduce thiol levels in
hypoxic cells.   Because of the 12-hour half-life of misonidazole, this would mean that the concentration in hypoxic
cells at the time of irradiation would be lower and this
would reduce the enhancement due to the "fast" free-radical
component of sensitization.   However, this could be more
than compensated by administering three-quarters of the drug
dose 12 hours before and the remainder about 3 hours before
radiotherapy.   The maximum cellular concentration would not

be very much lower and the much greater period of exposure
should lower thiol levels in the hypoxic cells.   Overall,
therefore, there should be a greater <u>net</u> amount of radiation
sensitization.   This is shown schematically in Figure 2.
This approach could be considered in exploring clinical uses
of electron-affinic sensitizers generally.

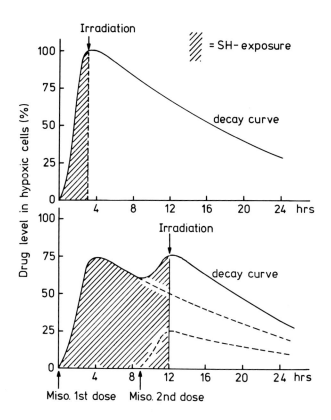

FIGURE 2.   Split-dose misonidazole.   Hypothetical
scheme for increasing sensitization efficiency.
Top: Normal scheme of administration of misonidazole
           3-4 hours before radiotherapy.

Bottom: Additional hypoxic cell exposure (indicated by
           shaded area) when 75% of the dose is given 12
           hours and 25% 3 hours before radiotherapy.

Influence of Thiol Binding Agents on Sensitization by Nitroimidazoles.

It is well known that various thiol reagents can sensitize both hypoxic bacterial and mammalian cells to radiation damage. While it is clear that fast free radical processes are responsible for a substantial component of radio-sensitization by the electron affinic agents, the demonstration of the slow pre-incubation effect has led to various studies on the sensitizing effect of combinations of sensitizers with known thiol-depleting agents.
     The compound, diethylmaleate (DEM), is an efficient thiol-suppression agent and it has recently been shown that the sensitizing efficiency of misonidazole in vitro is greatly increased when the cells are pre-treated with DEM (17).   Figure 3A shows some of our data using this combination.

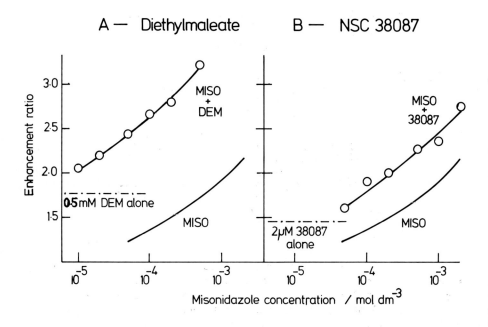

FIGURE 3. Enhancement of sensitization efficiency of misonidazole in irradiated hypoxic Chinese Hamster cells by A) 0.5mM DEM, B) 2μM NSC 38087.

The solid line in the figure shows the dependence of enhancement ratio on misonidazole concentration for hypoxic V79 cells irradiated <u>in vitro</u>.   DEM alone gives an ER of about 1.75 and together with misonidazole gives enhancement ratios which ultimately exceed the maximum value of the oxygen enhancement ratio in this system.   The parellel behaviour of the two curves is as expected on the basis of the two sensitizers acting by independent mechanisms.

Figure 3B shows data (taken from ref. 18) for combination of misonidazole with the compound NSC 38087.   This is a 4-nitroimidazole, 5-substituted with an electrophilic group.   It is able to deplete cellular thiols very efficiently under both hypoxic and aerobic conditions (19) and when used in the combination experiment increases the sensitizing efficiency of misonidazole in a <u>similar</u> manner to that shown by DEM.

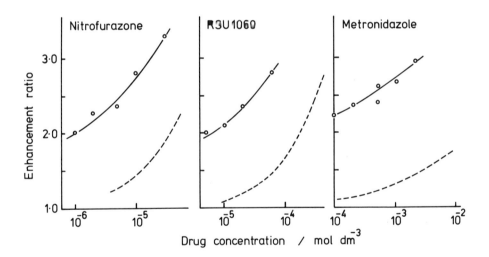

FIGURE 4.   Enhancement of sensitizing efficiency of three electron affinic compounds in irradiated Chinese Hamster cells by 0.5 mM DEM.   Cells were incubated with DEM for 2 hours at 37°C prior to addition of second drug, deaeration and irradiation.

DEM also enhances the sensitizing efficiency of other electron-affinic agents and this is illustrated in Figure 4. Data in the figure are for radiosensitization by the compounds metronidazole, nitrofurazone and RSU 1069, a 2-nitroimidazole with an alkylating function in the side chain. Nitrofurazone sensitizes over a concentration range about two orders of magnitude lower than that necessary for sensitization by metronidazole, which is in keeping with the large difference in electron affinity between the two compounds. RSU 1069 shows abnormal sensitizing efficiency and this is related to the presence of the alkylating group. Reasons for this are discussed later. For all three compounds there is a similar enhancement of sensitizing efficiency in the presence of DEM. Few such combination experiments have yet been done in vivo. However, if they are shown to be successful, the combination approach may be of value clinically, particularly if the agents chosen do not have additive toxicities.

Abnormally High Sensitizing Efficiency of Some Nitroimidazoles.

The existence of a class of electron-affinic sensitizers with efficiencies much higher than would be predicted from their redox properties has been referred to earlier. This group includes a range of 4-nitroimidazoles substituted in the 5-position with various electrophilic groups (10,18,20). It is known that some of these compounds react fairly rapidly with thiols in aqueous solution (19,21,22) and also suppress non-protein-bound SH levels intracellularly (19,22). It is not yet known, however, to what extent their abnormally high sensitizing efficiencies are due to enhanced thiol suppression. There is support, however, for this hypothesis derived from studies of isomeric pairs of 4(5)nitro-5(4)-substituted imidazoles (22,23). These studies show that the $4NO_2$ isomers are the more efficient sensitizers, react more rapidly with thiols in aqueous solution, but have lower one-electron reduction potentials.

Table 2 shows some of our recent data for 4- and 5-nitroimidazoles substituted in the 2, 4 or 5 position with an electrophilic leaving group.

For each compound the table lists the one-electron reduction potential (E_7^1), the sensitizing efficiency in irradiated cultures of hypoxic Chinese Hamster cells ($C_{1.6}$) and the bimolecular rate constant (k) for reaction of the compound with dithiothreitol, determined in aqueous solution

TABLE 2

SENSITIZING EFFICIENCY AND THIOL REACTIVITY
OF SOME 1-METHYLNITROIMIDAZOLES CONTAINING
A SECOND ELECTROPHILIC GROUP

Compound	Substituents*	E_7^1/mV	$C_{1.6}$/mol dm^{-3}	$\underline{k}$/dm^{3}mol^{-1}s^{-1}
RSU 3057	4-NO$_2$, 5-R	-302	1 - 2 x 10^{-6}	84
RSU 3047	5-NO$_2$, 2-R	-351	2.0 x 10^{-6}	32
RSU 3053	5-NO$_2$, 4-R	-324	2.0 x 10^{-5}	2.2
RSU 3069	4-NO$_2$, 5-R	-523	5.0 x 10^{-5}	0.31
RSU 3071	5-NO$_2$, 4-R	-460	1.3 x 10^{-4}	0.021
RSU 3089	5-NO$_2$, 2-R	-467	5.0 x 10^{-4}	0.0032

*Ring positions of substituents

at 37°C and pH 7.5. For this limited group of compounds
the values of $C_{1.6}$ are substantially higher than would be
predicted from the E_7^1 values. Further, there is a clear
trend of increasing sensitizing efficiency with increasing
thiol reactivity.

While compounds of this type are highly efficient
sensitizers in vitro, most show little, or no, activity in
vivo. This is most probably due to their metabolic instability which can be attributed to the susceptibility of
the imidazole ring to nucleophilic attack by RS⁻. However,
it has recently been shown (24) that the drug Azathioprine
(Imuran), a member of this class of compound, has considerable activity as a radiosensitizer both in vitro and in vivo.
Figure 5a reproduces some data showing the concentration-
dependence for sensitization of hypoxic Chinese Hamster cells
irradiated in vitro.

Sensitization efficiency in vitro is comparable to that
of misonidazole (dotted line in Figure 5a). Sensitization
by Imuran also occurs in vivo: data for sensitization of
the radiation response of the tumor MT in WH mice is shown
in Figure 5b (24). Tumor response was measured by clonogenic assay of tumor cells 18 hours after irradiation. A
dose of 0.43 mmoles/kg of Imuran given at various times
before 18 Gy of X-rays reduces the surviving fraction with
the greatest effect occurring when the drug was given 60

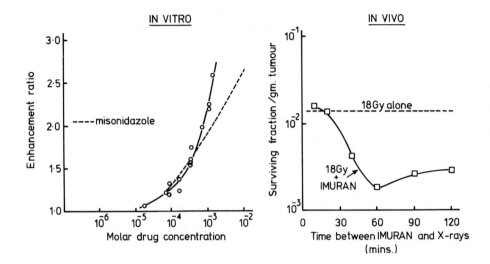

FIGURE 5.   Sensitization by Azathioprine (Imuran)
in vitro: Dependence of enhancement ratio on Imuran
concentration for hypoxic mammlian cells.
in vivo: Effect of time between administration of 0.43
mmoles/kg Imuran and irradiation on the response of the MT
tumor.

minutes before irradiation.   Under these conditions, the
enhancement ratio is 1.4.
     Imuran itself has no practical value as a clinical
radiosensitizer because one of its metabolic products is
6-mercaptopurine which is highly toxic.   However, the
development of suitably non-toxic analogues which display
fairly high thiol reactivity but are sufficiently metabolically stable to allow sensitization in vivo may prove a worthwhile route to follow.

Sensitizers with Activity as Alkylating Agents.

     Interest in this class of compound stems from the find-
ing that 2,4-dinitro-5-aziridinylbenzamide (CB 1954), a
monofunction alkylating agent, also functions as a hypoxic

cell radiosensitizer <u>in vitro</u> (25). Although the electron
affinity of this compound is similar to that of misonidazole,
its sensitizing efficiency <u>in vitro</u> is considerably greater
(26). The agent phenyl-AIC (2-phenyl-4-(5)-amino-5(4)-
carboxamide) which protects against the cytotoxic action of
CB 1954 (26,27) also reduces its sensitizing efficiency to
that found for misonidazole (26). This suggested therefore
that the additional sensitization normally found with CB 1954
is associated with the cytotoxic (presumably alkylating)
activity of this compound.

Studies are in progress with other sensitizers containing alkylating functions. These include analogues of
CB 1954, nitroimidazoles (28) and quinone derivatives.

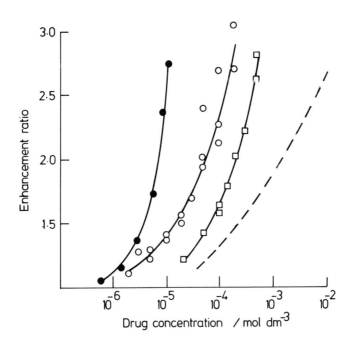

FIGURE 6. Sensitization of hypoxic Chinese Hamster
cells by electron affinic agents containing alkylating
groups. Dependence of enhancement ratio on drug concentrations.
Dashed line : misonidazole   ——□—— : RSU 1062
   ——○——   : CB 10-021   ——●—— : NSC 17262

Figure 6 shows some sensitization efficiency data for three representative compounds expressed as the concentration dependence of the enhancement ratios for sensitization of hypoxic mammalian cells in vitro. Compound RSU 1062 is a 2-nitroimidazole analogue of misonidazole with the N1 sidechain -CH$_2$CH-CH$_2$. Although its electron affinity is compar-

$$\underset{O}{\diagdown\diagup}$$

able to that of misonidazole, its sensitizing efficiency is greater. The compound CB 10-021, a dinitrobenzenoid analogue of CB 1954, is even more efficient, although again, its electron affinity is the same as that of misonidazole. The third compound, NSC 17262, a quinonoid derivative is over two orders of magnitude more efficient than misonidazole although in this case, its greater electron affinity must be a contributory factor.

Another compound in this series which is of considerable interest is an aziridinyl 2-nitroimidazole, RSU 1069. This compound, while also more efficient than misonidazole as a sensitizer in vitro, is remarkably efficient in vivo also. Studies in vivo show that this compound gives enhanced ratios similar to those with misonidazole at drug doses about a factor of ten less (Sheldon, unpublished). Toxicology studies with this, and related compounds, are in progress but are not yet sufficiently advanced to give any information relevant to possible therapeutic advantage over misonidazole. However, the considerably enhanced activity of sensitizers of this type offer real prospects for development of new clinical radiosensitizers.

ACKNOWLEDGMENTS

Our thanks to Drs. Clarke, Dawson, Hardy, Hoe and Sheldon for provision of unpublished information.
This work was supported by Grants from the NCI (Contract no. NO1-CM-17485) and an MRC Program Grant.

REFERENCES

1. Wasserman TH, Phillips TL, Van Raalte GV, Urtasun RC, Partington J, Kozio A, Schwade JG, Ganji D, Strong JM (1980). The neurotoxicity of misonidazole: Potential modifying role of phenytoin sodium and dexamethasone. Brit J Radiol 53:172.

2. Bleehen NM (1980). The Cambridge glioma trial of misonidazole and radiation therapy with associated pharmacokinetic studies. In Brady LW (ed): "Radiation Sensitizers" Cancer Management Vol. 5, New York: Masson, p 374.

3. Workman P, Bleehen NM, Wiltshire CR (1980). Phenytoin shortens the half-life of the hypoxic cell radiosensitizer misonidazole in man: Implications for possible reduced toxicity. Brit J Cancer 41:302.

4. White RAS, Workman P (1980). Phenytoin sodium-induced alterations in the pharmacokinetics of misonidazole in the dog. Cancer Treat Rep 64:360.

5. Brown JM, Lee WW (1980). Pharmacokinetic considerations in radiosensitizer development. In Brady LW (ed): "Radiation Sensitizers" Cancer Management Vol. 5, New York: Masson, p 2.

6. Conroy PJ, Shaw AB, McNeill TH, Passacacqua W, Sutherland RM (1980). Radiation sensitizer neurotoxicity in the mouse. In Brady LW (ed): "Radiation Sensitizers" Cancer Management Vol. 5, New York: Masson, p 397.

7. Clarke C, Dawson KB, Sheldon PW, Ahmed I (1982). Neurotoxicity of radiation sensitizers in the mouse. Int J Radiat Oncol Biol Phys 8:787.

8. Dische S, Saunders MI, Stratford MRL (1981). Neurotoxicity with desmethylmisonidazole. Brit J Radiol 54:156.

9. Coleman CN, Wasserman TH, Phillips TL, Strong JM, Urtasun RC, Schwade JG, Johnson RJ, Zagars G (1982). Initial pharmacology and toxicology of intravenous desmethylmisonidazole. Int J Radiat Oncol Biol Phys 8:371.

10. Adams GE, Ahmed I, Fielden EM, O'Neill P, Stratford IJ (1980). The development of some nitroimidazoles as hypoxic cell sensitizers. In Brady LW (ed): "Radiation Sensitizers" Cancer Management Vol. 5, New York: Masson, p 33.

11. Smithen CE, Clarke ED, Dale JA, Jacobs RS, Wardman P, Watts ME, Woodcock M (1980). Novel (nitro-1-imidazolyl)-alkanolamines as potential radiosensitizers with improved therapeutic properties. In Brady LW (ed): "Radiation Sensitizers" Cancer Management Vol. 5, New York: Masson, p 22.

12. Adams GE, Flockhart IR, Smithen CE, Stratford IJ, Wardman P, Watts ME (1976). Electron-affinic sensitization. VII. A correlation between structures, one-electron reduction potentials and efficiencies of nitroimidazoles. Radiat Res 67:9.

13. Wong TW, Whitmore GF, Gulyas S (1978). Studies on the toxicity and sensitizing ability of misonidazole under conditions of prolonged incubation. Radiat Res 75:541.

14. Hall EJ, Biaglow J (1977). Ro 07-0582 as a radiosensitizer and cytotoxic agent. Int J Radiat Oncol Biol Phys 2:521.

15. Stratford IJ, Adams GE, Horsman MR, Kandaiya S, Rajaratnam S, Smith E, Williamson C (1980). The interaction of misonidazole with radiation, chemotherapeutic agents or heat: a preliminary report. In Brady LW (ed): "Radiation Sensitizers" Cancer Management Vol. 5, New York: Masson, p 276.

16. Chapman JD, Ngan-Lee J, Stobbe CC, Meeker BE (1982). Radiation-induced and metabolism-induced reactions of hypoxic sensitizers with cellular molecules. In Breccia A, Rimondi C, Adams GE (eds): "Advanced Topics on Radiosensitizers of Hypoxic Cells", Nato Advanced Study Series Vol. A43, New York and London: Plenum, p 91.

17. Bump EA, Yu NY, Brown JM (1982). The use of drugs which deplete intracellular glutathione in hypoxic cell radiosensitization. Int J Radiat Oncol Biol Phys 8:439.

18. Adams GE, Fielden EM, Hardy C, Millar BC, Stratford IJ, Williamson C (1981). Radiosensitization of hypoxic mammalian cells in vitro by some 5-substituted-4-nitroimidazoles. Int J Radiat Biol 40:153.

19. Biaglow JE, Varnes ME, Astor M, Hall EJ (1982). Nonprotein thiols and cellular response to drugs and radiation. Int J Radiat Oncol Biol Phys 8:719.

20. Watts ME, Jacobs RS (1978). Some examples of anomalous radiosensitizing behaviour of electron-affinic compounds in vitro. Brit J Cancer 37 (Suppl III):80.

21. Wardman P (1982) The kinetics of the reaction of 'anomalous' 4-nitroimidazole radiosensitizers with thiols. Int J Radiat Biol 41:231.

22. Astor M, Hall EJ, Martin J, Flynn M, Biaglow J, Parham JC (1982). Radiosensitizing and cytotoxic properties of orthosubstituted 4- and 5-nitroimidazoles: Role of NPSH reactivity. Int J Radiat Oncol Biol Phys 8:409.

23. Stratford IJ, Hoe S, Adams GE, Hardy C, Williamson C (1982). Abnormal radiosensitizing and cytotoxic properties of ortho-substituted nitroimidazoles. Int J Radiat Biol (submitted).

24. Adams GE, Sheldon PW, Stratford IJ (1982). Evaluation of novel radiation sensitizers in vitro and in vivo. Int J Radiat Oncol Biol Phys 8:419.

25. Chapman JD, Raleigh JA, Pedersen JE, Ngan J, Shum FY, Meeker BE, Urtasun RC (1979). Potentially three distinct roles for hypoxic cell sensitizers in the clinic. In Okada S, Imamura M, Terasima T, Yamaguchi H. (eds): "Proc 6th Int Cong Radiat Res", Tokyo 1979. Tokyo: JARR, p 885.

26. Stratford IJ, Williamson C, Hoe S, Adams GE (1981) Radiosensitizing and cytotoxicity studies with CB 1954 (2,4-dinitro-5-aziridinylbenzamide). Radiat Res 88:502.

27. Hickman JA, Melzack DH (1976). Studies on the protection by imidazoles against the cytotoxicity of the antitumour alkylating agents melphalan and CB1954. Biochem Pharmacol 25:2489.

28. Stratford IJ (1982). Mechanisms of hypoxic cell radiosensitization and the development of new sensitizers. Int J Radiat Oncol Biol Phys 8:391.

Rational Basis for Chemotherapy, pages 407–422
© 1983 Alan R. Liss, Inc., 150 Fifth Avenue, New York, NY 10011

RADIOSENSITIZERS, CHEMOSENSITIZERS, AND
THEIR ACTION IN VIVO[1]

John F. Fowler, Nicolas J. McNally, Margaret Hinchliffe,
Juliana Denekamp, Varinder S. Randhawa and Fiona A. Stewart

Gray Laboratory of the Cancer Research Campaign,
Mount Vernon Hospital, Northwood, Middlesex HA6 2RN,
England

INTRODUCTION

Hypoxic cells are present in most tumours and are relatively resistant to X-rays. They therefore represent a
problem in the treatment of cancer by radiation, as described by Adams in this volume.

Drugs which radiosensitize hypoxic cells in tumours are
biologically active because they are strongly electron
affinic, as is oxygen, and therefore modify electron transfer
processes in the cell. Radiosensitizers are metabolized
within cells, the products being cytotoxic. This metabolism
is a slow biochemical process, requiring minutes or hours,
in constrast to the fast physico-chemical radiosensitizing
action which is complete within milliseconds. Table 1 lists
these other processes.

The process most relevant to the present symposium is
the potentiation of chemotherapeutic drugs. We shall
discuss this process in detail after describing other
actions briefly.

We wish to emphasize that the radiosensitization of
hypoxic cells depends only upon those hypoxic cells in a
tumour which are viable and which may therefore regrow the
tumour after radiotherapy. Chemosensitization, on the other

[1]This work was supported by the Cancer Research
Campaign, London SW1 5AR.

hand, depends upon any cells in the tumour that are hypoxic, even if they are doomed to die, because they can metabolize the sensitizer into its chemosensitizing state. Nitro reductase enzymes metabolize nitroimidazoles faster in hypoxic conditions than in the presence of oxygen.

TABLE 1

WHAT HYPOXIC-CELL SENSITIZERS CAN DO

1. RADIOSENSITIZATION OF HYPOXIC CELLS *

2. ENHANCEMENT OF CHEMOTHERAPY

3. Direct cytotoxicity

4. Reduce repair of sublethal X-ray injury

5. Reduce repair of PLD after X-rays or chemo

6. Change of respiration rate

7. Metabolic fix'n of cpd by hypoxia

* (1) Depends on concentration of sensitizer
       in cell at time of irradiation.

  (2)-(7) Depend on time of exposure in
       hypoxia, more than on concentration.

HYPOXIC CELLS IN TUMOURS

Over fifty different types of experimental animal tumour have been shown to contain hypoxic cells, with only two exceptions, both being very slowly growing carcinomas in which the blood supply was presumably able to keep pace with the growing bulk of tumour (1). Tumour masses as small as 2 mm in diameter contain significant numbers of hypoxic cells. The histological evidence from human tumours is that they have similar necrotic regions to those in mouse tumours, at more than about 150 μm from vascular capillaries. The physiological dimensions are similar in murine and in human tumours. The proportion of hypoxic cells varies from 1% to over 50% in different types of animal tumour. Calculations of the proportions in human subcutaneous nodules, secondary to Ca cervix, were possible from a significant clinical sensitization by misonidazole (2). The resulting hypoxic proportion was between 5 and 40%.

The most important relevant question in radiotherapy is whether the hypoxic cells in the tumour become reoxygenated fully during the several weeks of conventional treatment. If they do, the potentially large advantage of hypoxic cell sensitizers is reduced. Tumours which behave in this way should not be treated with hypoxic-cell sensitizers or high-LET radiation. The property of electron-affinic compounds of being fixed in cells by the hypoxic metabolism (No 7 in Table 1) may provide an important method of measurement of hypoxic cells in tumours, as described below.

RADIOSENSITIZATION

The radiosensitization of hypoxic cells has been dealt with thoroughly in several reviews (3, 4, 5 and Adams, this volume). We wish only to illustrate that it is a large effect <u>in vivo</u> in tumours in mice, when tested with a large single dose of X-rays (Fig. 1).

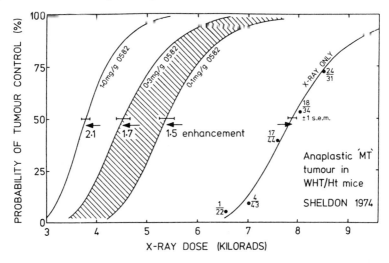

FIGURE 1.   Local tumour control as a function of X-ray dose (6). Right hand curve for X-rays alone. Left hand curve for X-rays given 30 min after 1000 mg/kg misonidazole given i.p., showing a large degree of radiosensitization, SER = 2*. The shaded indicates SER values obtained in multiple fractions as used clinically.

* See footnote on next page.

This large amount of radiosensitization is for single
doses of X-rays. However, less sensitization can be
achieved with multiple fractions, because lower drug doses
must be given with each fraction in order to keep within the
total toxic limit for misonidazole, $(12 \ g/m^2$ in 3 to 6
weeks due to peripheral neurotoxicity). Fig. 2 shows the
maximum radiosensitization achievable with misonidazole, for
various numbers of fractions. The actual values in practice
will be lower because not all the cells in tumours are
hypoxic.

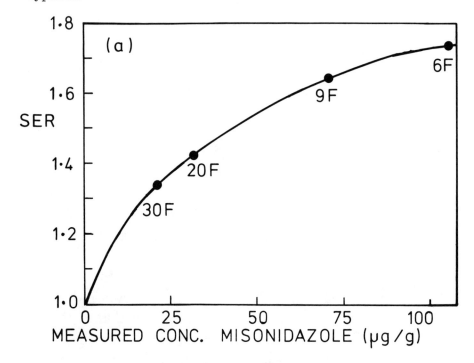

FIGURE 2.   SER* measured in vitro as a function of miso-
             nidazole concentration. The points are marked
             at the concentrations measured in the blood
             of patients being treated with the numbers of
             fractions indicated. It is assumed that the
             concentration in the tumours is equal that in
             blood (7).

* SER, Sensitizer Enhancement Ratio = X-ray dose without
  sensitizer divided by X-ray dose with sensitizer
  required to produce the same effect.

Even though smaller values of SER are obtained for 20 and 30 than for 6 and 9 fractions, these are likely to represent better radiotherapy to start with, so the final result will be better than a large SER applied to only six big dose fractions, which is a poor radiotherapy schedule (8). It is now known that six big fractions of X-rays kill fewer cells in the tumour than 30 small fractions, for the same amount of damage to normal tissues.

Better radiosensitizers than misonidazole have been synthesized and are being evaluated in pre-clinical tests (Table 2). Some of them may be more effective than misonidazole because the ratio of concentration which causes chronic aerobic cytotoxicity to concentration that yields an SER of 1.6 is greater, i.e. the compounds are relatively less toxic.

TABLE 2

NEW RADIOSENSITIZERS OF HYPOXIC CELLS

COMPOUND	CONC. REQ'D FOR		RATIO OF
	SER = 1.6 (μM)	CHRON. AEROBIC CYTOTOX.	LAST TWO In vitro index
Misonidazole	1,000	1,300	1.3
Ro 05-9963	1,000	1,300	1.3
Ro 07-1051	240	750	3.1
Ro 12-5272	200	480	2.4
Ro 31-0054	140	750	5.4
Ro 03-8799	100	500	5.0
Ro 31-0052	80	710	8.9
Ro 31-1030	350	3,000	8.6
SR 2508	- low lipophilicity		---
RSU 1047	- similar to 8799		---
RSU 1069	- double acting cpd		---

However, the effectiveness of such compounds in tumours appears to depend as much on whether or not hypoxic cells are reoxygenated as on the efficacy of the radiosensitization (8).

DIRECT CYTOTOXICITY

The nitroimidazoles are toxic to hypoxic cells which are exposed to them for several hours, and to oxic cells exposed for several days. This cytotoxic effect would add significant cell killing in tumours if the same hypoxic cells were present in tumours for many hours (9). However, if hypoxia is a cyclic phenomenon, due to intermittent closing and re-opening of capillary vessels, the effect is of course reduced (10). Nevertheless, some cytotoxic effect was seen even in mice, with a relatively short plasma half life of misonidazole (1h compared with 10h in human patients). This means that the cytotoxic effect cannot be neglected, although it is not as large as radiosensitization.

REDUCED REPAIR OF SUBLETHAL X-RAY INJURY AND OF POTENTIALLY LETHAL DAMAGE AFTER X-RAYS

The reduction in "shoulder repair" by misonidazole first reported by Wong et al (11) does indeed help in killing hypoxic cells but requires long exposure of hypoxic cells to the drug. Adams has proposed "two-shot" injections of radiosensitizer, aimed at keeping the plasma concentration reasonably high in patients for about two days, during which time three or four dose fractions of radiotherapy could be given, instead of the five small doses per week that are conventional. It is interesting that the clinical trial with misonidazole that is showing a positive effect (head and neck cancer, Bataini, 1982, pers. comm.) does operate in this mode.

CHANGES OF RESPIRATION RATE

Biaglow and Durand (12) have shown that respiration rate can be increased by some nitroimidazoles and decreased by others (Fig 3).

Misonidazole causes little change in respiration, but if a drug were selected which slows down the respiration rate of cells, more oxygen would then become available to radiosensitize the previously hypoxic cells. Durand and

Olive (13) have calculated that more radiosensitization of
hypoxic cells might be achieved in this way than by striving
to get better and better radiosensitizers if toxic side-
effects run parallel with increased sensitizing efficiency.
This approach remains to be exploited;   again its value
depends on how many hypoxic cells are not eliminated by
reoxygenation during conventional treatment.

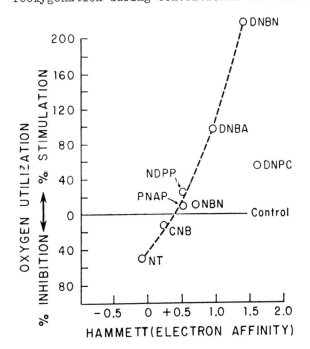

FIGURE 3.
Change of oxygen
utilization rate
as a function of
electron affinity
(12).

METABOLIC FIXATION OF NITROIMIDAZOLES

       In their preferential action on hypoxic cells, nitro-
imidazoles are themselves altered by reduction processes.
This can lead to fixation in the hypoxic cells. Chapman et
al (14) have demonstrated that radioactively labelled misonidazole is concentrated in the regions of tumours most
likely to be hypoxic (10-30 times greater uptake).   He has
proposed this as a method of attempting to measure which
tumours have large hypoxic volumes (14).

       A different approach is to use the fluorescence of some
nitroimidazoles, after their reduction, to indicate which
cells in a population were hypoxic Although much progress

remains to be made before this fluorescence method can be applied to human tumours, encouraging differentials between the fluorescence in hypoxic and oxic cells in spheroids have been reported by Durand and Olive at Baltimore (pers. comm., 1981) using the compound AF2 and by Hodgkiss, Begg and McNally in our laboratory with cells in culture using a nitroacridine (pers. comm). The method requires the presence of the nitroimidazole dye in the hypoxic cells for at least an hour at 37°C, so that the effect is not quickly reversible during processing.

When a method becomes available for measuring the extent of hypoxia in human tumours before and during therapy it will then be possible to allocate those tumours which contain most hypoxic cells, and do not reoxygenate, to methods of treatment such as radiosensitizers or high LET radiotherapy. This would be a very important selection to be able to make.

ENHANCEMENT OF CHEMOTHERAPY BY HYPOXIC CELL RADIOSENSITIZERS

Fig 4 illustrates the misonidazole-induced enhancement

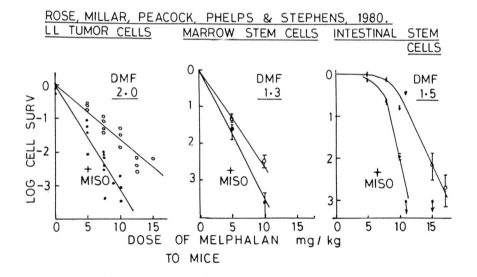

of chemotherapeutic drugs in tumours by a factor of 2 (left-
hand panel) and the enhancement of normal tissue injury by
smaller factors (Rose et al., (15)). The enhancement
requires hypoxic metabolism via the action of nitro
reductases. The mechanism of action has been discussed by
Brown (16) and by Adams in the present volume. Several
other laboratories are investigating the phenomenon. One
of the present authors reviewed the number of experiments in
which both an animal tumour and a normal tissue had been
investigated to determine whether the enhancement of damage
to the tumour was greater than the enhancement of normal-
tissue damage, with the results shown in Table 3 (17).

TABLE 3

MISO ENHANCEMENT OF CHEMOTHERAPY

MISO DOSE 500-1000 mg/kg TO MOUSE
GIVEN 0 - 1 hr BEFORE CHEMO DRUG

DRUG	No. OF TUMOURS WITH		
	ER ≥ 1.5	TGF ≥ 1.1	
CYCLOPHOS	9/14	7/10	(TGF = ER
MELPHALAN	8/9	7/8	of tumour ÷
CCNU	6/8	7/8	ER of normal
ADM	1/5	1/5	tissue)

It is clear that a therapeutic advantage is a rather
general, but not a universal, finding for the bifunctional
alkylating agents and nitrosoureas. Under circumstances like
this, more experimental effort is required to investigate
effects on normal tissues, especially late damage. Little
enhancement has been seen for adriamycin or bleomycin.

Examples of our own results which illustrate the phenomenon of chemosensitization in vivo are shown in Fig 5 which
summarises a large number of experiments (18).

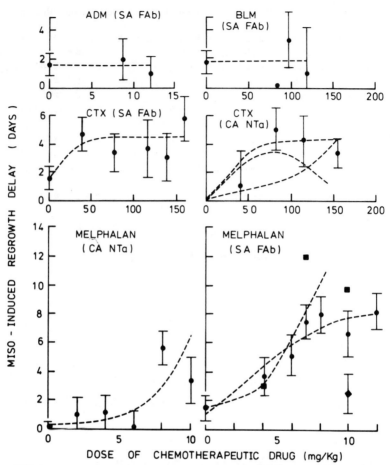

FIGURE 5. Regrowth delay as a function of drug dose of melphalan, cyclophosphamide, bleomycin or adriamycin concentration. The drug was given i.p. simultaneously with 1000 mg/kg of misonidazole for the sarcoma SAFAb tumour in WHT mice and with 800 mg/kg of misonidazole for the carcinoma CANTa in CBA/Gy mice. A large enhancement is demonstrated for melphalan and cyclophosphamide in both types of tumour.

The results are typical of others which show large enhancement ratios, in the range 1.8 - 5.3, for the bifunctional alkylating agents or the nitrosoureas, but little effect for adriamycin or bleomycin. (See the proceedings of the meeting at Key Biscayne in Sept 1981 for further details (e.g. 16, 17, 18)).

Recent experiments have been carried out to simulate the pharmacology in human patients. The half life of misonidazole is ten times longer than in mice, and lower concentrations must be used, as explained above in the paragraph on radiosensitization. Two of us have given repeated low doses of misonidazole, at 20 minute intervals for 8 hours, to see whether a large enhancement is still achieved (Hinchliffe and McNally, pers. comm.). The plasma level of misonidazole was maintained at about 100 µg/ml. The tumours were excised 24 hours after the last injection.

The results are interesting and important and will be published in full elsewhere. Briefly, for cyclophosphamide, the single-dose enhancement due to misonidazole was 1.8 and the "infused dose" value was 2.1. For melphalan the values were 2.7 and 1.8 respectively. It is clear that substantial enhancement ratios are still achieved at low plasma concentrations which can be used clinically.

It was further demonstrated that the half-life of the alkylating agents was not altered by the repeated small injections of misonidazole. The induction of a longer half-life could therefore not be a mechanism of this enhancement, as has been suggested by some authors.

An interesting illustration of the misonidazole induced enhancement of drug damage in a partial simulation of a realistic clinical schedule is shown in Fig 6. Weekly doses of cyclophosphamide were given to 30 mice bearing the WHFIB tumour. Ten of these mice were also injected repeatedly with misonidazole over a 3 hour period before the cyclophosphamide was given, so as to maintain about 100 µg/ml in the plasma. Ten other mice were given 500 mg/kg single dose of misonidazole 1 hour before the CY.

The weekly doses of cyclophosphamide alone could only cure 1 out of 10 mice. With a single large dose of misonidazole each time, the proportion of mice cured rose to 7/10, which is a significant difference (17). With the repeated injections of misonidazole maintained for 3 hours each time, the result was also 7/10 (McNally, de Ronde and Hinchliffe, pers. comm.).

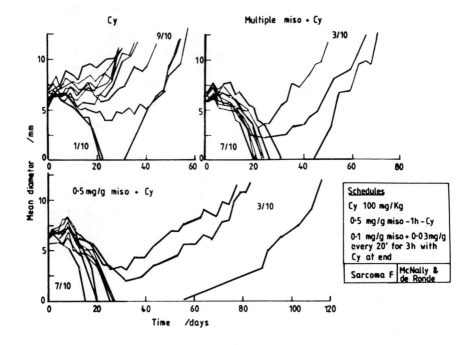

FIGURE 6.   Diameter of individual mouse tumours given
weekly doses of 100 mg/kg of cyclophosphamide i.p.
(a) cyclophosphamide (CY) alone, 1/10 cures.
(b) CY + 500 mg/kg misonidazole, 7/10 cures.
(c) CY + 3 hours 100 µg/ml plasma miso, 7/10
cures.

It is encouraging that these results are as good for the
simulated human pharmacology as for the single-large-dose
mouse experiments. This was not the case for the radiosensitization phenomenon, which depends upon the instantaneous concentration of sensitizer during the actual irradiation.

THE TOXICITY OF NORMAL TISSUES

As shown in Fig 4 and Table 3 above, the enhancement of
toxicity in normal tissues is usually, but not always, less
than in tumours. This would indeed be expected if the enhancement depends upon the presence of hypoxic cells, or
strictly upon the presence of nitroreductase enzymes, which
act faster in hypoxic conditions.

However, the magnitude of the enhancement in normal tissues requires further investigation, especially for late damage. Lethal toxicity is a poor endpoint for two reasons. First, it is an ambiguous endpoint, the cause of death in mice not necessarily being relevant to the tissue damage that is limiting in the clinical situation. Secondly, it requires very large doses which add pharmacological perturbations that are not relevant to the clinical use of lower drug doses. Nevertheless, lethal toxicity is usually the quickest endpoint to obtain and each laboratory has to obtain such data before further experiments can be safely carried out with its animals.

Our LD_{50} data for misonidazole plus melphalan agree with those of Siemann et al (19) in finding ER's of 1.3 - 1.4, i.e. less miso enhancement than was seen in 3 out of 4 of our tumour experiments (18).

It was shown by Millar et al (20) that the bone marrow toxicity from single doses of melphalan could be reduced by a small priming dose of the same drug given 48 hours before the main dose. The mechanism underlying this effect is not known, but it can lead to a therapeutic advantage (20). We have carried out tumour experiments to see whether a priming dose of 5 mg/kg of melphalan gave any protection against the combined dose of misonidazole plus melpalan, or against melphalan alone. There was no tumour protection.

For melphalan alone, the priming dose did protect normal tissue. It was possible to give double the dose of melphalan and thus to obtain longer tumour growth delay.

For melphalan plus miso, the priming dose of melphalan also enabled a somewhat higher dose to be given, although only about 20% higher. There was however no additional regrowth delay, perhaps because a very large effect was already being obtained with the melphalan plus misonidazole.

CONCLUSIONS

The enhancement of chemotherapy by hypoxic-cell radiosensitizers is of current interest. It may provide a larger gain factor than in the case of the radiosensitizers in radiotherapy for two reasons.

Firstly, the radiosensitization of hypoxic cells is only useful insofar as <u>surviving</u> hypoxic cells are present during conventional radiotherapy. Successful reoxygenation - which must be present in some tumours or radiotherapy would not be as successful as it is now - detracts from the advantage of radiosensitization. While reoxygenation must also detract from chemosensitization, chemosensitization does not depend only on the <u>surviving</u> hypoxic cells. Any hypoxic cells, or strictly <u>any active nitroreductase enzymes</u>, whether in cells or simply present in hypoxic or necrotic volumes, contribute to the metabolic processes which enhance chemotherapy.

Secondly, the presence of low concentrations of the sensitizer for many hours is easier to obtain in clinical practice than a high concentration for a short time. This is the mode required for these relatively slow metabolic processes, which take several hours at 37°C to produce significant enhancement at practical concentrations.

Important questions for the future include:

(a)   How much better enhancements than those obtained with misonidazole will other sensitizers give?

(b)   What are the limiting tissues for toxicity of the combinations in man? Especially for late injury.

(c)   Can altering the temperature by hyperthermia contribute more enhancement in tumours than in normal tissues?

REFERENCES

1.   Denekamp J, Hirst DG, Stewart FA and Terry NHA (1980). Is tumour radiosensitization by misonidazole a general phenomenon? Br J Cancer 41:1. See Table III p7. See also ref (5) Table 8, p 440.
2.   Denekamp J, Fowler JF and Dische S (1978). The proportion of hypoxic cells in a human tumour. Int J Rad Oncol Biol Phys 2:1227.
3.   Adams GE (1977). Hypoxic cell sensitizrtd for radiotherapy. In F F Becker (ed) "Cancer: A Comprehensive Treatise". New York: Plenum Press, p 181.
4.   Denekamp J and Fowler JF (1978). Radiosensitization of solid tumours by nitroimidazoles. Int J Rad Oncol Biol Phys 4:143.

5. Fowler JF and Denekamp J (1979). A review of hypoxic cell radiosensitizers. J Pharmac Ther 7:413.

6. Sheldon PW and Hill SA (1977). Hypoxic cell radiosensitizers and tumour control by X-ray of a transplanted tumour in mice. Br J Cancer 35:795.

7. Denekamp J, McNally NJ, Fowler JF and Joiner MC (1980). Misonidazole in fractionated radiotherapy: are many small fractions best? Br J Radiol 53:981.

8. Fowler JF (1979). Possibilities and limitations in the use of hypoxic sensitizers and hyperbaric oxygen for the improvement of fractionated radiotherapy of cancer. In Moore M (ed): "Advances in Medical Oncology, Research and Education", Vol 6, Basis for Cancer Therapy 2, p 191. Oxford: Pergamon Press.

9. Stratford IJ and Adams GE (1978). The toxicity of the radiosensitizer misonidazole towards hypoxic cells in vitro: a model for mouse and man. Br J Radiol 51: 745.

10. Denekamp J (1978). Cytotoxicity and radiosensitization in mouse and man. Br J Radiol 51:636.

11. Wong TW, Whitmore GF and Gulyos S (1978). Studies on the toxicity and radiosensitizing ability of misonidazole under conditions of prolonged incubation. Rad Res 75:541.

12. Biaglow J and Durand RE (1976). The effects of nitrobenzene derivatives on oxygen utilization and radiation response of an in vitro tumor model. Radiat Res 65:529.

13. Durand RE and Olive PL (1981). Evaluation of nitroheterocyclic radiosensitizers using spheroids. Advances in Rad Biol 9:75.

14. Chapman JD, Franko AJ and Koch CJ (1982). The fraction of hypoxic clonogenic cells in tumor populations. In Fletcher GH, Nervi C, Withers HR, Arcangeli G, Mauro F and Tapley N (eds): "Biological Bases and Clinical Implications of Tumor Radioresistance", New York: Masson Publ Co.

15. Rose CM, Millar JL, Peacock JH, Phelps T and Stephens TA (1980). Differential enhancement of melphalan toxicity in tumour and normal tissue by misonidazole. In Brady LW (ed): "Radiation Sensitizers", New York: Masson Publ Co. p 250.

16. Brown JM (1982). Mechanisms of cytotoxicity and chemosensitization. Int J Rad Oncol Biol Phys. Keynote lecture at CROS Conference, Key Biscayne, Florida, Sept 17-20, 1981 (in press).

17. McNally NJ (1982). The enhancement of chemotherapy
     agents. Int J Rad Oncol Biol Phys. Keynote lecture at
     CROS Conference, Key Biscayne, Florida, Sept 17-20, 1981
     (in press).
18. Randhawa VS, Stewart FA, and Denekamp J (1982). Chemo-
     sensitization of mouse tumours by misonidazole. Int J
     Rad Oncol Biol Phys. Poster pressentation at CROS Con-
     ference, Key Biscayne, Florida, Sept 17-20, 1981 (in
     press).
19. Siemann D (1981). The in vivo combination of the nitro-
     imidazole misonidazole and the chemotherapeutic agent
     CCNU. Brit J Cancer 43:367.
20. Millar JL, Clutterbuck RD and Smith IE (1980). Improving
     the therapeutic index of two alkylating agents. Br J
     Cancer 42:485.

Rational Basis for Chemotherapy, pages 423–426
© **1983 Alan R. Liss, Inc., 150 Fifth Avenue, New York, NY 10011**

THE BIOCHEMICAL BASIS FOR SELECTIVE FREE RADICAL INJURY

Charles E. Myers, M.E., Clinical Pharmacology Branch,

Clinical Oncology Program, Division of Cancer Treatment,
National Cancer Institute
Bethesda, Maryland

Free radical formation has been envoked as a
mechanism of drug induced injury for a wide range of
chemicals including the anti cancer drugs adriamycin
and bleomycin (1). Generally, the damage which results
is attributed to either the reactivity of the drug
radical or the subsequent production of the superoxide
radical. The latter has been commonly cited, especially
when injury is effected by oxygen concentration. There
are, however, reasons to be skeptical about the toxic
consequences of superoxide generation. First, it is
a normal bi-product of intermediary metabolism and
there exist enzymatic pathways which efficiently convert
superoxide to water and molecular oxygen (2). Second,
superoxide itself is fairly unreactive in aqueous
solution (3). As a result, there is no clear evidence
that superoxide can directly cause injury to living
organisms. Superoxide can react with itself to yield
hydrogen peroxide and with hydrogen peroxide to yield
the hydroxyl radical. The latter is extremely reactive
and, to the extend that tissue injury occurs after
superoxide generation, it is most likely via the
intermediacy of the hydroxyl radical. Hydroxyl radical
production does, however, require the simultaneous
presence of hydrogen peroxide, superoxide and a transition
metal ion catalyst, usually iron (4).

Under ordinary circumstances, metabolically generated superoxide does not yield significant hydroxyl radical generation because the enzyme superoxide dismutase causes rapid conversion of superoxide to hydrogen peroxide and the latter is also rapidly eliminated via the concerted action of catalase and glutathione peroxidase. Finally, transition metal ions such as copper and iron, which might be capable of catalyzing the formation of hydroxyl radical, are by and large bound rather than free and thus rendered unavailable. The net result is that the ambient concentrations of superoxide, hydrogen peroxide and metal catalyst are held to sufficiently low levels so as to minimize hydroxyl radical formation.

In view of the above considerations, it is important to consider how drugs might circumvent these defenses so as to cause oxygen radical injury. First, the magnitude of oxygen radical production may be so great as to simply overwhelm these defenses. Second, a drug might act to liberate transition metal ions so as to catalyze the above reaction. Third, a drug could inactivate one or more of the detoxification enzymes outlined above. It turns out that there are now examples of each of these. I will focus on examples of the second and third processes.

TRANSITION METAL CATALYSIS

The best documented example of this phenomenon is the action of bleomycin. Horwitz and others (5) have shown that bleomycin chelates iron. The resulting chelate catalyzes a complex redox reaction between thiols and oxygen which leads to cleavage of DNA. This reaction appears to require that the bleomycin bind to both iron and to the macromolecular target, in this case DNA. Recently Halliwell and coworkers (6) have shown that bleomycin can successfully trap iron from biologic fluids and others have shown that the cytotoxicity of a bleomycin analog is lessened by EDTA, presumable through competition for iron. A second example of this pattern may be adriamycin. May and coworkers (6) have recently demonstrated that adriamycin is an avid chelator of ferric ion with step association constants of 10^{18},

10^{11} and $10^{4.4}$ for the binding of the first, second and
third adriamycin to iron. We have subsequently shown
that the resulting complex will bind to DNA and cell
membranes (7). In the latter case, the membrane bound
complex catalyzes a reaction between the thiol glutathione
and oxygen with resultant destruction of the cell
membrane. The parallels between adriamycin and bleomycin
in this regard are interesting. In both cases
(1) the electron donor is an endogenous thiol whose
normal role is protection against oxidative damage and
(2) the iron complex binds to a macromolecular target
which is then destroyed. This binding to the target
may gain importance because reactive radicals such as
the hydroxyl radical have short half lives and, therefore,
diffusion distances.

ABROGATION OF ENDOGENOUS DEFENSES

There are a number of examples of this phenomenon.
One of the most interesting in terms of specificity of
injury occurs with adriamycin. We and others (8,9)
have shown that cardiac tissue lacks catalase and thus
is dependent upon glutathione peroxidase for disposal
of hydrogen peroxide. Adriamycin, however, rapidly
decreases cardiac glutathione peroxidase levels at the
same time as it induces oxygen radical production (8).
The result is that cardiac tissue, after adriamycin
exposure, is presented with hydrogen peroxide at a time
when it possesses inadequate mechanisms to detoxify the
hydrogen peroxide. This process has been documented in
both the acute and chronic adriamycin cardiac toxicity
models (8,10).

Two other examples of abrogation of existing
defenses are well documented. BCNU at low concentrations
effectively inactivates glutathione reductase, the
enzyme needed to keep glutathione in a reduced state.
The result is that cells pretreated with BCNU became
very sensitive to oxidative stress (11). Acetaminophen
offers yet offers yet another example. This compound
is metabolically activated in the liver into a reactive
electrophilic compound which depletes hepatic glutathione.
The result is that the liver suddenly becomes much more
susceptible to oxidative damage by drugs such as
adriamycin (12).

SUMMARY

The conclusion to be reached from the above discussion is that many normal tissues are well defended against oxygen radical injury and that special circumstances must prevail for tissue specific injury to occur. First, the biochemical machinery must be present to initiate drug mediated radical reactions. Second, injury is more likely if the tissue in question lacks one of the defenses per premium or such a defect can be created by another agent. These principles may well have therapeutic as well as toxicologic implications.

REFERENCES

1. Mason, R.P: In Reviews in Biochemical Toxicology. Hodgsin, R., Bend, C. Philpot, E. (Eds.) Elsevier-North Holland, Inc., 1979, pp. 151-200.
2. Chance, B., Sies, H. and Boveris, A.: Physiological Reviews 59: 527-589, 1979.
3. Valentine, J.S., and Sawyer, D.T.: Acc. Chem. Res. 14: 393-400, 1981.
4. Halliwell, B.: FEBS Lett. 92: 321-326, 1978.
5. Sausville, E.A. and Horwitz, S.B.: In Effects of Drugs on the Cell Nucleus. Crooke, S. (Ed), Academic Press, N.Y. 1979.
6. Gutteridge, J.M.C., Rowley, D.A. and Halliwell, B.: Biochem. J. 199: 263265, 1981.
7. Myers, C.E., Gianni, L., Simone, C.B., Klecker, R. and Greene, R.: Biochemistry 21: 1707-1713, 1982.
8a. Dorowshow, J.H., Locker, G.Y and Myers, C.E.: J. Clin. Invest. 65: 128-135, 1980.
8b. Doroshow, J.H., Locker, G.Y., Ifrim, I. and Myers, C.E.: J. Clin. Invest. 68: 1053-1054, 1981.
8c. Katki, A.G., and Myers, C.E.: Biochem Biophys Res. Comm. 96:85-91, 1980.
9. Thayer, W.S.: Chem. Biol. Interact. 19: 265-278, 1977.
10. Revis, N.W. and Marusic, N.: J. Mol. Cell Cardiol. 10: 945-950, 1978.
11. Babson, J.R., Abell, N.S. and Reed, D.J.: Biochem. Pharm. 30: 2299-2304, 1981.
12. Wells, P.G., Boerth, R.C., Tates, J.A. and Harbison, R.D.: Tox. and App. Pharm. 54: 197-209, 1980.

Rational Basis for Chemotherapy, pages 427–436
© 1983 Alan R. Liss, Inc., 150 Fifth Avenue, New York, NY 10011

HYPERTHERMIA TO ENHANCE DRUG DELIVERY

George M. Hahn, Ph.D.

Department of Radiology, Stanford University
Stanford, California   94305

INTRODUCTION

Chemotherapy of cancer, in order to be successful,
requires at least some degree of specificity. Such specificity can be of two types. The classical approach is to
attempt to find drugs that attack preferentially some or
all malignant cells, while sparing normal tissue, either
for biochemical or immunological reasons. Alternatively
one can look for agents whose cytotoxicity is enhanced in
the specific microenvironment that exists in many tumors,
particularly in large solid masses. While the first of
these approaches, "the magic bullet", is clearly the ultimate goal, in its absence the latter approach does offer
considerable hope for improving the current treatment techniques. The interiors of many tumors are characterized by
relatively low pH, low oxygen tension, and low concentration of nutrients required for cellular metabolism. Drugs
surely exist that are particularly effective against cells
forced to exist in such surroundings, and their inclusion
in multidrug treatments should improve the clinicans'
ability to deal with some neoplasms.
A different and potentially useful approach is to
create, artifically, a microenvironment inside tumors, but
not elsewhere, that increases the efficacy of currently
used anticancer drugs. One way of doing this is to elevate
the intratumor temperature of specific lesions. Many drugs
kill cells at appreciably higher rates at temperatures that
can be induced safely in the tumor volume. Equipment for
such heating is currently being developed by several institu-
tutions, and minimally or non-invasive methods of determining
the achieved level of temperature are being investigated by a
variety of universities and commerical firms, although formidable technical obstacles remain. In this paper I will ex-

amine the cytoxicity of several drugs at elevated temperatures. While my major emphasis is on drugs that have shown
efficacy in the clinic, I will also describe the temperature
dependences of the cytotoxicity of drugs not of use against
cancer when such data throw light on aspects of thermal
biology.

Cytotoxicity of Drugs at Elevated Temperatures

On strictly phenomenological grounds, drugs showing
increased activity at elevated temperatures can be sub-
divided into three groups. In the first of these, increased
death rates strictly reflect the incrased rate of reaction
of one or more critical processes. The major temperature
range of interest is between 37 and 45 degrees. For such a
small temperature change to have a major effect on a rate
constant, the activation energy (or enthalpy) involved must
be high. A single reaction might be affected, in which
case an Arrhenius plot desired from cell killing data is
linear; alternately different molecules may become critical
at different temperatures. In the latter case the Arrhenius
plot is nonlinear. Both situations have been observed.
Temperature dependent cell killing data from several nitrosoureas, BCNU and CCNU for example yield Arrhenius plots
whose shape is linear, at least within the accuracies of the
experiment, and the activation energy determined from that
slope is consistent with that of an alkylation process.
Curiously, the monofunctional alkylating agent, methylmethane
sulfonate, when similarly tested, demonstrates temperature-
dependent cell-killing curves whose Arrhenius plot is anything but linear (1).
Cell killing by another major group of agents shows
a marked threshold effect near 42.5°C. For these drugs,
raising the temeprature from 37°C to 41°C or 42°C hardly increases their cytotoxic efficiency. At 43°C, however, cell
killing increases appreciably. The reason for this threshold
effect is poorly understood. Some data implicate a marked
thermotropic transition that the plasma membrane (or at least
portions of the membrane) undergo at that temperature.
Alternate explanations evoke a cooperative process at the
level of the cytoskeleton. In any case, experiments show
that the influx into cells of adriamycin nd of misonidazole
is greatly facilitated at temperatures above 43°C over that
seen at lower temperatures (2,3).
Permeability consideration cannot explain results for
bleomycin (4). Cell killing curves here also show the threshold at 42.5°C; permeability studies, however, could not

detect any differences in flux at temperatures above 43°C to that below 43°C. The best explanation here, although one based on inferential results, implicates inhibition of a repair process at the higher temperatures (4).

Finally, there appears to be a group of drugs whose actions in many ways mimic that of heat. These drugs might be termed temperature modifiers. Cell killing by heat alone results in survival curves that show a distinct change in shape at about 43°C. Above that threshold cell killing proceeds rapidly, below that temperature inactivation is at a much reduced rate. Survival curves of cells heated in the presence of ethanol, lidocaine, DMSO etc. show both an increase in the slopes of the curves as well as a reduction in the temperature threshold for increased killing. For these drugs it is possible to equate a given concentration to an effective temperature equivalent. For example, for ethanol, an increment of 0.15 in molarity corresponds to about 1°C temperature change (5). For these drugs one might suspect that whatever critical lesion is induced by the elevated temperature, that lesion is also somehow affected by the drugs involved.

Table 1 lists most of the drugs whose cell killing ability has been tested over a range of temperatures; they are classified according to the three categories listed above, at least as far as their cytotoxicity in tissue culture is concerned. Furthermore, I have indicated whether or not the increased cytotoxicity in vitro is also reflected by increased activity against murine tumors in vivo. Culture and animal data don't necessarily agree, of course, because in vivo drug pharmaco-kinetics, and excesssive normal tissue toxicity of the combination treatment may mask cytotoxic effects. Nevertheless several agents show considerable clinical promise. In particular, the nitrosoureas, bleomycin, and cis-platinum appear to be excellent candidates for the combination of localized hyperthermia and generalized chemotherapy. Once the formidable problems of inducing and measuring optimum temperature distributions are solved, this type of combined modality treatment might greatly facilitate the management of some cancers. Large masses that traditionally do not respond well to chemotherapy, might well become susceptible to the combination of heat and drug.

Thermotolerance and Drug Response

One of the most fascinating aspects of thermal biology is the finding that cells that have been heated once acquire a transient resistance to subsequent heating(6,7). This phenomenon has been termed thermotolerance (5,6). The effect of thermotolerance can be quite dramatic, leading to changes of survival by several orders of magnitude. Of perhaps even greater interest is the ability of many drugs to mimic heat in their ability to involve thermotolerance. Several such drugs are listed in Table 2. Induction of thermotolerance by heat is accompanied by the preferential synthesis of a series of proteins termed heat-shocked proteins (hsp)(8). Similarly, when drugs induce thermotolerance, hsp's are synthesized preferentially. Whether or not the development of thermotolerance requires hsp's is not as yet established. In thermotolerant cells a variety of metabolic and functional processes are protected against heat. These include macromolecular synthethesis, for example protein synthesis. It is not easy to see how a relatively small amount of newly synthesized proteins could act to protect all these functions.

Not only do cells respond differently to heat after initial heat treatments, but the initial thermal exposures also modifies the cells' later response to some drugs (2,9). Such results are shown in Table 3. Immediatley following heating periods of 43°C for one hour, the activity of all the listed drugs, with the possible exception of actinomycin-D, is appreciably enhanced. This is shown by the upward arrow in the column headed "zero hour". However, by six hours, a very different pattern emerges. If exposure is at 37°C, cells now have developed resistance to adriamycin and actinomycin-D; this is indicated by the arrow pointing downwards in column 2. At that temperature, cells respond to bleomycin as though the cells had not seen the previous heat exposure; however, if the bleomycin exposure is at 43°C, the drugs' efficiency is greatly reduced (10). For the nitrosoureas, by six hours all interactions seem to have disappeared. The cells, although they are thermotolerant at both six and twenty-four hours, show no induced resistance to BCNU. A rather remarkable behavior is evoked by methylmethanesulfonate (10). Six hours after the initial heating, the drugs' efficacy is increased if exposure is at either 37°C or 41°C; however it is reduced if the temperature exposure is at 43°C or 45°C.

A very interesting and potentially clinically useful finding is that the influx into cells of misonidazole is greatly enhanced at 43°C over that seen at lower temperatures. At 37°C the extracellular concentration of this radiation sensitizer of hypoxic cells exceeds the intracellular concentration by a factor of 4 or 5; at 43°C the gradient disappears and the intracellular concentration rises to match the extracellular level. Concomitantly, sensitization to X-rays of cells in their hypoxic state is greatly enhanced (3).

Discussion

I have indicated that data in the literature demonstrate that the cytotoxicity of many agents is strongly temperature dependent. Dose modification factors to achieve a
given level of cell kill in vitro can be as high as 10-15
fold (11). Clearly these are large effects and even if only
partially achieved in vivo should substantially increase
anti-tumor effects. Temperatures of 43°C or higher are
necessary for maximum enhancement of drug kill. These are
too high for whole-body hyperthermia. Therefore the most
reasonable application of "thermochemotherapy" would be for
the ablation of large masses, i.e., localized hyperthermia
and systemic chemotherapy. Because chemotherapy is given
in repeated applications, the effects of previous heating
on drug response must be considered, as well as the possibility that some of the agents themselves introduce drug and
heat resistance. At our present state of knowledge it
would likely to be wisest to restrict clinical applications
to those drugs that kill thermotolerant cells as efficiently
as unheated cells. Finally it might be considered that
hyperthermia employed in conjunction with drugs not currently
used as anti-cancer agents might open a new area of thermochemotherapy.

TABLE 1
CELL SURVIVAL AND TUMOR RESPONSES

Agent	Effects In Vitro		Effects In Vivo	Refs
Nitrosoureas	Type	Magnitude		
BCNU	A_s	++	++	1, 12
CCNU	A_s	++	++	1, 12
MeCCNU	A_s	++	++	1, 12
Alkylating agents				
Thio-tepa	A_s	+	NP	13
MMS	A_m	++	-	1, 15
Antibiotics				
Actinomycin P	Th	+	?	14
Adriamycin	Th	+	?	16,17
Amphotericin B	Th	++	+	18, 1
Bleomycin	Th	++	++	16
Anti-metabolites				
5-FU		+	+	15
Methotrexate		-	NP	15
Ara-C		-	NP	15
Alkaloids				
Vinblastine		-	NP	15
Vinchristine		-	NP	15
Metalic Complexes				
cis-platinum	A_s(?)	++	+	1, 15
Thiol-rich compounds				
AET	Th	++	-	17,12
Cysteamine	Th	++	-	17,15
Local Anesthetics				
Lidocaine	TM	++	+	
Procaine	TM	++	NP	
Aliphatic Alcohols				
Ehtanol	TM	++	NP	9
n-pentanol	TM	++	NP	15
Miscellaneous				
DMSO	?	++		
Di-methylformamide	?	++	NP	

Table 1 (Cont'd)

Explanations: ++ - marked effect; + - effect; - no increased cell killing; NP - not performed;
? - questionable or contradictory findings;
A_s - Arrhenius plot consistent with one single,
temperture sensitive step rate-determining for
cell death; Am - Arrhenius plot consistent
with multiple steps of different heat sensitivities responsible for cell death; Th - marked
threshold at or near 43°C (see text); TM -
temperature modifiers (see text).

TABLE 2

Thermotolerance and drug responses: drugs that induce thermotolerance and/or synthesis of heat shock proteins

| | Induction of | | Refs |
	Tolerance	hsp's	
Ethanol	+ +	+	5, 8
n-pentanol	+++	NP	15
Dimethyl fluoride (DMF)	+ +	NP	15
Dimethylsulfoxide (DMSO)	+ -	NP	15
Diiodonitrophenol (DNP)		+	8
Cadmium	+	+	18, 8
Sodium Arsenite	+ +	+ +	19, 8
Lidocaine	+ +	+	15,18
Procaine	+ -	+	15,18
Tetracaine	-	?	15

Explanations: +, ++, +++ positive effects with increasing
potency; + questionable effect; - no effect;
NP   not performed.

TABLE 3
Thermoltolerance and drug response: effect of
tolerance on drug cytoxicity

Hours after exposure to 43°:		0h	6h	24h	Refs
Adriamycin		↑	↓	↓	16
Actinomycin D		↑	↓	↓	14
Amphotericin B		↑	-	-	1,18
Bleomycin	37°C	↑	-	-	15,16
	43°C	↑	↓	↓	15,16
BCNU	37°C	↑	↑	↑	1,15
	41°C	↑	↑	NP	1,15
	43°C	↑	-	-	1,15
Methylmethane					
Sulfonate	37°C	↑	↑	NP	9,15
	41°C	↑	↑	NP	9,15
	43°C	↑	↓	NP	9,15
	45°C	↑	↓	NP	9,15

Explanations: ↑ increased cytotoxicity; ↓ decreased
cytotoxicity; - cytotoxicity indistinguisha-
ble from that seen against unheated controls.

REFERENCES

1. Hahn GM (1977). Interactions of drugs and hyperthermia in vitro and in vivo. Proc. 2nd Int. Symp. on Hyperthermia in Cancer Treatment, Essen, Germany, In: Cancer Therapy by Hyperthermia and Radiation (C. Streffer, et al. ed). Urban & Schwartzenberg, Inc. Baltimore-Munich (1978), 72-79.
2. Hahn GM, Strande DP (1976). Cytotoxic effects of hyperthermia and adriamycin on Chinese hamster cells. J. Natl. Cancer Inst. 57:1063-1067.
3. Sagerman RH, Brown DM, Gonzalez-Mendez R, Cohen MS, Brown JM, Hahn GM (1982). Enhancement by Hyperthermia of the Intracellular Uptake of 2-Nitroimidazole Radiosensitizers In Vitro. Abstract, 13th Meeting of Radiation Research Society, Salt Lake City, Utah.
4. Braun J, Hahn GM (1975). Enhanced cell killing by bleomycin and 43° hyperthermia and the inhibition of recovery from potentially lethal damage. Can. Res. 35:2921.
5. Li GC, Hahn GM (1978). Ethanol-induced tolerance to heat and to adriamycin. Nature 274:699-701.
6. Henle KJ, Leeper DB (1976). Interaction of hyperthermia and radiation in CHO cells: Recovery kinetics. Radiat. Res. 66:505-518.
7. Gerner EW, Schneider MJ (1976). Induced thermal resistance in HeLa cells. Nature 256:500-502.
8. Ashburrow M, Bonner JJ (1979). The Induction of Gene Activity in Drosphila by heat shock. Cell 17:241-245.
9. Hahn GM and Li GC (in press). The Interactions of Hyperhtermia and Drugs: treatments and probes. J.N.C.I.
10. Hahn GM, Li GC, Van Kersen I (in preparation). Responses of thermotolerant cells to drugs.
11. Hahn GM (1979). Potential for Therapy of Drugs and Hyperthermia. Cancer Res. 39:2264-2268.
12. Marmor JB (1979). Interactions of Hyperthermia and Chemotherapy in Animals. Can. Res. 39:2269-2276.
13. Johnson HA and Pavelec M (1973). Thermal enhancement of thio-TEPA cytotoxicity. J. Natl. Canc. Inst. 50: 903-908.
14. Donaldson SC, Gordon C, Hahn GM (1978). Protective effect of hyperthermia against the cytotoxicity of actinomycin D on Chinese hamter cells. Cancer Treatment Reports 62(10):1489-1495.
15. Hahn GM (unpublished).

16.   Hahn GM, Braun J, Har-Kedar I (1975). Thermochemother-
       apy: Synergism between hyperthermia (42-43°) and adri-
       amycin (or bleomycin) in mammalian cell inactivation.
       Proc. Natl. Acad. Sci. U.S. 72:937-940.
17.   Kapp DS, Hahn GM (1979). Thermosensitization by sulf-
       hydryl compounds of exponentially growing Chinese
       hamster cells. Cancer Res. 39:4630-4635.
18.   Li GC (unpublished)
19.   Li GC, Werb Z (1982). Correlation between synthesis
       of heat shock protein and the development of thermo-
       tolerance in Chinese hamster fibroblasts. Proc. Natl.
       Acad. Sci. U.S. 79:3218-3222.

Rational Basis for Chemotherapy, pages 437–439
© 1983 Alan R. Liss, Inc., 150 Fifth Avenue, New York, NY 10011

WORKSHOP SUMMARY:
LIPOSOMES ENCAPSULATION: DETERMINANTS OF
LOCALIZATION AND DRUG UPTAKE IN THE WHOLE ANIMAL

Timothy D. Heath and Demetrios Papahadjopoulos[*]

Cancer Research Institute,
and [*]Department of Pharmacology
University of California, San Francisco, CA 94143

This workshop was designed to consider the role which liposomes may play in improving the efficacy of cancer therapy. Encapsulation of antitumor agents within the aqueous or lipid portion of a liposomes may modify the in vivo characteristics of these drugs in a number of ways which may improve their antitumor effects. First, the liposomes may change the pattern of drug distribution leading to altered uptake by various in vivo sites. This effect may reduce toxicity to sensitive tissues such as bone marrow and the gatrointestinal tract. The altered distribution of the drug may also promote drug delivery to the tumor cells, particularly if the liposomes are able specifically to interact with those cells via a ligand-receptor interaction. The covalent attachment of antibodies to liposomes for which several methods now exist, may well prove useful in this respect. Liposomes may also improve the efficacy of some drugs by altering their pharmacokinetics. This arises because the liposomes act as a slow-release depot, leaking drug into the circulation as they break down due to cell or lipoprotein mediated lysis. Cytosine arabinoside shows improved antitumor effects in mice after encapsulation, possibly by such a slow-release effect.

Three speakers presented information; Jaque Barbet, Eric Forssen and Timothy Heath. Dr. Heath described work on the antibody targeting of liposomes and in particular concentrated on the selection of appropriate drugs. He demonstrated that antifolate-loaded liposomes conjugated to monoclonal antiH2K could be more toxic to L929 fibroblasts than antifolate-loaded liposomes which had a nonspecific antibody attached to them. If the antifolate was methotrexate, the free compound was more toxic than both liposome preparations. By using methotrexate- - aspartate, an antifolate which is poorly able to penetrate cells, the efficacy of anti $H2K^K$ targeted vesicles in improved in two respects. First, the targeted liposomes are more toxic, based on drug content than the equivalent free antifolate. Second, the difference in the toxicity of the anti $H2K^K$ bearing liposomes and the nonspecific-antibody bearing liposomes is greater than is seen for methotrexate. This is believed to be due to the reduced efficacy of drug which leaks from the liposomes.

Dr. Barbet discussed his work on the toxicity of methotrexate-containing liposomes, conjugated to a variety of monoclonal antibodies. Dr. Barbet's experimental model involved measuring the inhibition of deoxy-uridine incorporation by con A or LPS stimulated mouse spleen cells. He had compared the amount of liposomes bound to the cells with the toxic effects of the vesicles and found disparities in several cases. In particular a monoclonal anti IE^K antibody gave a much lower level of liposome association with lymphocytes than an anti $H2K^K$ antibody. However, the anti IE^K preparation was more effective on LPS stimulated cells than the anti $H2K^K$ preparation but was without effect on con A stimulated cells. In another example, Dr. Barbet had used a series of antibodies to the IA^K antigens and found 2 distinct classes when conjugated to liposomes. One group produced antibody conjugated vesicles that were much more effective in inhibiting UdR incorporation than liposomes conjugated to the other group. It seems likely that one group may react with IA and the other with IA . These experiments suggest that the effect of targeted liposomes for drug delivery depends on the extent and rate of interiorization of the antigen.

Dr. Forssen presented data which demonstrated the effect of encapsulation on adriamycin cardiotoxicity and in vivo distribution in mice. He had first found stearylamine:phosphatidylcholine vesicles to be the most useful for drug encapsulation. Histological examination of cardiac tissues by 2 independent examiners has clearly shown a reduction in adriamycin damage to cardiac tissues to result from liposome encapsulation. Surprisingly, an examination of levels of adriamycin in the heart showed little difference between mice receiving encapsulated drug and mice receiving free drug. The reduction of cardiotoxicity may therefore arise from the rate of adriamycin uptake by heart muscle, which is presumably slower for the encapsulated drug. Several groups have examined adriamycin antitumor efficacy in liposomes and have found no change or a slight improvement in effects.

The discussion which followed these three presentations considered the potential of antibody-targeted liposomes in antitumor therapy, and the factors which should be considered in selecting antitumor agents for encapsulation. The in vitro experiments described by Drs. Heath and Barbet clearly demonstrate that targeted liposomes can deliver their contents to specific cells in vitro. However, the in vivo use of such a strategy is potentially more complex and may depend on parameters such as the accessibility of the target cells, the availability of tumor-specific antibodies, and the ability of the target cells to internalize the vesicles. Most discussants seemed to feel that it is unrealistic to hope that targeted liposomes could reach solid tumors sequested behind the barrier of the endothelial cells of the blood vessels. More practicable targets considered for this system, at least initially, were the leukemias, and hematogenously spread metastatic disease.

The selection of appropriate drugs for encapsulation was seen as both complex and a potentially very fruitful area of investigation. When liposomes were first suggested as carriers of chemotherapeutic agents, their role was viewed in a very simple way. The carrier would take the drug to the tumor cell and deliver it in greater amounts than were mornally able to enter cells. Subsequent investigations have shown that this generally does not happen for several reasons. First, most antitumor agents are selected because they are quite well able to enter cells. Secondly, liposomes do not reach tumor cells in sufficient quantity to accelerate drug accumulation by these cells. Two of the best examples of drugs for which liposomes mediated an improvement of drug efficacy are ara C and adriamycin. The improvements which are seen are probably not due to delivery but to slow release and the concomitant prolongation of the drug half-life. One interesting possibility raised, was the potential importance of evaluating antitumor agents other than those known to be of clinical relevance. The work described by Dr. Heath on the use of methotrexate- -aspartate demonstrated the possibility of using compounds which are delivered only by the liposomes to the target cells. Clearly many other parameters, such as clearance rates, metabolism and sites of activation might make agents which were poorly effective in the free form effective liposome-dependent antitumor agents.

Rational Basis for Chemotherapy, pages 441–473
© 1983 Alan R. Liss, Inc., 150 Fifth Avenue, New York, NY 10011

TARGET-DIRECTION OF LIPOSOMES:
FOUR STRATEGIES FOR ATTACKING TUMOR CELLS

John N. Weinstein

Laboratory of Mathematical Biology, Division of Cancer
Biology and Diagnosis, National Cancer Institute, NIH
Bldg 10, Rm 4B-54, Bethesda, MD 20205

ABSTRACT The pharmacokinetic properties of a drug, a
biological agent, or a diagnostic marker can be changed
radically by encapsulating it in liposomes. However,
many projected clinical and research applications will
require that liposome contents be selectively directed
to a target. Described here is our work on four
conceptually different approaches to that task: (i)
Ligand-mediated targeting -- in particular, the
attachment of antigen and/or antibody to liposomes for
specific cell surface recognition; (ii) Natural
targeting -- i.e., to the phagocytic cells which
normally take up naked liposomes; (iii) Physical
targeting -- the design and testing of
"temperature-sensitive liposomes," which self-destruct
and release drug in a heated tumor; (iv) Compartmental
targeting -- the delivery of liposomes to lymph nodes
from the peritoneal cavity or a subcutaneous injection
site.

INTRODUCTION

Conventional tumor chemotherapy rests on a knife-edge
balance between therapeutic and toxic effects -- hence the
dream of Ehrlich's magic bullet, the target-directed carrier
lending sight to blind drugs. The list of molecules and
particles studied as carriers is a long one: synthetic
polymers, albumin, protein aggregates, monoclonal
antibodies, lectins, hormones, microcapsules, nucleic acids,

liposomes. For diagnostic purposes the payload will likely be a gamma-emitter, a positron-emitter, or a nuclear magnetic resonance marker; for therapy, it may be a toxin, a drug, or a biological agent. Liposomes[1] have been the most extensively studied of the carriers, beginning with the work of Bangham and his colleagues in the mid-1960's (1). For a recent review of the use of liposomes in cancer, see ref. (2). My plan here is briefly to introduce the types of liposomes, their interactions with cells, and the rationale for their use, then to describe our efforts at four different ways of "targeting" them to particular cell types or anatomicaal locations.

Fig. 1 shows the three major types of liposomes. Multilamellar vesicles (MLV) develop spontaneously upon hydration of bilayer-forming lipids such as those found in natural biological membranes. The usual formulations are based on phosphatidylcholines or sphingomyelins, with cholesterol added to "toughen" the vesicle and often with a charged lipid species included in smaller amounts. The bilayer formers have two fatty acid chains and a balance between hydrophilic headgroup and hydrophobic tail. Predominance of the hydrophobic part would inhibit hydration; predominance of the hydrophilic would lead to micelles, not bilayers. The MLV range in diameter from 500 A to perhaps 10 μm. Hydrophilic molecules can be trapped in the aqueous spaces between bilayers; hydrophobic agents partition into the lipid. MLV are the equilibrium form, stabler and simpler to make than the other types of liposome. These are major factors in their favor as pharmaceuticals, even if they do tend to be heterogeneous -- and inelegant for experimental studies because of the variable numbers of layers. Small unilamellar vesicles (SUV) are formed from MLV by an input of energy, usually ultrasonic. They are about 200 - 300 A in diameter, the

[1]The terms "liposome" and "lipid vesicle" will be used synonymously. Abbreviations: CF, carboxyfluorescein; DNP, dinitrophenyl; DPPC and DSPC, dipalmitoyl and distearoyl phosphatidylcholines; LUV, large unilamellar vesicle; MLV, multilamellar vesicle; MTX, methotrexate; NBD, N-4-nitrobenzo-2-oxa-1,3-diazole)-aminocaproyl phosphatidyl-choline; PE, phosphatidylethanolamine; SUV, small unilamellar vesicle; T_m, lipid phase transition temperature; TNP, trinitrophenyl

Small Unilamellar Vesicle

 Multilamellar Vesicle

O Large unilamellar Vesicle

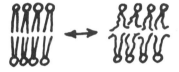

"SOLID"   "FLUID"

FIGURE 1. Three types of liposome. Each line represents a lipid bilayer. Also shown schematically is the phase transition from "solid" to "fluid" bilayer. After ref. (12).

lower limit being set by strains in packing of the bilayer. They are smaller and remain in the circulation longer than do the other types. The price is a small volume/surface ratio, hence inefficient trapping of water-soluble drugs. They are also less stable and somewhat more complex to make than are the MLV. The large unilamellar vesicles (LUV), 800 A to several microns in diameter, are relative newcomers. They can trap water-soluble agents more efficiently than the others but are less stable and are hard to make reproducibly. Though very good for basic pharmacological studies, it is unclear whether they will be practical as pharmaceuticals. Szoka and Papahadjopoulos (3) have recently reviewed the various methods for forming and characterizing liposomes.

Liposomes can interact with cells in at least four different ways: (i) fusion with the cell membrane bilayer, thereby injecting water-soluble contents into the cytoplasm and elements of the liposome bilayer into the cell membrane; (ii) endocytosis, by phagocytic or coated pit mechanism; (iii) binding to the cell surface, either non-specifically or through a ligand; (iv) lipid exchange, that is the transfer of lipid components to the cell membrane without incorporation of the liposome as a structure into the cell.

Fusion was initially seen as a way of bypassing membrane permeability barriers. However, we found, using fluorescence techniques, that little (if any) fusion takes place spontaneously between vesicles and cells (4). That makes good teleological sense, since cells only occasionally have reason to fuse their membranes with neighboring external ones. Several newer techniques, using polyethylene glycol (5) or viral coat proteins (6), have been developed for precipitating, fusion in vitro, and there remains an active interest in the use of lipid vesicles for insertion of nucleic acids into cells. However, there is currently no known way to use these methods in vivo. Hence, for practical purposes, the present generation of liposomes are processed in vivo by one of the other cellular mechanisms listed, or else by dissolution in the serum (7).

Table 1 lists some of the anti-tumor agents encapsulated in either the lipid or the aqueous space of liposomes. In some cases, the studies done with those liposomes have been based simply on the wish that encapsulation would somehow magically change the pharmacokinetic rules to advantage. Better formulated reasons have included (i) prolongation of drug effect due to lengthened circulation time, especially with cell cycle specific agents; (ii) possible passage of liposomes through leaky endothelia selectively in tumors; (iii) reduction of toxicity where liposomes do not accumulate (e.g., reduction of adriamycin toxicity for cardiac muscle (8)); (iv) protection of a drug from metabolism or immune attack until its target has been reached; (v) amplification of drug effect by encapsulation of numerous drug molecules in each liposome; (vi) circumvention of permeability barriers by endocytosis or fusion; (vii) finally, target-direction by one of the four generic types of "targeting" listed in Table 2.

ANTIBODY-MEDIATED TARGETING OF LIPOSOMES

TABLE 1. ANTI-TUMOR DRUGS ENCAPSULATED IN LIPOSOMES[a]

Drug	Sample references
Methotrexate	Colley and Ryman (1975); Kimelberg (1976); Kosloski, et al. (1978); Weinstein, et al. (1980)
5-Fluorouracil	Gregoriadis (1973)
L-Asparaginase	Neerunjun and Gregoriadis (1976)
6-Mercaptopurine	Tsujii, et al. (1976)
8-Azoguanine	Fendler and Romero (1976)
Melphalan	Gregoriadis, et al. (1977)
Mechlorethamine	Rutman, et al. (1976)
Cytosine arabinoside	Mayhew, et al.(1976); Kobayashi, et al. (1977); Hunt, et al. (1979)
Bleomycin	Gregoriadis and Neerunjun (1975)
Adriamycin	Forssen and Tokes (1979); Rahman, et al. (1980); Parker and Sieber (1981); Maslow, et al. (1980)
Vinblastine	Juliano and Stamp (1978)
Actinomycin D	Gregoriadis (1973); Poste and Papahadjopoulos (1976); Juliano and Stamp (1978)
Daunorubicin	Juliano and Stamp (1978)
Cis-platinum	Deliconstantinos, et al. (1977); Yatvin, et al. (1981)
Actinomycin D	Gregoriadis (1973); Rahman, et al. (1974) Papahadjopoulos, et al. (1976)
Bischloroethyl- nitrosourea (BCNU)	Rutman, et al. (1976)

a. Adapted from Table 2 of ref. (2). See that source for the original references. The list is by no means exhaustive.

The work of Gregoriadis and his colleagues in the mid-1970's (9,10) suggested a slight selectivity of association if liposomes were treated with antisera to tumor lines and then allowed to interact with those cells. We wanted to determine directly whether liposomes could be bound to cell surfaces and to develop methods for assessing

TABLE 2
TYPES OF "TARGETING"

---

1. LIGAND-MEDIATED
   (by antibody, hormone, lectin, carbohydrate, etc.)

2. NATURAL
   (i.e., to phagocytic cells)

3. PHYSICAL
   (e.g., temperature-sensitive, pH-sensitive,
   photosensitive liposomes)

4. COMPARTMENTAL
   (in lung, peritoneal cavity, lymphatics, etc.)

---

a. After ref. (12).

the consequences of any binding achieved. Figure 2(I) shows schematically the first experimental system in which antigen-antibody interaction was directly shown to bind vesicles to cells (11).[2] Subsequent work from other laboratories on antibody-mediated targeting is reviewed in ref. (2).

We made small unilamellar vesicles whose lipids included a dinitrophenyl (DNP)-modified phosphatidyl-ethanolamine. When those vesicles were incubated with anti-nitrophenyl sheep IgG and with lymphocytes chemically modified with trinitrophenyl hapten (TNP), they became cross-linked to the cells in large numbers. The evidence for specificity was obtained from a combination of fluorescence microscopy, fluorescence measurements on cell suspensions in a cuvette, and flow microfluorimetry.

---

[2] Here I will describe our published experimental systems only in broad outline; the reader should consult original references for details of liposome composition and for protocols, as well as for more complete surveys of the relevant literature.

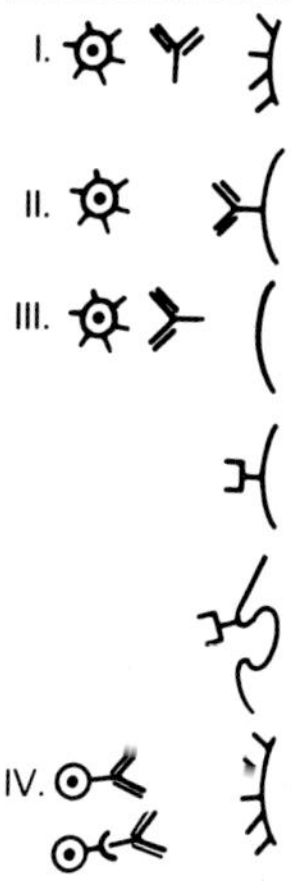

	Binding	Incor- poration	MTX Effect
I. Hapten-Modified Lymphocyte	+	−	N.D.
II. Myeloma Cell	+	−	−
III. Fc-Receptor Negative	−	−	−
Fc-Receptor Positive "Non-Phagocytic"	+	+/−	+/−
Fc-Receptor Positive Phagocytic	+	+	+
IV. Lymphocyte	+/− −	+/− −	

FIGURE 2. Summary of experiments on antibody-mediated targeting. Circles at left represent SUV modified with DNP. I. DNP-liposomes are bound to TNP-modified lymphocytes by anti-nitrophenyl IgG (11); II. Liposomes bearing DNP or phosphorylcholine hapten are bound to mouse myeloma cells bearing the corresponding surface immunoglobulin (14,15); III. Opsonized DNP-liposomes are incubated with cells differing in presence/absence of Fc receptor and in capacity for phagocytosis (16); IV. Lymphocyte surface antigens are targets for IgG linked to liposomes covalently or through protein A (17). Incorporation and drug effect depend on the target antigen and cell type. N.D.: not done. See text and references for details. After ref. (12).

To distinguish between liposome contents bound on the surface of the cell and those internalized and released in the cytoplasm, we used a technique based on fluorescence self-quenching. High concentrations of a fluorescent dye, carboxyfluorescein (CF), were encapsulated in the liposomes. At such high concentrations, the fluorescence emission is largely suppressed, but it reappears upon release of the dye and its dilution into the much larger cytoplasmic space (4,13). Thus, fluorescence measurement monitors dye released into the cytoplasm, whereas measurement after disruption of intact vesicles with detergent monitors total cell-associated dye. The difference between the two reflects intact, bound vesicles. Figure 3 shows the result obtained: binding of thousands of vesicles to the surface of each cell but no suggestion that antibody-mediated binding increased release into the cytoplasm. Those findings are mirrored in the flow microfluorimetric results in Fig. 4. In the experiments of Figure 4a the vesicles contained 10 mM dye (a non-quenched concentration); in those of Figure 4b, 200 mM dye (a self-quenched concentration). Again, there was binding but no increased entry. Fluorescence microscopy showed patchy surface binding of targeted vesicles but corroborated the lack of an increase in uptake over spontaneous background levels.

We were left, then, asking three questions: Can antibody be used to bind vesicles to cells? Clearly, the answer was "yes," and no more is required for some pharmacological applications -- for example, the use of

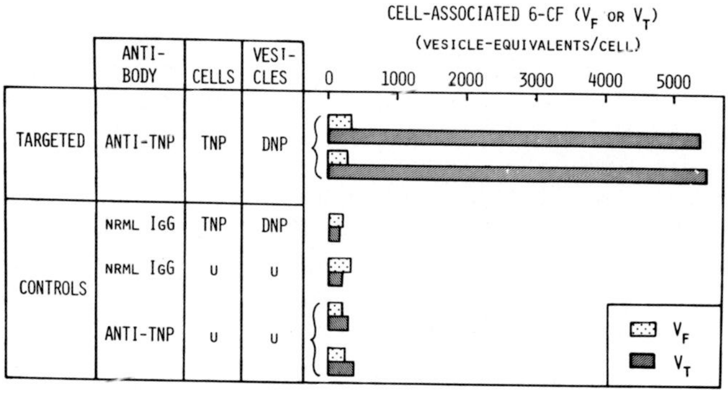

FIGURE 3. Fluorometric demonstration of antibody-mediated binding of small unilamellar vesicles to human lymphocytes. Total cell CF (V_T -- determined from fluorescence after treatment with Triton X-100 detergent) was increased more than ten-fold by targeting; free intracellular CF (V_F -- determined from initial fluorescence) was not increased over background levels. U, unmodified. After ref. (11).

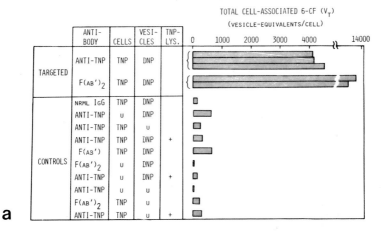

a

b

FIGURE 4. Flow microfluorimetric analysis of human peripheral blood lymphocytes incubated with antibody-targeted liposomes containing CF. (a) Vesicles containing 10 mM CF -- to indicate total cell fluorophore; (b) vesicles containing 200 mM CF -- to monitor release into the cell cytoplasm. TNP-lys., TNP-lysine (a soluble competitor for binding). U, unmodified. Bars represent means computed from histograms such as those in Fig. 5 below. After ref. (11).

gamma-emitters for diagnostic imaging or alpha-emitters for cell killing. But for therapy with internally acting agents, the second and third questions are vital: "Does binding lead to entry into the cell? And if entry is achieved by endocytosis, does the drug escape the endosomal apparatus?"

It seemed possible that the lack of entry was due to our chemical modification of the cell surface. To avoid that possibility, we turned to the system shown in Figure 2(II), using the mouse myeloma MOPC 315, which secretes and surface-expresses an IgA with high affinity for DNP. The answer was the same: considerable binding of DNP-bearing vesicles but no discernible entry into the cell. The same conclusions held for vesicles bearing phosophorylcholine hapten incubated with TEPC 15 cells, which bear anti--phosphorylcholine antibody.

Since endocytosis appeared necessary for internalization, we tried opsonizing hapten-modified liposomes with rabbit IgG for interaction with Fc receptors (16), as diagrammed in Fig. 2(III). This approach was similar in principle to studies by Weissmann and co-workers (18,19) in which liposomes were opsonized by non-specifc attachment of aggregated immunoglobulin. We compared three murine tumor cell lines: EL4 (Fc receptor-negative, non-phagocytic), P388 (Fc receptor-positive, non-phagocytic), and P388D$_1$ (Fc receptor-positive, highly phagocytic). Figure 5 shows one set of results from flow microfluorimetry, and Table 3 summarizes an extensive series of such studies. The 10,200,000 CF molecules associated on average with each P388 cell in the targeted case represented approximately 800,000 vesicles per cell. Non-specific backgrounds were very low, and (as an aside) liposomes appear useful as high signal/noise markers for sparse antigens or receptors on cell surfaces. Vesicles failed to bind to the Fc receptor-negative EL4 cells. Also as expected, there was no binding to any of the cells with F(ab')$_2$ or IgA anti-nitrophenyl.

Fluorescence microscopy (Figure 6) supported the idea that endocytosis is necessary for entry into the cell. The system with P388D$_1$ cells showed massive uptake of opsonized vesicles but comparatively little of "naked" vesicles under the conditions of incubation. Internalization could be largely blocked by azide and 2-deoxyglucose or by carrying out the incubations at 2°C. P388 is not classically phagocytic, but there was clearly a small amount of

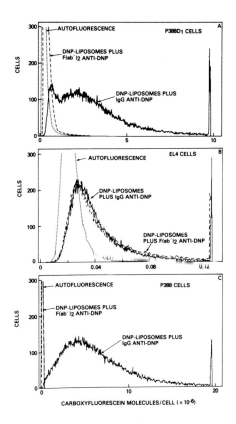

FIGURE 5. Flow microfluorimetric profiles of (A) P388D$_1$ cells, (B) EL4 cells, and (C) P388 cells after incubation with opsonized vesicles. Incubations were for 20 minutes with vesicles containing 10 mM (i.e., not self-quenched) CF. Note the difference in abscissa scales for A,B, and C. From ref. (16).

Fc-receptor-mediated uptake, blockable by metabolic inhibitors or incubation on ice.

To examine escape from the endosomal apparatus, we encapsulated methotrexate (MTX) in the vesicles along with CF. We could then monitor the fluorescence properties and also use cellular uptake of tritiated deoxyuridine as an

TABLE 3.
SUMMARY OF FLOW MICROFLUORIMETRY ON TUMOR CELLS INCUBATED WITH DNP-LIPOSOMES AND RABBIT ANTI-DNP IMMUNOGLOBULIN G

		Mean cell fluorescence			
Cell line	Temp., °C	No Ig*	IgA anti-DNP (MOPC 315)	$F(ab')_2$ anti-DNP	IgG anti-DNP
$P388D_1$	4	55	37	27	3,130
	37	183	171	86	4,530
P388	4	19	12	8	4,520
	37	17	17	17	10,200
EL4	4	3	3	3	6
	37	25	22	29	27

Mean cell fluorescence expressed as CF molecules x 10^{-3}/cell
* Background autofluorescence: $P388D_1$, 334; P388, 60; EL4, 38. These values have been subtracted to obtain the above entries. After ref. (16).

assay for the ability of MTX to reach its cytoplasmic target, dihydrofolate reductase. The results are indicated in Figure 7. Encapsulation of MTX in opsonized liposomes effectively protected EL4 cells from the drug (B); in contrast, encapsulation increased MTX effect on $P388D_1$ cells (A); an intermediate result was obtained for P388 (C). As with the fluorescent marker, the MTX effect showed all of the appropriate immunological specificities. At this point we do not know how efficiently MTX escaped to the cytoplasm. We also do not know whether that escape depended on the character of MTX as a weak anion (which would be expected to partition out of an acid compartment such as that thought to precede entry into lysosomes).

As a natural continuation of this work, one would want to couple immunoglobulin to liposomal lipid covalently. Over the last several years a number of methods have been devised for doing so, as reviewed in ref. (2). Our method (17) was the first to take advantage of the relative specificity of heterobifunctional cross-linking. The reagent used was N-hydroxy-succinimidyl 3-(2-pyridyldithio)--propionate (SPDP). Liposomes containing phosphatidylethanolamine (PE) are formed and then coupled to the antibody (or protein A) through the primary amino groups on the PE. Most of the other methods also couple either via PE

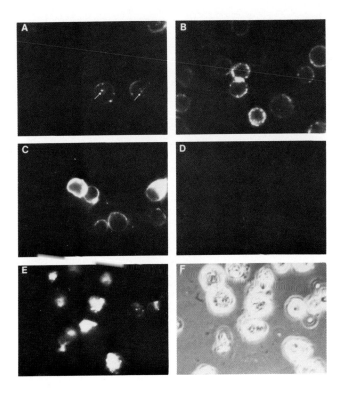

FIGURE 6. Fluorescence micrographs of tumor cells incubated with DNP-liposomes containing 10 mM CF. (A) P388 cells with rabbit IgG anti-DNP at $37^{o}C$. Arrows indicate internalized CF in some vesicular system near the nucleus. (B) Same as A but with 0.2% azide and 50 mM 2-deoxyglucose. (C) Same as A but at $4^{o}C$. (D) Same as A but with $F(ab')_2$ instead of whole IgG. (E) P388D$_1$ cells with IgG anti-DNP at $37^{o}C$. (F) Same field as (E) but phase-contrast. From ref. (16).

or via glycolipids included in the liposome formulation. This sort of target-direction clearly makes possible selective killing of cells in vitro and perhaps in vivo. L.D. Leserman, J. Barbet, and P. Machy (20,21,22) are going on to identify which surface antigens mediate sufficient uptake to permit killing or other alterations of cellular physiology. Opsonization can be considered a way of

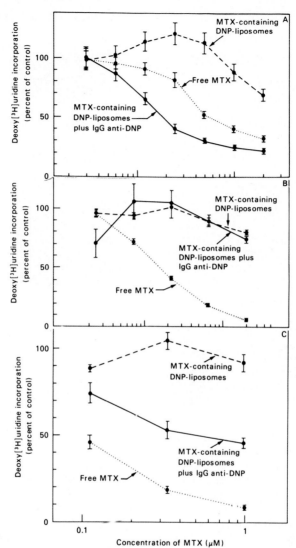

FIGURE 7. Dose response curves for MTX in solution or in DNP-liposomes, assayed by inhibition of ^{3}H-deoxyuridine incorporation into (A) P388D$_1$, (B) EL4, and (C) P388 cells. An MTX effect indicates access of the drug to the cytoplasm. Bars are S.E.M. From ref. (16).

enhancing, and perhaps directing, the "natural" targeting of liposomes for highly endocytic cells.

TEMPERATURE-SENSITIVE LIPOSOMES

The use of antibody (or any other ligand) to target vesicles faces a number of obvious limitations: the requirement for a usable antigenic determinant; modulation of the antigen; clonal heterogeneity; the possible antigenicity and immunogenicity of the antibody itself; the question of delivery to the cytoplasm or nucleus after binding. These problems pertain to any pharmacological use of antibodies, but there is an additional issue unique to large carrier particles: they do not readily cross continuous (or even fenestrated) endothelia (23). Permeation through the intercellular junctions is restricted to particles less than about 200 A in diameter (24), slightly less than the size of most SUV. Vesicular transport across endothelial cells appears not to be possible for them either. It would do no good to coat a liposome with antibody to a determinant on a solid tumor if i v. injection did not provide access. If liposomes are to reach solid tumors from the bloodstream, they must do so by passing through areas of vascular damage, by hitch-hiking on diapedesing cells (23), or, more speculatively still, by bearing the "open sesame" signal used by cells to open intercellular junctions. At present, the endothelial barrier is a major limitation.

We have developed a conceptually quite different approach, "physical targeting" (see Table 2). It has its own list of limitations, as will be discussed later, but at least none of those listed above. The first and most highly developed version is the "temperature-sensitive liposome" (25-28), developed and applied in close collaboration with a number of others, principally with M.B. Yatvin and R. Magin. The idea is not to obtain specific localization of the liposomes themselves but rather to have them release their contents in a specified capillary bed, for example, that of a tumor. It has been known since the early 1970's that liposomes release encapsulated water-soluble contents more quickly near their liquid-crystalline phase transition temperature (T_m) than at other temperatures (29,30). Figure 8 shows the principle in operation with liposomes designed to have transition temperatures at about $42^{\circ}C$, a temperature achievable by techniques of moderate local hyperthermia. Obviously, selectivity might also be obtained with appropriately designed liposomes by such maneuvres as cooling parts of the body to be spared or injecting

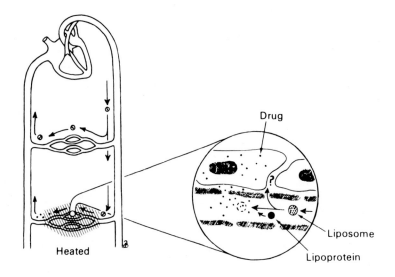

FIGURE 8. Schematic view of drug release from temperature-sensitive liposomes in a tumor heated to the transition temperature. Serum components, principally the lipoproteins, induce rapid release, and drug equilibrates with the extracellular space. This "physical targeting" does not require that liposomes be able to leave the capillaries or interact directly with tumor cells. From ref. (26).

anaesthetics locally to influence properties of the liposome bilayer.

Our first task was to design liposomes with the right release properties. We used mixtures of dipalmitoyl (T_m=41°C) and distearoyl (T_m=56°C) phosphatidylcholines. Since these two are miscible in all proportions in both fluid and quasi-crystalline phases, the mixture has a single major transition; by varying the ratio of the two lipids, one can manipulate the transition within a broad range of values. To assay release we again used the self-quenching of CF fluorescence. Dye released from a high concentration inside the vesicle increases its fluorescence approximately twenty-fold; release can therefore be monitored by placing a cuvette containing vesicles in the well of a fluorometer and heating through the transition. We term this method "phase transition release" (PTR) and have used it to explore details of the interaction between proteins and lipid bilayers. Initial results in physiological saline were discouraging: the release at transition was small and relatively slow. We also worried that the presence of serum would doom our efforts in any case. Serum components were well known to exchange with those of the vesicle, altering its properties. To the contrary, and a pleasant surprise: liposomes were essentially impervious to serum below T_m, but broke down in an all-or-nothing fashion very rapidly at T_m. This observation made the whole enterprise appear feasible. Quantitatively, the largest releasing effect of serum is due to high density lipoprotein (HDL), but the other lipoproteins and at least one non-lipoprotein component also play roles. Figure 9 shows a set of PTR scans for HDL. There is little release in the absence of protein, but essentially 100% release within at most a few seconds at sufficiently high concentrations. If the vesicle concentration is increased, the stoichiometric disruptive

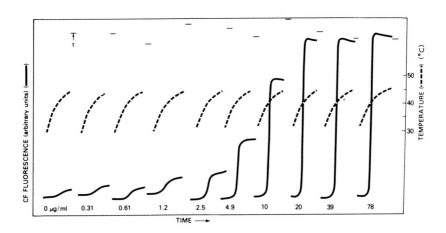

FIGURE 9. Phase transition release profiles for small unilamellar 7:3 (molar) DPPC:DSPC vesicles, as a function of human HDL concentration. (t) indicates 100% release point. The vesicle lipid concentration was kept constant at 60 µM for each scan, and HDL concentration was varied as indicated at bottom of figure. From ref. (31).

capacity of serum can be exceeded, potentially an important factor in the design of therapy with temperature-sensitive liposomes. These studies have since been extended to MLV and LUV liposomes, as well as to the release of drugs (32,33). Figure 10 shows a temperature profile for release of cytosine arabinoside from LUV. The experiments were done by sealing liposomes in a 100-µl capillary tube, which was then plunged into a bath at the desired temperature and into a cold bath to stop release. In this way, time resolutions on the order of a second could be achieved. Release proved to be fast, taking at most a few seconds to completion at T_m.

Our next question was whether large fractional release could be achieved in single pass through a capillary bed. To answer the question, we injected anaesthetized rats i.v.

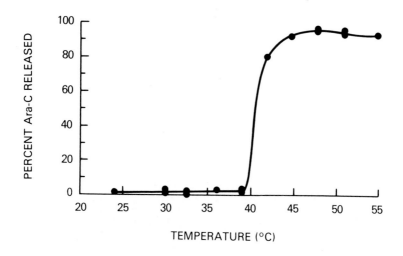

TEMPERATURE (°C)

FIGURE 10. Temperature-sensitive release of ^{3}H-cytosine arabinoside from 5.5:1 (molar) DPPC:DSPC large unilamellar vesicles in 50% mouse serum. Vesicles were incubated in capillary tubes for rapid temperature equilibration and then were pelleted. Incubations were for 1 minute, but time course studies showed full release within 1-2 seconds. The lipid concentration was 3 mg/ml. After ref. (32)

with temperature-sensitive liposomes containing quenched CF, withdrew a loop of small intestine through an abdominal incision, and submerged it in a temperature-controlled saline bath. By sampling from the arcades of mesenteric arteries and veins serving the loop (or adjacent ones at other temperatures), we could determine from the degree of self-quenching how much CF had been released, as a function of bath temperature. The arterial-venous difference in total CF concentration was small, indicating low fractional clearance. However, most of the CF had in fact been released from the vesicles during single pass, as indicated in Figure 11. These results were encouraging but did not, of course, indicate what fraction was released in the arteries, areterioles, and capillaries; drug released in the veins would simply be washed out of the area and redistributed.

The next step was to look for in vivo clearance, and localization in a tumor. We first used Lewis lung tumors implanted in the flanks of mice and heated with microwaves.

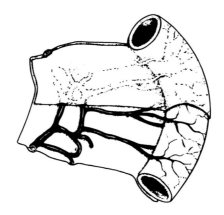

37° → 9% Release

42° → 70% Release

FIGURE 11. Temperature-sensitive release in single pass through capillaries of the small intestine, as monitored by CF fluorescence in arterial inflow and venous outflow. SUV were as in Figure 9.

However, here I will describe only the similar results obtained with L1210 implanted in the footpad and heated by water bath. Tumors were placed in each foot and one was heated. This design provided an internal control for any effect of heating on the circulatory system as a whole. We chose to use ^{3}H-MTX as the principle marker for these studies for three major reasons: (i) it is water-soluble; (ii) the extensive information available on its pharmacokinetics and interaction with L1210 cells (34) was useful in designing experiments; (iii) once bound (at tracer levels) to its target enzyme dihydrofolate reductase, it remains in place for many hours. Thus, we could wait long enough for blood MTX levels to recede and still measure how much had entered the tumor without worrying about efflux. Figure 12 gives the first suggestion of selective local MTX release: heating a tumor-containing foot more than doubled the rate at which liposomal MTX (and CF) were released and

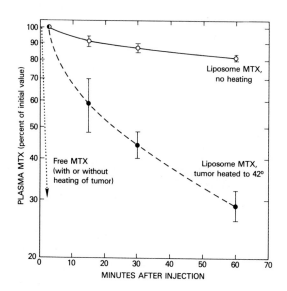

FIGURE 12. Clearance from blood of ^{3}H-MTX in temperature-sensitive SUV. Clearance is accelerated by heating one foot. The MTX dose was 3 mg/kg, and MTX levels were determined by high pressure liquid chromatography. Liposomes were as in Figure 9. From ref. (27).

cleared from the bloodstream. When tumors were heated for one hour after intravenous injection and the animals sacrificed 3 hours later, the amount of ^{3}H-MTX found in the tumors was as shown in Figure 13. The heated tumors contained an average of 14 times as much tritium as did the unheated ones (a). Analysis by high pressure liquid chromatography confirmed that the tritium counts represented primarily intact MTX. Empty liposomes did not affect the uptake of free MTX (b), which was increased 3-fold by heating (c). Simply immersing the left foot in water without heating (d) did not affect uptake. Co-injection of excess free, unlabeled MTX (e) and dl-L-Ca leucovorin (f) effectively blocked tumor incorporation of ^{3}H-MTX,

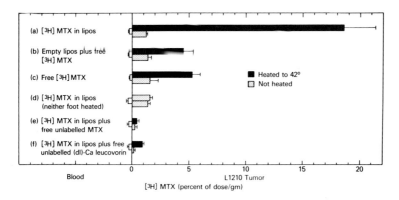

FIGURE 13. Incorporation of ^{3}H-MTX into L1210 tumors of double-tumored mice after injection free or encapsulated in 7:3 (molar) DPPC:DSPC small unilamellar vesicles. Left tumors were heated to 42°C. (a) Heating increased MTX incorporation 14-fold; (b) empty liposomes (i.e., containing only buffer) did not affect uptake of free MTX; (c) heating increased uptake of free MTX 3-fold; (c) immersion of the left foot in water at body temperature had no effect; (e) co-injection of excess free unlabeled MTX (300 mg/Kg) effectively inhibited incorporation; (f) free dl-L-Ca leucovorin (300 mg/Kg) also inhibited incorporation. Open bars to left indicate blood levels. Error bars are S.E.M. for groups of 4 mice. From ref. (27).

indicating that the differences seen with heating did not simply represent liposomes sequestered intact in the tumor. As expected, the uptake of ^{14}C lipid label did not show the differences seen in MTX uptake (data not shown), another point against sequestration of vesicles.

Given the large increases in tumor uptake of ^{3}H–MTX from temperature-sensitive liposomes, our next step clearly was to try therapy. However, we knew from the outset that the MTX system, while excellent for tracer studies, would not be optimal for therapy: First, the relatively high concentrations of MTX-containing SUV required would saturate the ability of mouse serum to disrupt the vesicles. Second, entry into the tumor cell cytoplasm depends largely on a saturable transport system. Hence, increasing the ambient concentration locally and temporarily (at concentrations above the Michaelis constant for transport) does not have a proportionate effect on delivery into the cell. However, given all of the kinetic information we had developed on the MTX-SUV-L1210 system from work at the tracer level, we decided to go ahead and try therapy anyway. The essential results were as follows: (i) liposome-encapsulated MTX delayed tumor growth more than did an equivalent concentration of free MTX, with or without heating (not shown); (ii) heating alone to 42°C for one hour delayed tumor growth about 0.7 days, whereas heating increased by 2.8 days the growth delay obtained with temperature-sensitive liposomes containing MTX (Fig. 14). The "non-additive" effect (about 2.1 days) corresponds to an extra cell kill of only 4- to 16-fold beyond that attributable to the separate effects of heating and of the encapsulated MTX (27). As expected, the effect was not large, and its mechanism cannot be considered established beyond doubt. Current efforts, in collaboration with R. Magin, are aimed at (i) use of LUV and MLV to increase the amount of drug releasable within the constraints of serum combining power, and (ii) investigation of more favorable choices of drug.

Heating a tumor had no discernible effect on the uptake of ^{3}H–MTX by other tissues from temperature-sensitive liposomes, and the uptake elsewhere was also approximately the same as for a bolus of free ^{3}H–MTX (26). Hence, it is reasonable to expect, though we have not demonstrated it directly, that increases in therapeutic index could be achieved. With regard to toxicity, it would usually not matter if the margins of the heated field included normal tissues, unless those tissues were sites of toxicity for the

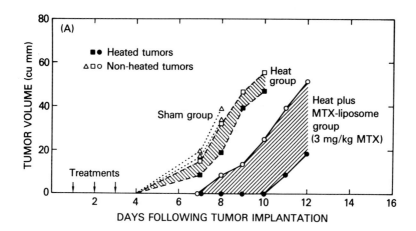

FIGURE 14. L1210 tumor growth in mouse feet after i.v. treatment with hyperthermia (42°C) and/or temperature-sensitive liposomes. Points are medians for groups of 8 mice. A generalized Wilcoxon test showed the non-additive effect of heat and liposomal MTX to be significant at p = 0.015. From ref. (27).

drug used. Most of the bone marrow would lie outside of the heated field, so marrow cells would not be depleted.

The major limitation of temperature-sensitive liposomes for cancer therapy is that they do not address the problem of widespread metastates. In this regard, they are similar to x-radiation and to hyperthermia itself. Hyperthermia received new attention in the 1970's after reports appeared suggesting that tumor cells are more sensitive to heat than are normal cells (35). Its use in combination with drugs is under study for possible synergistic effects (36). Temperature-sensitive liposomes can be thought of a providing an additional amplification through selective localization of the chosen drug. They are clearly a long way from the clinic. Whether or not they will be of practical use depends in part on the future of hyperthermia itself, especially on developments in the medical physics of heating.

LIPOSOMES IN THE LYMPHATICS

The inability of liposomes to cross anatomical linings such as the vascular endothelium is a considerable limitation. But it can also be an advantage if the aim is to sequester liposomes in a chosen compartment. Because of its importance in oncology, the lymphatic system has been examined in several laboratories (37-46). Our own work in the area began a number of years ago with two portals of entry in mind: peritoneal administration for delivery to nodes of the thorax, and subcutaneous administration for

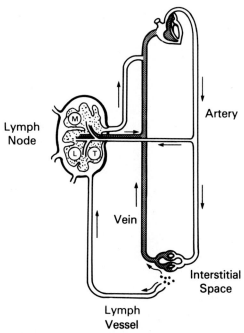

FIGURE 15. Schematic view of the passage of a liposome from an injection site into the lymphatics. Given the size, very few will pass into the bloodstream directly. Small unilamellar vesicles are mobilized from the site much more quickly than are large ones. In transit through lymph nodes, liposomes may be taken up by macrophages (M), lymphoid and other normal cells (L), or tumor cells (T).

tracking to regional nodes. The basis for entry of liposomes into the lymphatics is indicated in Figure 15. Small molecules injected interstitially or intraperitoneally tend to pass directly into the bloodstream; large molecules and particles tend to enter the lymphatics through clefts in the terminal vessels (47).

An important question is whether liposomes can pass intact from peritoneal cavity to bloodstream and, if so, by what route. Simply finding a vesicle label in the blood is not sufficient to answer either question. The fluorescent dye CF provided a convenient test for latency of liposome contents and therefore a sufficient criterion for integrity of the liposome as a structure. In a collaboration a number of years ago with L. Leserman, SUV containing three labels -- CF, ^{14}C-inulin, and ^{3}H-DPPC -- were injected into the peritoneal cavities of mice and a series of blood samples taken thereafter by retroorbital puncture. The two radiotracer labels and self-quenched CF appeared commensurately in the bloodstream over a period of hours, indicating passage of intact vesicles. The route of at least a major part of that flux was established in collaboration with R. Parker and S. Sieber. They cannulated the thoracic ducts of rats and found that a considerable fraction of an intraperitoneal load of SUV passed by that route, with CF still self-quenched (39).

Fluorescence techniques have also been helpful in monitoring the progress of liposomes from subcutaneous sites of injection. Figure 16 shows the progression of images seen as fluorescent SUV (made with NBD-phosphatidyl-ethanolamine) pass toward and into an inguinal lymph node of a mouse. The initial photographs were taken in vivo by anaesthetizing the mouse, opening a flap of skin, and focusing a microscope on the node or its ducts. For high magnification, a drop of oil was added. At early times (b) an afferent lymphatic could be seen to contain fluorescence. Occasional larger vesicles contaminating the sonicated preparation could be seen in Brownian motion within the duct; the node itself was lit up (c), presumably by passage of large numbers of vesicles through marginal and medullary sinusoids; within an hour, a more granular pattern developed, suggesting cellular uptake (d). Uptake was confirmed by higher magnification images (e), in which aggregated fluorescent material appeared in individual cells, with a pattern of nuclear sparing. Panel (f) shows a right inguinal node after injection in the ipsilateral

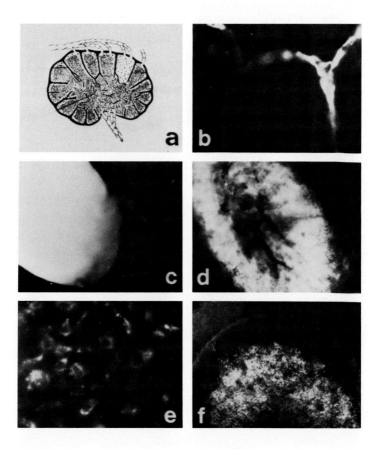

FIGURE 16. Fluorescence micrographs of inguinal lymph
nodes in mice after subcutaneous injection of NBD-labeled
liposomes in the thigh and base of the tail. (a) Schematic
representation of a lymph node, showing afferent vessels
emptying into the marginal sinus. Lymph flows in sinusoids
through the medullary region and out through an efferent
vessel at the hilum; (b) afferent vessel 30 minutes after
injection; (c) node 40 minutes after injection; (d) node 2
hours after injection; (e) higher magnification image of
node similar to that in (d), showing cellular uptake with a
"nuclear sparing" pattern; (f) inguinal node 2 hours after
injection in the ipsilateral hind foot pad. Frames (b) and
(c) were taken in vivo on anaesthetized mice; (d) - (f) were
on nodes after sacrifice of an animal.

footpad, rather than the thigh and base of the tail. The uptake is clearly localized within the node.

The next task was to determine which cells of the node had taken up the vesicles. After in vivo labeling from the footpad, popliteal nodes were disrupted to yield suspensions of single cells. These were then analyzed by flow microfluorimetry, with the results shown in Fig. 17.

Only a few percent of the cells were labeled significantly beyond control levels. Upon fluorescence microscopy (not shown), the images were consistent with endocytosis of the fluorescent lipid by macrophages. Given the fate of other types of particles in the node, that is not unexpected. Left open is the question whether liposomes can reach other cell types, normal or abnormal, in the node.

Since this is a conference on novel approaches to chemotherapy, it seems appropriate to conclude with the following flight of fancy -- even more fanciful than what

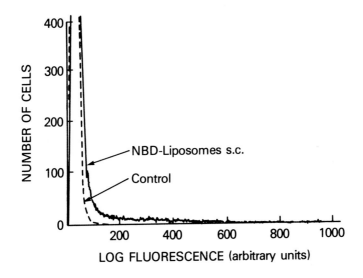

FIGURE 17. Flow microfluorimetric profile of popliteal lymph node cells 2 hours after footpad injection of NBD-liposomes. Control cells were obtained from the contralateral node. Only a small percentage of cells labeled significantly beyond control levels.

has preceded: Perhaps the conceptually different modes of targeting can profitably be combined. For example, antibody-bearing liposomes might be used in the lymphatics, and temperature-sensitive, antibody-bearing liposomes could perhaps yield rapid, local effect. Another possibility is shown schematically in Fig. 18. Temperature-sensitive liposomes flowing through a node could be disrupted by local heat (with the aid of lipoproteins in the lymph). In the case of mammary tumors, for example, a hot compress in the axilla or over the sternum might perhaps release quite large amounts of drug selectively in the nodes after subcutaneous injection.

In the wake of this "brain-storming," however, it must be clearly stated that targeted liposomes appear still to be a long way from practical clinical application

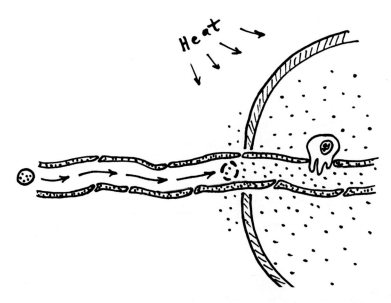

FIGURE 18. Local release from temperature-sensitive liposomes in the lymphatics.

ACKNOWLEDGMENTS

The work described here has involved the efforts of a large number of others, as indicated in the references below. Principal among them on the work with antibody have been R. Blumenthal, P.A. Henkart, L.D. Leserman, and S.O. Sharrow; on temperature-sensitive liposomes, R.L. Magin and M.B. Yatvin; on lymphatic delivery, R.J. Parker and S.M. Sieber.

REFERENCES

1. Bangham A.D. and Horne R.W. (1964). Negative staining of phospholipids and their structural modification by surface-active agents as observed in the electron microscope, J. Mol. Biol. 8:660.
2. Weinstein JN, and Leserman LD (1982). Liposomes as drug carriers in cancer chemotherapy. Pharmacology and Therapeutics, in press.
3. Szoka F, and Papahadjopoulos D (1980). Comparative properties and methods of preparation of lipid vesicles (liposomes). Ann. Rev. Biophys. Bioeng. 9:465-506.
4. Weinstein JN, Yoshikami S, Henkart PA, Blumenthal R, Hagins WA (1977). Liposome-cell interaction: transfer and intracellular release of a trapped fluorescent marker. Science 195:489.
5. Szoka F, Magnusson K-E, Wojcieszyn J, Hou Y, Derzko Z, Jacobson K (1981). Use of lectins and polyethylene glycol for fusion of glycolipid-containing liposomes with eukaryotic cells. Proc. Natl. Acad. Sci. U.S.A. 78:1685.
6. Cabantchik ZI, Volsky DJ, Ginsberg H, Loyter A (1980). Reconstitution of the erythrocyte anion transport system: in vitro and in vivo approaches. Ann. N.Y. Acad. Sci. 341:444.
7. Scherphof G, Roerdink F, Waite M, Parks J (1978). Disintegration of phosphatidylcholine liposomes in plasma as a result of interaction with high density lipoproteins. Biochim. Biophys. Acta 542:296-307.
8. Forssen EA and Tokes ZA (1979). In vitro and in vivo studies with adriamycin liposomes. Biochem. Biophys. Res. Commun. 91:1295.
9. Gregoriadis G, and Neerunjun DE (1975). Homing of liposomes to target cells. Biochem. Biophys. Res. Commun. 65:537.

10. Gregoriadis G, Neerunjun DE, Hunt R (1977). Fate of liposome-associated agents injected into normal and tumour-bearing rodents: attempts to improve localization in tumour lines. Life Sci. 21:357.
11. Weinstein JN, Blumenthal R, Sharrow SO, Henkart PA (1978). Antibody-mediated targeting of liposomes: binding to lymphocytes does not ensure incorporation of vesicle contents into the cells. Biochim. Biophys. Acta 509:272.
12. Weinstein JN (1981). Liposomes as "targeted" drug carriers: a physical chemical perspective. Pure and Appl. Chem. 53:2241.
13. Hagins WA and Yoshikami S (1978). In Barlow HB and Fatt P (eds): "Vertebrate Photoreception," New York: Academic Press, p. 97.
14. Leserman LD, Weinstein JN, Blumenthal R, Sharrow SO, Terry WD (1979). Binding of antigen-bearing fluorescent liposomes to the murine myeloma tumor MOPC 315. J. Immunol. 122:585.
15. Leserman LD, Weinstein JN, Moore JJ, Terry WD (1980). Specific interaction of myeloma tumor cells with hapten-bearing liposomes containing methotrexate and carboxyfluorescein. Cancer Res. 40:4768.
16. Leserman LD, Weinstein JN, Blumenthal R, Terry WD (1980). Receptor-mediated endocytosis of antibody opsonized liposomes by tumor cells. Proc. Natl. Acad. Sci. U.S.A. 77:4089.
17. Leserman LD, Barbet J, Kourilsky FM, Weinstein JN (1980). Targeting to cells of fluorescent liposomes covalently coupled with monoclonal antibody or protein A. Nature 288:602.
18. Weissmann G, Bloomgarden D, Kaplan R, Cohen C, Hoffstein S, Collins T, Gotleib A, Nagle D (1975). A general method for the introduction of enzymes, by means of immunoglobulin-coated liposomes, into lysosomes of deficient cells. Proc. Natl. Acad. Sci. U.S.A. 72:88.
19. Cohen CM, Weissmann G, Hoffstein S, Awasthi YC, Srivastava SK (1976). Introduction of purified hexosaminidase A into Tay-Sachs leucocytes by means of immunoglobulin-coated liposomes. Biochemistry 15:452.
20. Leserman LD, Machy P, Barbet J (1981). Cell-specific drug transfer from liposomes bearing monoclonal antibodies. Nature 293:226.

21. Barbet J, Machy P, Leserman LD (1981). Monoclonal antibody covalently coupled to liposomes: Specific targeting to cells. J. Supramolec. Struct. and Cell Biochem. 16:243.

22. Machy P, Barbet J, and Leserman LD (1982). Differential endocytosis and T and B lymphocyte surface molecules evaluated with antibody-bearing fluorescent liposomes containing methotrexate. Proc. Natl. Acad. Sci. USA, in press.

23. Poste G, Bucana C, Raz A, Bugelski P, Kirsh R, Fidler IJ (1982). Analysis of the fate of systemically administered liposomes and implications for their use in drug delivery. Cancer Res. 42:1412.

24. Simionescu N, Simionescu M, Palade GE (1975). Permeability of muscle capillaries to small heme-peptides -- evidence for the existence of patent transendothelial channels. J. Cell Biol. 64:586.

25. Yatvin MB, Weinstein JN, Dennis WH, Blumenthal R (1978). Design of liposomes for enhanced local release of drugs by hyperthermia. Science 202:1290.

26. Weinstein JN, Magin RL, Yatvin MB, Zaharko, DS (1980). Liposomes and local hyperthermia: Selective delivery of methotrexate to heated tumors. Science 204:188.

27. Weinstein JN, Magin RL, Cysyk RL, Zaharko DS (1979). Treatment of solid L1210 murine tumors with local hyperthermia and temperature-sensitive liposomes containing methotrexate. Cancer Res. 40:1388.

28. Magin RL and Weinstein JN (1980). Selective delivery of drugs in "temperature-sensitive" liposomes. In Tom B. and Six H.R. (eds): "Liposomes and Immunobiology," Amsterdam: Elsevier,p. 315.

29. Papahadjopoulos D, Jacobson K, Nir S, Isac T (1973). Phase transitions in phospholipid vesicles: Fluorescence polarization and permeability measurements concerning the effect of temperature and cholesterol. Biochim. Biophys. Acta 311:330.

30. Blok MC, van der Neut-Kok ECM, van Deenan LLM, de Gier J (1975). The effect of chain length and lipid phase transition on the selective permeability of liposomes. Biochim. Biophys. Acta 406:187.

31. Weinstein JN, Klausner RD, Innerarity T, Ralston E, Blumenthal R (1981). Phase transition release, a new approach to the interaction of proteins with lipid vesicles: Application to lipoproteins. Biochim. Biophys. Acta 647:270.

32. Magin RL, and Weinstein JN (1982). Delivery of drugs in temperature-sensitive liposomes. In Gregoriadis G and Papahadjopoulos D (eds):"Targeting of drugs," New York, Plenum, in press.

33. Yatvin MB, Muhlensiepen H, Porschen W, Weinstein JN, Feinendegen LE (1981). Selective delivery of liposome encapsulated cis-dichlorodiammineplatinum (II) by heat: Influence on tumor drug uptake and growth. Cancer Research 41:1602.

34. Chabner BA, and Young RC (1973). Threshold methotrexate concentration for in vivo inhibition of DNA synthesis in normal and tumorous target tissues. J. Clin. Invest. 52:1804.

35. Giovanella B, Stehlin J, Morgan A (1976). Selective lethal effect of supranormal temperatures on human neoplastic cells. Cancer Res. 36:3944.

36. Hahn G (1979). Potential for therapy of drugs and hyperthermia. Cancer Res. 39:4630.

37. Segal AW, Gregoriadis G, Black CDV (1975). Liposomes as vehicles for the local release of drugs. Clin. Sci. Mol. Med. 49:99.

38. Osborne MP, Richardson VJ, Jeyasingh K, Ryman BE (1979). Radionuclide-labelled liposomes: a new lymph node imaging agent. Int. J. Nucl. Med. Biol. 6:75.

39. Parker RJ, Sieber SM, Weinstein JN (1981). Effect of liposome encapsulation of a fluorescent dye on its uptake by the lymphatics of the rat. Pharmacology 23:128.

40. Kaledin VI, Matienko NA, Nikolin VP, Gruntenko YV, Budker VG (1981). Intralymphatic administration of liposome-encapsulated drugs to mice: possibility for suppression of the growth of tumor metastases in the lymph nodes. J. Natl Cancer Inst. 66:881.

41. Kaledin VI, Matienko NA, Nikolin VP, Gruntenko YV, Budker VG, Vakhrusheva TE (1982). Subcutaneously injected radiolabeled liposomes: transport to the lymph nodes in mice. J. Natl Cancer Inst. 69:67.

42. Jackson AJ (1980). The effect of route of administration on the disposition of inulin encapsulated in multilamellar vesicles of defined particle size. Research Communications in Chemical Pathology and Pharmacology 27:293.

43. Jackson AJ (1981). Intramuscular absorption and regional lymphatic uptake of liposome-entrapped inulin. Drug Metabolism and Disposition 9:535.

44. Khato J, Priester ER, Sieber SM (1982). Enhanced lymph node uptake of melphalan following liposomal entrapment and effects on lymph node metastasis in rats. Cancer Treat. Reports 66:517.

45. Parker RJ, Hartman KD, Sieber SM (1981). Lymphatic absorption and tissue disposition of liposome-entrapped ^{14}C-adriamycin following intraperitoneal administration to rats. Cancer Res. 41:1311.

46. Parker RJ, Priester ER, Sieber SM (1982). Comparison of lymphatic uptake, metabolism, excretion, and biodistribution of free and liposome-entrapped ^{14}C-cytosine β-D-arabinofuranoside following intraperitoneal administration to rats. Drug Metabolism and Disposition 10:40.

47. Leak LV (1971). Studies on the permeability of lymphatic capillaries. J. Cell Biol. 50:300.

Rational Basis for Chemotherapy, pages 475–485
© 1983 Alan R. Liss, Inc., 150 Fifth Avenue, New York, NY 10011

COMPARATIVE REACTIVITY OF CYCLIC AMINO ACIDS WITH
SYSTEM L IN MURINE L1210 LEUKEMIA CELLS AND
MURINE BONE MARROW PROGENITOR CELLS (CFU-C):
A POTENTIAL BASIS FOR SELECTIVE DRUG DESIGN

David T. Vistica, Richard Fuller, Nancy Dillon,
and Barbara J. Petro

Laboratory of Medicinal Chemistry and Biology
National Cancer Institute, Bethesda, Maryland   20205

ABSTRACT. Seven aromatic and aliphatic cyclic amino acids were evaluated for their interaction with system L, the sodium-independent amino acid carrier system responsible for the uptake of selected branched chained and aromatic amino acids. Inhibition analysis of both the initial rate of transport of the model substrate 2-aminobicyclo[2,2,1]heptane-2-carboxylic acid (BCH) and the reduction of melphalan cytotoxicity indicated that the aliphatic cyclic amino acids 2-aminoadamantane-2-carboxylic acid and BCH and the aromatic bicyclic amino acid 2-amino-2-carboxylic acid naphthalene were potent competitive substrates for that transport system. The observed failure of any of the cyclic amino acids to reduce melphalan cytotoxicity to a sensitive host tissue, the bone marrow progenitor cells (CFU-C), suggests that system L may be absent or altered in affinity for cyclic amino acids in this cell type. These observations raise the possibility that synthesis of cytotoxic derivatives of the cyclic amino acids which are transported with highest affinity by system L into tumor cells may result in chemotherapeutic agents which exhibit less myelosuppression.

INTRODUCTION

The host toxicity of alkylating agents severely limits their usefulness in the treatment of neoplastic disease and

presents the experimental chemotherapist with the difficult
task of attempting to design more selectively toxic chemotherapeutic agents. The toxicity of one nitrogen mustard,
L-phenylalanine mustard (melphalan), presents itself primarily as hematopoietic toxicity (1) and involvement of the
intestinal epithelium (2). Melphalan transport into a
number of different tumor cells has been shown to be mediated by two separate high-affinity amino acid transport
systems (3-6). One system is system L since it exhibits no
dependence on sodium and is sensitive to 2-aminobicyclo-
[2,2,1]heptane-2-carboxylic acid (BCH), a synthetic L system
amino acid (7) and L-leucine. Melphalan transport by the
second amino acid transport system is sodium-dependent,
exhibits its highest affinity for L-leucine (8) but is
insensitive to BCH and α-aminoisobutyric acid (AIB), an
alanine (A system) amino acid (9). In an attempt to examine
amino acid transport systems present in murine hematopoietic
precursor cells it became apparent that standard transport
studies with radiolabelled drug could not be performed since
these cells constitute such a small fraction (1 in 1000)
of nucleated cells isolated from femur preparations. An
approach was taken which utilized the cytotoxicity of melphalan as an indicator for discerning the presence of
specific amino acid transport systems in hematopoietic
precursor cells (10). These results indicated that in this
cell type system L may be absent or altered in affinity for
BCH, the model L system substrate, and raises the possibility that this may be a potentially exploitable difference
between tumor cells and sensitive host tissue. As an
extension of these studies we have examined a series of
aliphatic and aromatic cyclic amino acids for their reactivity with system L in murine L1210 leukemia cells and, in
this communication, we report on these observations.

METHODS

1-Amino-1-carboxylic acid naphthalene, 1-aminocyclo-
pentane-1-carboxylic acid, 1-aminocyclohexane-1-carboxylic
acid, 1-aminocycloheptane-1-carboxylic acid and 2-aminoada-
mantane-2-carboxylic acid were obtained from the Drug
Synthesis and Chemistry Branch of the National Cancer
Institute, Bethesda, Maryland. Unlabelled and DL-[carboxyl-
^{14}C] labelled 2-aminobicyclo[2,2,1]heptane-2-carboxylic
acid were obtained from New England Nuclear, Boston, MA.
β-Tetralone-hydantoin was purchased from the Aldrich

Chemical Co., Milwaukee, WI and was converted to 2-amino-2-carboxylic acid naphthalene by the following procedure.

Ten grams of β-tetralone hydantoin (.046 mole) was added to a refluxing mixture of 30% aqueous barium hydroxide and heated for thirty hours. The resulting mixture was cooled and carbon dioxide bubbled into the mixture for 30 minutes. The mixture was then filtered and the water soluble fraction cooled overnight. The precipitate was collected and dried (yield 6.7g). Excess barium was removed by treating 0.5 g of the crude product with two equivalents of 1.0 N NaOH for 15 minutes. The solution was filtered, layered on to a sodium ion exchange column and the ultra-violet active fractions combined following elution with water. The combined fractions were acidified to pH 4.0 with 1.0 N HCl. The solution was cooled overnight and the resulting precipitate was filtered and dried. Elemental analysis was acceptable. Overall yield 55%, purity > 98%.

Cellular Transport and Cytotoxicity Studies.

The methodology used in the present communication has been extensively described for tumor cell transport studies (3), tumor cell cytotoxicity studies (3) and bone marrow toxicity assays (10). Cellular transport studies with labelled BCH were performed in sodium-free transport medium as previously described (3). Inhibition constants were derived from Dixon plots (11).

RESULTS

Melphalan Transport by Neoplastic Cells.

Melphalan transport into a number of neoplastic cells is mediated by 2 separate high-affinity amino acid transport systems (3-6). The effect of selected model substrates for system L (2-aminobicyclo[2,2,1]heptane-2-carboxylic acid, BCH) and system A (α-aminoisobutyric acid) upon melphalan transport by murine L1210 leukemia cells is illustrated in Figure 1. 2-Aminobicyclo[2,2,1]heptane-2-carboxylic acid is capable of reducing the initial velocity of melphalan transport to a limiting maximum value of 50%. α-Aminoiso-butyric acid, in the presence of BCH, is incapable of further reducing the initial velocity of melphalan trans-port. The remaining 50% of melphalan transport is effectively reduced by L-leucine at concentrations of 5-10 μM.

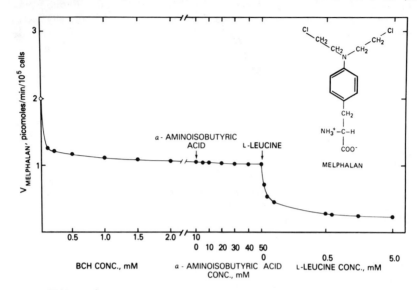

FIGURE 1. L-Phenylalanine mustard transport by murine L1210 leukemia cells. L-Phenylalanine mustard (MELPHALAN; L-PAM), an aromatic amino acid nitrogen mustard, is an effective chemotherapeutic agent whose primary host toxicity is myelosuppression. Melphalan transport into a number of neoplastic cells is mediated equally by two separate high-affinity amino acid transport systems (3-6). One system is the classical sodium-independent system L as melphalan transport is reduced by the model system L substrate, 2-aminobicyclo[2,2,1]heptane-2-carboxylic acid (BCH). The remainder of melphalan transport is mediated by a monovalent cation-dependent system which exhibits its highest affinity for the branched chained amino acid leucine (8).

Comparison of Amino Acid Carrier Systems in Murine L1210 Leukemia Cells and Murine CFU-C.

2-Aminobicyclo[2,2,1]heptane-2-carboxylic acid reduces the cytotoxicity of melphalan to murine L1210 leukemia cells to a limiting maximum value of 50% (Figure 2), a value identical to its reduction of the initial velocity of melphalan transport (Figure 1). α-Aminoisobutyric acid is incapable, in the presence of BCH, of further reducing melphalan cytotoxicity at concentrations of 25-50 mM. The reduction in melphalan cytotoxicity toward murine L1210 leukemia cells contrasts markedly with that observed with murine CFU-C. As can be seen in Figure 2, BCH does not reduce melphalan cytotoxicity toward this sensitive host tissue and suggests that murine CFU-C lack system L or

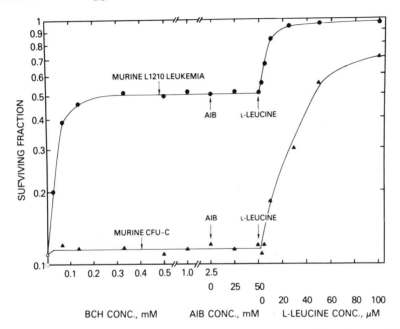

FIGURE 2. Comparison of the ability of amino acids to reduce melphalan cytotoxicity to murine L1210 leukemia cells and murine bone marrow progenitor cells (CFU-C). 2-Aminobicyclo[2,2,1]heptane-2-carboxylic acid (BCH), the system L specific-substrate, is capable of reducing mel-phalan cytotoxicity to tumor cells but not to host CFU-C (10). This observation suggested that CFU-C lack system L or possess a system L with reduced affinity for the bi-cyclic amino acid.

possess a system L with reduced affinity for the bicyclic amino acid. This observation prompted additional studies with a number of aliphatic and aromatic cyclic amino acids (Figure 3) to determine whether (1) there were differences in their respective affinity for system L in tumor cells and (2) whether any were capable of reducing melphalan cytotoxicity to host CFU-C. These two features, the ability

to be transported with high-affinity by system L into a
tumor cell and the inability to reduce melphalan cytotoxicity to host CFU-C were established as criteria for selecting an amino acid substrate which could be utilized to
introduce the cytotoxic bis(chloroethyl)amine group into
the tumor cell.

CYCLIC AMINO ACIDS

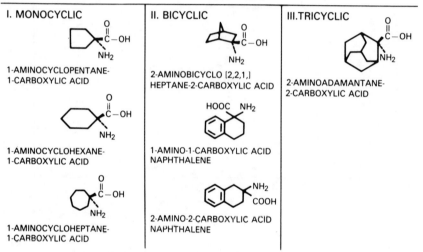

I. MONOCYCLIC

1-AMINOCYCLOPENTANE-
1-CARBOXYLIC ACID

1-AMINOCYCLOHEXANE-
1-CARBOXYLIC ACID

1-AMINOCYCLOHEPTANE-
1-CARBOXYLIC ACID

II. BICYCLIC

2-AMINOBICYCLO [2,2,1,]
HEPTANE-2-CARBOXYLIC ACID

1-AMINO-1-CARBOXYLIC ACID
NAPHTHALENE

2-AMINO-2-CARBOXYLIC ACID
NAPHTHALENE

III. TRICYCLIC

2-AMINOADAMANTANE-
2-CARBOXYLIC ACID

FIGURE 3. Structures of selected aliphatic and aromatic cyclic amino acids.

Inhibition of 2-Aminobicyclo[2,2,1]heptane-2-carboxylic
Acid Transport by Murine L1210 Leukemia Cells by Cyclic
Amino Acids.

Little difference was observed in the ability of 1-
aminocyclopentane-1-carboxylic acid, 1-aminocyclohexane-1-
carboxylic acid or 1-aminocycloheptane-1-carboxylic acid to
inhibit the transport of the system L specific substrate,
BCH, by murine L1210 leukemia cells (Table 1). A striking
difference in the ability of 2 aromatic bicyclic amino
acids, 1-amino-1-carboxylic acid naphthalene and 2-amino-2-
carboxylic acid naphthalene to inhibit BCH transport by

murine L1210 leukemia cells was observed (Table 1). 1-
Amino-1-carboxylic acid naphthalene was incapable of

TABLE 1

INHIBITION OF 2-AMINOBICYCLO[2,2,1]HEPTANE-2-CARBOXYLIC
ACID TRANSPORT BY MURINE L1210 LEUKEMIA CELLS BY CYCLIC
AMINO ACIDS

	Inhibition Constant
Monocyclic Amino Acids	
1-Aminocyclopentane-1-carboxylic acid	25 μM
1-Aminocyclohexane-1-carboxylic acid	35 μM
1-Aminocycloheptane-1-carboxylic acid	40 μM
Bicyclic Amino Acids	
2-Aminobicyclo[2,2,1heptane-2-carboxylic acid	10-15 μM $km = 10$ μM
1-Amino-1-carboxylic acid naphthalene	>10 mM
2-Amino-2-carboxylic acid naphthalene	5 μM
Tricyclic Amino Acid	
2-Aminoadamantane-2-carboxylic acid	15 μM

reducing BCH transport by these cells whereas 2-amino-2-
carboxylic acid naphthalene was found to be an effective
competitive substrate for system L as evidenced by its
inhibition constant of 5 μM. The aliphatic tricyclic amino
acid, 2-aminoadamantane-2-carboxylic acid, also is an
effective competitive substrate for system L although its
inhibition constant of 15 μM is somewhat less than that of
2-amino-2-carboxylic acid naphthalene.

Failure of Cyclic Amino Acids to Reduce Melphalan Cytotoxicity to Murine CFU-C.

None of the cyclic amino acids utilized in the present
study reduced melphalan cytotoxicity to murine CFU-C.

TABLE 2
FAILURE OF CYCLIC AMINO ACIDS TO REDUCE MELPHALAN
CYTOTOXICITY (LD_{90}) TO MURINE BONE MARROW
PROGENITOR CELLS (CFU-C).

Amino Acid	Surviving Fraction
None	0.1
Monocyclic Amino Acids	
1-Aminocyclopentane-1-carboxylic acid	0.1
1-Aminocyclohexane-1-carboxylic acid	0.1
1-Aminocycloheptane-1-carboxylic acid	0.1
Bicyclic Amino Acids	
2-Aminobicyclo[2,2,1]heptane-2-carboxylic acid	0.1
1-Amino-1-carboxylic acid naphthalene	0.1
2-Amino-2-carboxylic acid naphthalene	0.1
Tricyclic Amino Acid	
2-Aminoadamantane-2-carboxylic acid	0.1

Reduction in Melphalan Cytotoxicity Toward Murine L1210 Leukemia Cells by Cyclic Amino Acids.

In general the efficacy of aliphatic cyclic amino acids in reducing melphalan cytotoxicity was tricyclic > bicyclic > monocyclic (Figure 4). The aromatic bicyclic amino acid, 2-amino-2-carboxylic acid naphthalene was found to be slightly superior to the aliphatic tricyclic amino acid 2-aminoadamantane-2-carboxylic acid in reducing melphalan cytotoxicity to murine L1210 leukemia cells.

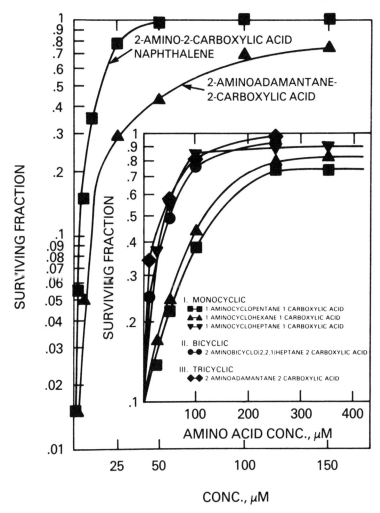

FIGURE 4. Reduction in melphalan cytotoxicity toward murine L1210 leukemia cells by cyclic amino acids. In general the efficacy of aliphatic cyclic amino acids in blocking melphalan cytotoxicity was tricyclic > bicyclic > monocyclic (inset of figure). The aromatic bicyclic amino acid 2-amino-2-carboxylic acid naphthalene was found to be superior to the aliphatic tricyclic amino acid 2-amino-adamantane-2-carboxylic acid in both blocking melphalan cytotoxicity and in blocking BCH transport. Experiments were performed in sodium-free transport medium (3).

DISCUSSION

The results described in the present communication indicate that the efficacy of aliphatic cyclic amino acids in
reducing melphalan cytotoxicity to murine L1210 leukemia
cells is tricyclic > bicyclic > monocyclic and, in general,
correlates with their affinity for system L, the sodium-
independent transport system. The observation that cyclic
amino acids do not reduce melphalan cytotoxicity to a sensitive host tissue, the CFU-C, indicates that, in this cell
type, system L may be absent or altered in affinity for
cyclic amino acids and suggests that preparation of new
amino acid nitrogen mustards which are transported by system
L may result in chemotherapeutic agents which are less
myelosuppressive than melphalan. Likely candidates would
be the bis(chloroethyl)amine derivative of the aliphatic
cyclic amino acids (2-aminobicyclo[2,2,1]heptane-2-carb-
oxylic acid and 2-aminoadamantane-2-carboxylic acid) and
the aromatic bicyclic amino acid 2-amino-2-carboxylic acid
naphthalene.

These new amino acid nitrogen mustards, if transported
by system L, may be efficacious in the treatment of brain
neoplasia since the amino acids which pass rapidly across
the blood brain barrier are system L substrates (12).

REFERENCES

1. Young RC, Canellos GP, Chabner BA, Schein PS, Hubbard
    SP, DeVita VT (1974). Chemotherapy of advanced ovarian
    carcinoma: A   prospective   randomized   comparison   of
    phenylalanine mustard and high dose cyclophosphamide.
    Gynecol Oncol 2:489.
2. Millar JL, Hudspith BN, McElwain TJ, Phelps TA (1978).
    Effect of high-dose melphalan on marrow and intestinal
    epithelium   pretreated   with   cyclophosphamide.   Br J
    Cancer 38:137.
3. Vistica DT (1979).   Cytotoxicity as an indicator for
    transport mechanism: Evidence that melphalan is trans-
    ported by two leucine-preferring carrier systems in the
    L1210 murine leukemia cell.   Biochim Biophys Acta 550:
    309.
4. Goldenberg GJ, Lam HYP, Begleiter A (1979).   Active
    carrier-mediated transport of melphalan by two separate
    amino acid transport systems in LPC-1 plasmacytoma
    cells in vitro.   J Biol Chem 254:1057.

5. Begleiter A, Lam HYP, Grover J, Froese E, Goldenberg GJ (1979). Evidence for active transport of melphalan by amino acid carriers in L5178Y lymphoblasts in vitro. Cancer Res 39:353.

6. Begleiter A, Froese EK, Goldenberg GJ (1980). Comparison of melphalan transport in human breast cancer cells and lymphocytes in vitro. Cancer Lett 10:243.

7. Christensen HN, Handlogten ME, Lam I, Tager AS, Zand R (1969). A bicyclic amino acid to improve discriminations among transport systems. J Biol Chem 244:1510.

8. Vistica DT, Schuette B (1979). Substrate specificity of a high-affinity, monovalent cation-dependent amino acid carrier. Biochem Biophys Res Commun 90:247.

9. Oxender DL, Lee M, Moore PA, Cecchini G (1977). Neutral amino acid transport systems of tissue culture cells. J Biol Chem 252:2675.

10. Vistica DT (1980). Cytotoxicity as an indicator for transport mechanism: Evidence that murine bone marrow progenitor cells lack a high-affinity leucine carrier that transports melphalan in murine L1210 leukemia cells. Blood 56:427.

11. Dixon M (1953). The determination of enzyme inhibitor constants. Biochem J 55:170.

12. Wade LA, Katzman R (1975). Synthetic amino acids and the nature of L-DOPA transport at the blood-brain barrier. J Neurochem 25:837.

Rational Basis for Chemotherapy, pages 487–489
© 1983 Alan R. Liss, Inc., 150 Fifth Avenue, New York, NY 10011

WORKSHOP SUMMARY: DRUG TRANSPORT AND ANTITUMOR RESPONSE

David T. Vistica

Laboratory of Medicinal Chemistry and Biology
National Cancer Institute, Bethesda, Maryland 20205

The workshop on drug transport and antitumor response attempted to address areas of importance to clinical cancer chemotherapy with respect to (1) improving the use of currently used chemotherapeutic agents, (2) developing more selectively cytotoxic chemotherapeutic agents and (3) addressing the problem of resistance of neoplastic cells to cytotoxic agents.

Dr. John Byfield discussed his division of clinically useful alkylating agents into two groups based on their mechanism of cellular transport. Alkylating agents such as nitrogen mustard, melphalan and activated cyclophosphamide which enter into neoplastic cells via carrier-mediated processes were shown to be most cytotoxic toward rapidly proliferating host and tumor cells, to be water soluble, relatively impermeable to the blood brain barrier and sparing of nonproliferating marrow stem cells. Alkylating agents which enter into cells via non-carrier mediated processes such as diffusion were shown to exhibit the opposite properties, i.e. higher lipid solubility, an ability to cross the blood brain barrier and higher activity against non-proliferating cells. An interesting observation was presented for cis-dichlorodiammine platinum (cis-Pt) in that this agent exhibits properties which are compatible with its being classified as an alkylating agent whose cellular transport is carried-mediated. This is a distinct possibility since studies were described which demonstrated that amino acids reduce cis-Pt cytotoxicity.

Dr. Vistica discussed a potentially useful combination of melphalan and Acinetobacter glutaminase:asparaginase in the treatment of metastatic ovarian carcinoma. The work described indicated that melphalan transport by human ovarian carcinoma cells is reduced 8-fold by ascitic fluid and that this can be attributed to the presence of the amino acids leucine and glutamine in the ascitic fluid. It was suggested that glutamine depletion using Acineto-bacter glutaminase:asparaginase prior to melphalan treatment may increase the uptake of melphalan by human ovarian carcinoma cells. Cytotoxicity data presented indicated that melphalan cytotoxicity to human ovarian carcinoma cells is dramatically increased by exposure of cells to melphalan in an amino acid free environment. Acinetobacter glutaminase:asparaginase (AGA) appears to be the optimal glutaminase:asparaginase preparation since maximum enzymatic activity is observed at physiological pH (7.4) and the apparent K_m of the enzyme for L-glutamine is very low (5 μM). This combination is feasible since melphalan cytotoxicity is not reduced by L-glutamic acid or ammonia, the products of L-glutamine deamination.

$$L\text{-glutamine} \rightarrow L\text{-glutamic acid} + NH_3$$

Dr. Vistica also discussed the rationale for preparation of new cyclic amino acid nitrogen mustards. These results appear elsewhere in the conference proceedings.

Dr. Kevin Scanlon discussed evidence which suggests that 2,4-diamino compounds such as methotrexate (MTX) may preferentially inhibit the ASC (alanine-serine-cysteine) amino acid transport system in growing lymphocytes. It was indicated that inhibition of cellular transport of essential amino acids such as methionine by MTX may be an additional mechanism of action of MTX cytotoxicity, particularly if the cells are auxotrophic for the respective amino acid.

Dr. Vistica discussed some recent work implicating the tripeptide glutathione as being the determinant factor in resistance of murine L1210 leukemia cells to L-phenyl-alanine mustard and other cytotoxic agents.

Dr. Hugues Ryser discussed work which indicated that membrane related resistance to MTX could be overcome by conjugating MTX to poly-L-lysine. Such conjugates enter cells via endocytosis and MTX is released intracellularly where it can achieve its pharmacological effect. Dr. Ryser also described work indicating that daunomycin and poly-D-lysine can be joined through a cis-aconityl linkage and, subsequent to intracellular accumulation, daunomycin can be released by the action of specific lysosomal enzymes. Such intracellular targeting of anticancer agents may result in improved selectivity.

Dr. Zoltan Tokes discussed work with adriamycin coupled to microspheres of polyglutaraldehyde. Such complexes are active against adriamycin resistant human leukemic cells. These adriamycin-polyglutaraldehyde complexes may be able to be used in instances where drug resistance is caused by decreased surface binding of the respective chemotherapeutic agents to neoplastic cells.

Dr. Norbert Kartner discussed the role of the P-glycoprotein in multiple drug-resistant Chinese Hamster Ovary cells. This membrane-associated glycoprotein (MW 170,000) appears in drug resistant neoplastic cells and disappears as cells regain sensitivity. The possibility that the presence of this glycoprotein may be useful in predicting the response of neoplastic cells to certain classes of chemotherapeutic agents was discussed.

Participants: Dr. David T. Vistica
                  Dr. John Byfield
                  Dr. Kevin Scanlon
                  Dr. Hugues Ryser
                  Dr. Zoltan Tokes
                  Dr. Norbert Kartner

INDEX